AIDS:
RAGE & REALITY

AIDS:
RAGE & REALITY
Why Silence is Deadly

GENE ANTONIO

ANCHOR BOOKS
Dallas

141167

With the exception of foreign terms and indicated notations, all italics and uppercase characters within quotations have been added by the author for emphasis.

Readers with personal questions or concerns regarding diagnosis or treatment of the health conditions described in this book should consult their physician.

AIDS: Rage and Reality
Copyright 1993 Gene Antonio
Published by Anchor Books
Dallas, TX
Book Distribution Service
(817) 294-6366

Available in Canada through:
Life Cycle Books
2205 Danforth Ave.
Toronto, Ontario M4C 1K4
Canada
(416) 690-5860

Available in Australia through:
J. 23 Cooperative
P.O. Box 22
Ormond, Victoria 3204
Australia
61-3-596-2323

ISBN 0-9634774-3-9

Printed in the United States of America

IMPORTANT WARNING AND DISCLAIMER

The federal "Americans with Disabilities Act" (ADA) prohibits the exclusion of individuals from an occupation or "public accommodation" based on their actual or *perceived* mental or physical impairment(s).

The ADA has a provision which permits employers to exercise some discretion in placing individuals whose mental or physical impairment(s) would pose a "direct threat to safety or health." Currently, it is not entirely clear how this provision would be interpreted by the courts with respect to communicable diseases such as active tuberculosis and AIDS. It is also uncertain to what extent, if any, employers may restrict individuals with mental impairments such as dementia, psychiatric disorders, etc., in occupations where such conditions could endanger workplace safety.

Regulations issued by the Equal Employment Opportunity Commission with respect to the ADA indicate that each situation will have to be handled on a "case-by-case" basis.

OBTAIN LEGAL ADVICE FIRST

Due to the high risk of litigation and heavy fines under the myriad of local, state and federal laws prohibiting discrimination against individuals with real or "perceived" mental or physical disabilities, EMPLOYERS AND PRIVATE BUSINESSES *MUST* OBTAIN PROFESSIONAL LEGAL COUNSEL *PRIOR TO* FORMULATING OR ATTEMPTING TO IMPLEMENT ANY POLICY REGARDING EMPLOYEES, CUSTOMERS, VISITORS AND PATIENTS WITH COMMUNICABLE DISEASES, INCLUDING AIDS AND TUBERCULOSIS or any other mental or physical conditions.

The public policy recommendations contained in this book do NOT in any way constitute a legal opinion as to which employment or public accommodation standards the courts may or may not deem to be lawful.

IGNORANCE IS NO EXCUSE

Refusing to hire or retain a prospective or present employee or accommodate a customer or visitor on the basis of their actual or "perceived" infectious disease would most likely be considered a violation of the ADA, unless the courts permit an exemption under the "threat to health or safety" proviso. Other local/state statutes may *not* provide an exemption based on the threat to safety or health. It would be prudent to have the legal counsel involved consult with appropriate public agencies, the Equal Employment Opportunity Commission (EEOC), local/state human rights commissions, etc., in order to obtain an opinion regarding the lawfulness of any proposed infectious disease policy for the occupation(s) or "public accommodation(s)" in question. The principle to bear in mind is: *Ignorantia legis neminem excusat* – ignorance of the law is not an excuse.

CONTENTS

FOREWORD

Future historians will look at the discovery of the AIDS epidemic during the 1980s and wonder how it was possible that so many opportunities to contain the disease were missed. Two years ago, *Barron's* published an article I wrote called "AIDS and Ostriches," which detailed projections of how AIDS would cost our country billions of dollars. At that time, some thought the figures were on the high side. Today, those projections appear conservative. If one reads official projected figures by various health agencies five years ago regarding the anticipated number of AIDS cases, one is shocked at how low these figures are in contrast to the actual number of AIDS cases reported and projected today.

AIDS is the most significant threat to the human race in the modern era. The potential for an infectious disease to cause the devastation of human life on a mass scale is not without precedent. The bubonic plague wiped out one third of the population of Europe before it was finally brought under control. AIDS has the potential of killing more people worldwide than those who died in both world wars. Some researchers now estimate that over 100 million people worldwide will be infected with HIV by the turn of the century.

In the twentieth century, great strides were made to control contagious diseases. Health departments throughout the country were empowered with special authority to prevent their spread. These rules were formulated with one highest priority: *to protect society as a whole*. No inconvenience to an individual, no individual right of privacy, no individual right to freedom could take priority over the need to protect society as a whole from the threat of contagious diseases.

What has happened in the 12 years since AIDS was recognized as a contagious disease? There has been an explosion of information and research. Everyone knows it is a sexually transmitted disease – but a disturbing skepticism remains. Can this virus be spread by less intimate levels of contact? This is a vitally important question because presently no attempt is being made to limit the activity of people infected with AIDS. There are a number of documented instances where AIDS has been spread by non-intimate contact, such as where a dentist spread the virus through casual contact to his patients.

More significantly, health officials by and large are not utilizing the basic measures for tracking and preventing the spread of the disease: reportability and contact tracing. In not utilizing such procedures, health officials violate the basic, precedented standards for contagious disease control. It is evident that *AIDS has become a politically protected disease. The basic priority of protecting the well-being of society as a whole has been completely subverted.* Simply put, the sexual comfort and privacy of those infected with AIDS have been given total supremacy over the rights of the uninfected members of society.

Thirty-five years ago when I entered medical school, there was much talk about finding cures for cancer within 10-15 years. Well, thirty-five years later, some cancers are curable but the majority are still incurable. At the present time there is no cure or effective vaccine on the horizon for AIDS.

In the year 2000, if current trends continue, we will have millions of Americans fatally afflicted with AIDS. By then most Americans will know that even casual contact with AIDS carriers can be deadly because of the risk of contracting drug-resistant TB. Social panic and chaos may occur well before then if the population as a whole begins to realize that things are getting out of control. This type of grim scenario does not have to take place if the public demands positive action before the situation reaches the point of no return.

How long must society tolerate HIV carriers not only spreading AIDS, but other contagious diseases such as TB, among health care workers and the general public? The perilous situation at present is one where the uninfected public–the overwhelming majority of the U.S. population–is unorganized. In contrast, the infected (and infectious) segment of the population has a constituency which is highly organized and maintains advocates who pressure politicians into approving public health policies that are against the overall best interests of society.

Is it really too much to test all susceptible individuals for AIDS and to inform those found to be infected that they are restricted from infecting others? At the present time, the answer by many in the public health establishment is yes, it is too much to ask. In my state you can be fined $10,000 to $50,000 for improper disposal of so-called medical waste. Incredibly, an individual knowingly infected with AIDS can willfully expose others without legal constraints.

There is a great body of misinformation and distortion which is being used to justify some of the current AIDS policies. The only way that the uninfected majority of this country can hope to stop the spread of AIDS is to become fully educated about the disease.

Gene Antonio has written a very important book which carefully documents many of the crucial facts about HIV disease and its related infections. By becoming truly informed, people will come to understand the necessity of maintaining an appropriate balance between the right of uninfected members of society to be provided proper protection from AIDS and its related infections, and the need to provide humane care and treatment for those with HIV disease.

AIDS: Rage and Reality provides essential information for educating society about AIDS and its dire health ramifications.

Joseph Feldschuh, M.D.
Fellow, American College of Physicians
Fellow, American College of Cardiologists

Dr. Feldschuh, an endocrinologist and cardiologist, has been associate clinical professor in both medicine and pathology at New York Medical College and has been assistant clinical professor at Cornell Medical School. He is the author of *Safe Blood – Purifying the Nation's Blood Supply in the Age of AIDS*, the definitive work on ways people can protect themselves when transfusions are needed. Dr. Feldschuh is Medical Director of Idant, the first public autologous blood program in the United States. Idant is headquartered in Manhattan, New York, but can enable the storage of blood for persons living throughout the United States.

INTRODUCTION

In 1985, as the AIDS pandemic began to be recognized as the dreadful global scourge which it would become, few people had enough insight to question the common wisdom of the health establishment "experts." Gene Antonio was one of the few. With the publication of his first book, *The AIDS Cover-Up?*, he stood on the front lines advocating sound health measures in spite of strident opposition. Those who are manipulating the AIDS agenda for their own social, political, and economic benefit are being given prominence, while the media and medical researchers pander to them and threaten our very existence as a society.

Despite facing incredible odds, Gene Antonio has continued to ask the tough questions. Time has proven the validity of many of his earlier conclusions as the medical establishment grudgingly admits the truth.

Antonio has tenaciously continued to press for rational management of the AIDS epidemic according to sound medical and public health practices. The astounding complexity of this deadly disease must be taken into account when determining public health policy.

After seven years of continued research, *AIDS: Rage and Reality* presents a frightening picture of the path which we have taken in failing to deal effectively with this plague. It is imperative that both the medical profession and the lay public grasp the medical and social realities that are painstakingly documented in this book. In times such as these, ignorance is death. Everyone in America needs to read this truly awesome book.

Raymond E. Brady, M.D.
Fellow, American Academy of Allergy and Immunology

A DEADLY IRONY

AIDS is likely to cause the U.S. economy—built on consumer growth—to stagnate. Hospitals will be desperately overcrowded, and many AIDS patients will die at home or be abandoned. . . . Fear of AIDS will affect a broad range of activities—even those non-intimate activities where contracting AIDS would seem very unlikely. The disease could ultimately shift the world's balance of power. Some countries will be destroyed by it, some badly hurt, and some almost unharmed. Those that suffer least will tend to dominate afterwards, as in previous epidemics. AIDS could make overpopulation, famine, environmental destruction, or the extinction of species seem like minor complaints.
  – Dr. John Platt, Ph.D. biophysicist in *The Futurist Magazine*, a publication of the World Future Society[1]

The world's vulnerability to the spread of AIDS is increasing not decreasing. The pandemic is spreading to new areas and communities. The disease has not peaked and will reach every country by the end of the century. . . .
  – Dr. Johnathan Mann, Director of the International AIDS Center at Harvard University. The Center estimates that as many as 110 million people will have contracted HIV disease by the year 2000.[2]

Lillian King used to flip the TV dial when shows about AIDS came on. Faithfully married, she felt the issue was largely irrelevant. King was rudely jolted out of her indifference when she and her 17-year-old son Jeffrey were notified that they had been treated by a health care worker with HIV disease. Lillian and her son were among 1,800 other patients exposed to the infected worker at a medical center in the town of Nashua, New Hampshire. King has become a galvanizing force in the drive to enact legislation requiring HIV testing of physicians and patients. "My son was furious, ready to kill over this. I think it's time to start treating AIDS like a deadly disease instead of a special secret."[3]

Many people feel a growing sense of uneasiness about the way the AIDS epidemic is being handled. There is a nagging consensus both in the lay public and among medical professionals that something is terribly amiss in public health policy regarding this disease. Dr. Edward Annis, former President of the American Medical Association, asserts that the government's overwhelming emphasis on the civil rights aspect of AIDS has stymied disease control efforts.[4]

PUBLIC STILL NOT BEING GIVEN THE FACTS

For years people have been told that AIDS doesn't kill a person; one only dies of other diseases caused by the weakening of the immune system. It has clearly been established that this is inaccurate. The AIDS virus itself does kill directly in many diverse ways. The direct lethal attack of HIV has critical implications for public policy in terms of occupational limitations, the prospect of developing a treatment or vaccine, and the potential for different modes of transmission.

THE AIDS VIRUS IS CONSTANTLY MUTATING

The author's first book, *The AIDS Cover-Up?* underscored the hazards associated with the ability of the AIDS virus to mutate.[5]

Dr. William Haseltine, a prominent investigator at Harvard's Dana-Farber Cancer Institute has stated:

> The kind of readout of genetic information we see in this system [of the AIDS virus] is absolutely astounding. Nobody would have thought this level of transcription [gene activity] was possible before we did these studies. We were shocked. It's about 1,000 times faster than the genes we know about.
>
> *This system is very potent in permitting viruses to replicate at a ferocious rate.* It's one of the reasons this is such a devastating disease. It's one of the reasons *this virus can be transmitted so easily from person to person.*[6]

According to Dr. Luc Montagnier, the French co-discoverer of the AIDS virus:

> The potential for genetic variation is perhaps the greatest danger in the future of the AIDS epidemic. It will make it difficult to design efficient vaccines against all strains, and *a further change of the virus* in its tropism [preference for different types of cells] and *ways of transmission* cannot be excluded.[7]

COVERT AIDS: AN OMINOUS TURN

At the Eighth International Conference on AIDS, scientists from different parts of the world reported "new" cases of AIDS appearing among people who tested negative for HIV-1 and HIV-2, the conventional strains of the AIDS virus. One of the cases involved a New York City male who admitted having multiple liaisons with known AIDS carriers. Another case reported from Spain involved a married man with no known risk factors who has suffered from

Kaposi's sarcoma and tuberculosis since 1990. Of six reported American patients with AIDS who tested negative for HIV-1 and HIV-2, three have histories of blood transfusions (two received blood *after* blood banks started screening for HIV), one has used drugs and *one is a health care worker.* Epidemiologist Thomas Spira of the U.S. Centers for Disease Control suggests, "HIV may not be the only infectious cause of immunosuppression in man."[8]

The medical establishment and the media reported the cases as though they were a startlingly novel turn of events. The public has been told that instances of patients with AIDS who are negative for HIV-1 and HIV-2 are "rare." In reality, *over 40 such cases were reported from New York City alone at a previous AIDS conference held in 1988.*[9] Those portentous findings still have not been widely circulated in the medical community or reported by the media.

Almost all of the covert AIDS cases reported back in 1988 occurred in high-risk patients. Now, a disconcertingly high percentage of reported covert AIDS cases are being seen among people with no known risk factors for HIV. [10]

In spite of the fact that several of the more recent cases involve persons whose only risk factor was a blood transfusion, health officials are continuing to reassure people that the blood supply is "safe."

DEADLY NEW MUTANTS

Although yet to be reported in the media, French researchers have isolated a mutant form of HIV from an AIDS patient *which is 100,000 times more powerful and more contagious* than previous AIDS viruses.[11]

Japanese scientists have identified a strain of HIV that kills more rapidly than previously known forms. The virus was found in the blood of a 24-year-old man who died within only eight months after he was infected. The same type of swift-killing virus has been found in France.[12]

AIDS AND TB TAXING HOSPITALS

In New York City, the hospital system is imploding under the crushing influx of AIDS patients. HIV-related TB has broken out among patients, staff and visitors at medical facilities and the population at large. The staggering impact of AIDS has helped reduce the medical system into near shambles. Medical facilities with residencies which were once among the most highly sought after in the nation are having difficulty in attracting physicians. As the AIDS epidemic expands, the situation in the Big Apple can be seen as a foreboding of things to come elsewhere.

In his insightful book *A Time for Truth*, written prior to the AIDS epidemic, William Simon, former Secretary of the Treasury, noted:

> If New York were a discrete political entity, disconnected from America and committing suicide in a unique way, it would be sad but not frightening. But it is frightening, for New York is not disconnected from America. It is America's premier city and its intellectual headquarters. It is America in microcosm – the philosophy, the illusions, the pretensions, and the rationalizations which guide New York City are those which guide the entire country.[13]

In two large New York City teaching hospitals, at least 100 patients caught the deadly drug-resistant form of TB and at least 19 health care workers developed the deadly strain on the job.[14]

Atlanta, Georgia has now surpassed New York as the city with the highest incidence of TB in the United States. Atlanta recently reported a colossal 50% increase in TB over one year. "We were startled to hear the news, we thought everything was getting better," said Joseph Wilber, M.D., director of the communicable disease branch of Georgia's Division of Public Health. Dr. Wilber attributes Atlanta's plight to the high rate of HIV infection in the city.[15] Outbreaks of TB have been occuring with rising frequency across the United States.

AIDS NOT REGARDED AS A COMMUNICABLE DISEASE

In a deadly twist of irony, the states which are besieged with AIDS do not recognize HIV infection as a communicable or sexually transmitted disease.[16] This has forestalled the most basic preventive health measures from being taken. The result has been the loss of untold lives and the continued spread of HIV disease and its related infections into the population.

Medical and dental workers, feared and fearful, are caught in the crossfire. In many cases they are not allowed to know which patients are carrying AIDS – an infectious, fatal disease which could destroy their careers, their lives and the lives of loved ones. Concurrently, they face apprehensive patients who are concerned about contracting AIDS from them and demanding that medical and dental workers be tested.

Dr. Philip Levitan, President of the New York Society of Surgeons, has stated:

> The entire AIDS problem has been politicized and we feel at this point it needs to be medicalized.[17]

It is with this goal that *AIDS: Rage and Reality* has been written.

CHAPTER ONE

WHY RAGE WILL NOT PRODUCE
A CURE OR VACCINE

*We have been lined up in front of a firing squad and it is called
AIDS. We must riot.*
 *The new phase is terrorism. . . . I don't know whether it means
burning buildings, or killing people or setting fire to yourselves. . . .*
 *A tremendous wrong is being done to us, and it makes me furious. I
think when I'm ready to go, I will take somebody with me.*
 – Larry Kramer, an HIV-infected homosexual and founder of the militant
   protest group, ACT-UP[1]

AIDS MILITANTS INCENSED AT LACK OF PROGRESS

The serenity of the majestic cathedral of Notre Dame in Paris,
France was shattered as scores of angry AIDS protestors invaded
the sanctuary to challenge the Church's opposition to condoms and
homosexual conduct.
 At St. Patrick's Cathedral in New York City, a mob of enraged
homosexuals shouting obscenities swarmed into the aisles and
pews during Mass and showered churchgoers with condoms. One
of the militants desecrated a consecrated communion host, believed by Catholics to be the body and blood of Christ. Thousands
of militant demonstrators paraded outside the sanctuary, ha-
ranguing the Church. Some carried obscenely altered posters of
the crucifixion of Christ.
 In Costa Mesa, California vociferous members of ACT-UP
(AIDS Coalition to Unleash Power) and Queer Nation disrupted
the worship services of Calvary Chapel, a large evangelical church.
The groups angrily opposed the church's outreach to homosexuals
in an area of the city with a high rate of AIDS.
 In another particularly vicious outburst elsewhere in the state,
homosexual militants smashed doors and flung shards of broken
glass like frisbees, slicing the kneecaps of police officers. None of
the offenders were arrested.
 In cities throughout the United States and Europe, aggressive
AIDS activists have conducted similar peppery demonstrations,
demanding that more money be spent on developing a cure or
vaccine for AIDS. Militant AIDS protest groups such as ACT-UP

1

and Queer Nation (whose trademark chant is "We're here, we're queer, we're fabulous, get used to it!") have staged countless guerilla street theater exhibitions and media events. These and allied organizations allege that antagonism toward homosexuals has been the root cause for the lack of progress in developing a cure or vaccine for AIDS. They accuse politicians, public health officials, religious leaders, physicians, et al., of letting anti-homosexual attitudes block adequate funding for AIDS research. Those who advocate conventional disease control measures are labeled "homophobes."

If AIDS was perceived to be a disease affecting mainly hetero-sexual middle-class Americans, AIDS activists claim, far greater sums of money would have been expended on research efforts and many lives spared. Some homosexuals angrily charge that the lack of progress in AIDS treatment stems from a campaign of anti-homosexual genocide.[2]

PER CAPITA FEDERAL SPENDING ON AIDS OVERSHADOWS OTHER ILLNESSES

In dealing with an emotionally charged issue like AIDS, it is essential to differentiate between rhetoric and reality. The report *Federal Research and Prevention Funding for AIDS and Other Diseases*[3] provides some sobering statistics:

FEDERAL SPENDING PER DEATH	
AIDS	$46,428 - $52,702
Cancer	$3,494
Heart Disease	$931
Diabetes	$8,194
Alzheimer's	$2,430
Breast Cancer	$2,314

The above figures document how per capita public spending on AIDS proportionately far outweighs that of any other life-threatening illness. Indeed, federal spending on other diseases pales in comparison to AIDS.

These figures do not include the additional hundreds of millions of public dollars spent on treating AIDS patients, a large number of whom rely on public funds such as Medicaid and Social Security for medical care and support.[4] In the mid-1990s, the cost of treating all people with HIV disease in the United States is estimated to exceed ten billion dollars annually ($10,000,000,000 per year).[5]

Contrary to the claims of homosexual and AIDS patient advocacy groups, public financing of AIDS research has been given a pre-eminence unequaled by any other disease in history.

ARGUMENTS FOR INCREASED AIDS FUNDING

AIDS advocates use several arguments to buttress their drive for increased spending.

1. The AIDS pandemic could result in more deaths than the Black Plague (a reference to the darkened discoloration of the skin of bubonic plague victims) making the death toll from other diseases seem small in comparison. On a worldwide basis, AIDS is overwhelmingly a heterosexual disease. In the face of untold numbers of mortally infected adults, adolescents and children, it is unconscionable not to spend more money and increase scientific efforts to fight the disease.

2. The official count of AIDS cases reflects only the tip of the iceberg. The number of reported cases of end-stage AIDS reflect infections acquired in the past; many more people are carriers of HIV disease and will develop "full-blown" AIDS.[6]

3. AIDS is a relatively new illness and there is a great deal of catching up to do in terms of research. While more people will develop cancer and heart disease than are currently diagnosed, scientists have been working on these other maladies for decades. Spending on AIDS research should therefore match if not exceed that of other illnesses.

4. Money is spent on other diseases caused by human behavior. Research for treatment of heart disease and various types of cancer continue even though there are substantial behavioral components such as smoking and a high-fat diet. Inducing people to radically alter entrenched behaviors is an extremely difficult task at best.

5. Barring an effective vaccine, HIV will reach catastrophic levels of infection in a vast proportion of the world's population. Consequently, greater resources should be devoted *post haste* to developing a way of protecting people at risk and curing those infected.

THE VALUE OF HUMAN LIFE

The question is *not* whether the lives of people with HIV disease are "worth" saving or "deserve" saving. Human life is intrinsically valuable in its worth. To measure the *essential value* of human life in terms of mental or physical handicap promotes a dangerous utilitarian ethic.

The crucial issue is whether there is a reasonable likelihood of developing an effective treatment or vaccine for AIDS anytime in the foreseeable future. Answering this question will help maximize limited scientific and financial resources.

FORMIDABLE OBSTACLES TO AIDS TREATMENT

Researchers attempting to find a remedy for HIV disease face a series of formidable challenges.

1. The AIDS virus permanently integrates into the genetic core material of human cells.

Various other viruses, such as those which cause the common cold or flu usually cause transient illness. After a period of time the immune system clears the virus out of the body.

In drastic contrast, *infection with the AIDS virus is a monumental catastrophe in the biological life of a human being.* HIV integrates itself into the human genetic blueprint (genome). This means that HIV becomes enmeshed within the genetic material of the cells of the infected individual. There is no way for the AIDS virus to be "flushed out" or cleared from the body. *Once infection with the AIDS virus occurs, the individual becomes a permanent genetically stamped HIV carrier.*

Dr. Jay Levy of the University of San Francisco explains:

THE AIDS VIRUS IS A RETROVIRUS WHICH INFECTS AND INTE-GRATES IN THE CHROMOSOMES OF INFECTED CELLS, rather than just staying in the cytoplasm and replicating. What that means is that a cell can go on replicating the virus for years and years as it replicates [reproduces] itself. THERE ARE NO DRUGS WHICH CAN ACTU-ALLY DISENTANGLE THE VIRUS FROM THE GENES OF THE CELLS IT IS HIDING INSIDE – so your option if you want to get rid of the virus for good is actually to kill all the infected cells.[7]

California physician William T. O'Connor, M.D., a strong advocate of progressive health measures to combat AIDS, writes:

Simply put, THE AIDS VIRUS CHANGES OR MUTATES THE IN-FECTED HUMAN'S GENETIC CODE PERMANENTLY.

Once incorporated into the person's chromosomes . . . that person's cells have the capacity to make more virus which can go on to infect other cells and other people. By virtue of that reality, it can be said that THERE IS NO FORESEEABLE MEDICAL TECHNOLOGY TO PRODUCE A CURE.

A cure would entail going inside a cell's nucleus and selectively incapaci-tating, removing or destroying the virus' DNA (which only differs from hu-man DNA by its arrangement or sequencing of molecules) while preserving the human DNA. Any medicine that damages the virus' DNA would be toxic to the infected person's DNA as well.[8]

In short, *there is no way of killing the AIDS virus without destroying the cells it infects.* As the body's HIV-infected cells reproduce, all subsequent "offspring" cells will be infected with the AIDS virus.[9]

A toxic anti-viral drug such as AZT may briefly relieve some of the symptoms caused by HIV disease. *Nevertheless, the AIDS virus remains entrenched within the genetic material of infected cells and vital organs throughout the body.* As stated by Swedish AIDS researcher Bo Oberg, "Blocking HIV multiplication will not eliminate the virus because of integration into cellular genes. . . . *A permanent cure remains a remote possibility.*"[10]

2.   HIV is a lentivirus.

HIV is a member of the lentivirus group of viruses.[11] "Lenti" is derived from the Latin, *lentus,* meaning sticky, tenacious, slow. Lentiviruses are known for their lengthy "slow" incubation period. Lentiviruses are extremely virulent and complex.* Chronic degenerative disorders involving the joints, nervous system and lungs are a common feature of lentivirus infections in humans and animals.[12]

Prior to HIV, lentiviruses were thought to exist only in animals such as sheep (maedi-visna), goats (caprine arthritis) and horses (equine infectious anemia or "swamp fever"). *Infections with these "slow" viruses in animals have proved unremittingly resistant to therapy.* As reported in the *Journal of the Royal Society of Medicine*:

> In domestic animals, lentivirus infections have proved so lethal and unresponsive to treatment, and vaccines have proved so useless, that slaughter of infected animals has been the universal means of control.[13]

"*I don't think one can think of a cure for a retrovirus,*" states Dr. Anthony Fauci, Director of the National Institute of Allergy and Infectious Diseases.[14]

3.   The AIDS virus incessantly mutates and multiplies within the body.

During most of the 1980s, the popular wisdom of the scientific community assumed that AIDS had a prolonged latency or "resting" period during which the virus remained inert. It was speculated that boosting the immune system of an HIV-infected individual might stave off the initiation of the virus multiplying itself and prevent depletion of the immune system.

Contemporary research has demonstrated, however, that the

---

*The remarkable similarities between human AIDS and AIDS-type diseases in cats, monkeys, sheep, mice, horses and cows are discussed in-depth in the book *Animal Models of Retroviral Infection and Their Relationship to AIDS,* by Lois Ann Salzmann of the National Institute of Allergy and Infectious Diseases (Orlando, Florida: Academic Press).

AIDS virus is never dormant or inactive.[15] "HIV has no quiescent stage of replication, *replication occurs at all stages of HIV disease*," according to Dr. Anthony Fauci.[16] *The virus is far more prevalent in the blood of infected individuals than previously thought.*[17]

The AIDS virus commences mutating and multiplying from the very earliest stage of infection, including the so-called "asymptomatic" period in which the infected individual appears outwardly healthy. HIV viruses rapidly multiply in the lymph nodes, thereby maintaining lethal reservoirs of virus throughout the body. This finding has dampened support for the idea that there would be a means of holding back the virus from being triggered into replicating; the AIDS virus mutates and multiplies continuously from the time it invades the body.

4.   HIV infection is a progressive degenerative disease.

During the early course of the AIDS epidemic, various medical authorities contended that the vast majority of people infected with HIV would remain healthy carriers. It was commonly held that only a small subset would develop AIDS.

The Truth About AIDS which was hailed in the *New England Journal of Medicine* as "by far the clearest and most insightful book published to date [1985]," asserted:

> *What should those who test positive expect?* Current estimates of progressing from positive to the next stage are between 5 and 19 percent. *The greatest likelihood is that nothing will happen.*[18]

The upbeat notion that "nothing will happen" to most HIV carriers was far removed from medical reality. Widespread dissemination of that outlook conveyed a dangerous false sense of security. Many people were led to believe that even if they contracted the AIDS virus, it was unlikely that they would ever get sick. Among other factors, this early false optimism may have contributed to HIV infection reaching pandemic levels among male homosexuals.[19]

Though initially criticized by some as unduly pessimistic, the long range mortality predicted in *The AIDS Cover-Up?* (published in 1986) has proved entirely tenable:

> Ultimately infection with the AIDS virus may leave no survivors. This means that the majority—perhaps all—of the persons already infected will probably die of AIDS-related disease.[20]

This grim prognosis has been repeatedly confirmed by studies tracking the progression of disease in HIV-infected individuals over time. These studies indicate that there is no slowdown in the progression to end-stage AIDS.[21]

Dashing early hopes that only a small percentage of HIV-infected people would get AIDS, epidemiologists at the San Francisco Health Department now believe it's possible that everyone who's infected will progress to the fatal disease. "*100% progression [to terminal AIDS] is our best guess. That's what we're using for planning purposes,*" says Dr. George Lemp, chief of the department's AIDS surveillance branch.

Dr. Donald Abrams, assistant director of the San Francisco General Hospital AIDS clinic, points out that in a subset of the San Francisco hepatitis B cohort, half of the patients with lymphadenopathy [swollen lymph glands] developed AIDS after five years. *The rate of progression was consistent until the five-year mark, when it accelerated dramatically.* "And there's no evidence that the curve will drop," says Dr. Abrams.[22]

HIV disease is a relentlessly progressive degenerative illness. Canadian researchers report that AZT-resistant strains of HIV have developed rapidly in the majority of asymptomatic AIDS patients treated with high doses of AZT, as well as those receiving low doses (300-400 mg/day) of the drug.[23]

Researchers from the AIDS Office of the San Francisco Health Department, the University of California (SF) and the U.S. Centers for Disease Control did a 13-year follow-up study comparing the health status of HIV-infected men treated with various prophylactic therapies (AZT, DDI, or *P. carinii* pneumonia prophylaxis) with men who did not receive such treatment. They found *no significant difference between men who underwent these therapies and those who did not in the time it took for them to progress to AIDS.*[24] They state, "The devastating impact of HIV infection on mortality is increasing."[25]

Dr. Paul Volberding, Director of the AIDS program at San Francisco Hospital, asserts: "*It is clear that HIV infection progresses inexorably despite the best therapies currently available.*"[26]

5.   HIV infection means AIDS is present.

The pronouncement, "A positive test for HIV does not mean someone has AIDS," has become axiomatic among public health officials, in AIDS education courses and the media.

Dichotomizing between HIV infection and AIDS can be misleading. The concept of a "healthy HIV carrier state" existing at any time during the course of infection with HIV is illusory. French AIDS researchers state emphatically:

Asymptomatic HIV-seropositive individuals are NOT healthy carriers [emphasis in original].[27]

Wide-ranging alterations of the immune system exist even when no clinical signs of HIV-1 infection are detectable.[28] The AIDS virus invades the brain and nervous system very early in the course of infection.[29] The vast majority of HIV-1 infected individuals harbor actively replicating virus in cerebrospinal fluid during all stages of infection.[30]

In his seminal work, *Safe Blood: Purifying the Nation's Blood Supply in the Age of AIDS*, Joseph Feldschuh, M.D., states:

> . . . medical experts across the country now concede that ALMOST ALL INDIVIDUALS WHO ARE HIV POSITIVE HAVE AIDS, EVEN IF THEY APPEAR HEALTHY because they are still at an earlier stage of the disease. There has been a great deal of public confusion about the distinction between HIV infection and AIDS. HIV INFECTION SIMPLY MEANS THAT ONE HAS AIDS WITH NO SYMPTOMS. If you have HIV, you are infected with the AIDS virus. RESTRICTING THE TERM ["AIDS"] TO THOSE WHO HAVE SYMPTOMS IS TANTAMOUNT TO SAYING THAT IF YOU HAVE CANCER WITH NO SYMPTOMS, YOU DON'T HAVE CANCER.[31]

Dividing the course of HIV infection into various stages such as asymptomatic carrier state, AIDS-related complex (ARC) and "full-blown AIDS" may help portray the worsening effects of HIV infection.[32] In actuality, the term "infection with the AIDS virus" denotes a continuum of HIV disease. "HIV disease" is currently the term used to refer to the spectrum of conditions associated with HIV infection.

Individuals infected with HIV do not simply "have the virus which causes AIDS." Every person infected with the AIDS virus has HIV disease. Scientists are not merely treating an infection; they are dealing with a degenerative, infectious disease with a 100% fatality rate.

6. The AIDS virus infects and destroys the cells which normally help to ward off disease.

The AIDS virus invades and takes over the cells which normally help to defend against invading organisms. The immune system is designed to ward off invading germs and organisms. HIV infects the T4 lymphocyte and monocyte-macrophage which serve as pivotal cells in the armada of the immune system.[33] The cells of the body's immune system are transformed into deadly biological accomplices for the infiltration of HIV throughout the body. "Boosting" the immune system of someone with HIV disease can at best have a transient effect because the virus remains entrenched and replicating within the cells of the immune system itself. *Instead of defending the body against HIV, the immune system becomes a means of furthering the onslaught of the virus.*

7. There is no means of reconstituting the human immune system.

It is well established that the AIDS virus infects and destroys cells which normally protect the body from disease and leaves the body vulnerable to deadly opportunistic infections (OIs) and cancers. These secondary cancers and diseases such as Kaposi's sarcoma, lymphoma, *P. carinii* pneumonia, disseminated herpes, CMV, tuberculosis, and the like, are usually cited as causing the death of AIDS patients. Even when these secondary diseases respond to treatment, there is no way of effectively rebuilding the debilitated immune system. The continuing immune deficiency leaves AIDS patients vulnerable to a host of chronic opportunistic infections and diseases.

According to Dr. Anthony Fauci:

> Although effective therapies are available for many of the infections and tumors that occur in patients with AIDS, NO THERAPY EXISTS FOR THE UNDERLYING IMMUNODEFICIENCY.[34]

8.   HIV can induce autoimmune disease.

In addition to crippling the immune system and devastating the central nervous system, mounting scientific evidence indicates that HIV induces autoimmune disease.[35] Autoimmunity is a condition in which the body attacks and rejects its own healthy tissues. The body mounts an immune response against its own normal, healthy tissue elements, attacking them as though they were a harmful substance. Autoimmunity causes severe inflammatory reactions and is associated with a variety of diseases, such as systemic lupus erythematosus (SLE) and rheumatoid arthritis.

The occurrence of autoantibodies is a common finding in HIV disease.[36] Researchers from the University of British Columbia report:

> *Autoimmunity often precedes the onset of ARC or AIDS,* and a number of autoantibodies have been described in AIDS patients and persons at risk for AIDS. . . . Titration of anti-collagen activity in positive sera revealed levels *100 times higher* than the levels in normal sera. . . . The *antibodies . . . are similar to those seen in graft versus host disease and leprosy.* . . . These results suggest that *all persons progressing to AIDS express anti-collagen antibodies* which may be useful markers of disease progression.[37]

Collagen is the protein substance of the white fibers of skin, tendon, bone, cartilage and all other connective tissue in the body. When HIV-induced anti-collagen antibodies attack collagen as though it were a harmful substance, it can produce serious disease of connective tissues.[38]

Researchers from the National Academy of Medicine in Buenos Aires, Argentina, state that their results suggest:

> . . . antibodies reacting with neurotransmitter receptors . . . might trigger cholinergic-like response in the heart and *could play an immunopathogenic role in the development of cardiac and neurologic disease in AIDS.*[39]

These findings mean that it is not only the AIDS virus itself which produces devastating illness. *The various types of autoantibodies which form in response to HIV infection also cause disease.* In addition to trying to develop ways to deal with the manifold assaults of the AIDS virus itself, scientists face the daunting prospect of contending with destructive autoantibodies both in treatment and in vaccine development.[40]

According to Dr. Luc Montagnier, the French co-discoverer of the AIDS virus, even if there was a way to curtail the growth of HIV, the autoimmune disease caused by AIDS would continue. He states:

> Autoimmune mechanisms that may be involved in AIDS could prove to be self-perpetuating even in the face of inhibition of virus multiplication.[41]

9. The AIDS virus kills directly.

The notion that "AIDS itself doesn't kill. People don't die of AIDS; they die of other diseases caused by their weakened immune systems," is found in most popular "AIDS education" materials, and is reiterated frequently in the media. This statement contains a substantial error of omission. It has been well established that *the AIDS virus itself invades vital organs in the body and directly causes disease.*

As far back as the Third International Conference on AIDS in 1987, Dr. Peter Piot of the Institute of Tropical Medicine in Antwerp, Belgium, stated:

> The clinical expression of HIV infection appears increasingly complex. It includes manifestations due to opportunistic disease, *as well as illness caused directly by HIV itself.* Neurological disease may include involvement of brain, spinal cord, and peripheral nerves, and is . . . *directly caused by HIV* as is lymphocytic interstitial pneumonia.[42]

The AIDS virus directly causes disease within vital organs, apart from the secondary illnesses related to immune suppression. If most AIDS patients were not dying first of other secondary diseases, they would fall prey to HIV's direct destruction of vital organs throughout the body. The direct attack of HIV on the body has grave implications for ever finding a "cure" for AIDS and has serious implications for public policy.

10. HIV invades the spinal cord and brain (CNS).

The author's first book on AIDS published several years ago predicted that HIV-induced brain deterioration (dementia) would become increasingly problematic among persons infected with the AIDS virus.[43] *The AIDS Cover-Up?* quoted the ominous warning by Dr. Paul Volberding:

It is entirely reasonable to speculate that *everyone* who is seropositive [infected with the AIDS virus] will develop central nervous system complications. We are seeing an increasing number of signs of this on our ward. They take the form of varying degrees of dementia.[44]

The history of mental decline evinced by many AIDS patients studied since then has borne out the worst fears of both those suffering with HIV disease and health care providers. HIV invades the central nervous system (CNS) soon after infection occurs.[45] A progressive, dementing illness is among the most common and devastating manifestations of HIV infection.[46] The vast majority of HIV-infected individuals will experience substantial brain deterioration during the course of the disease.[47] AIDS is a devastating disease of the brain and spinal cord. In some AIDS patients, the total brain mass shrinks to less than one half its normal size.[48] Attempting to purge HIV from the CNS is fraught with peril. Dr. Jay Levy states:

When the virus goes to the brain and you have infectious virus replicating in the brain, that obviously means you have serious problems in trying to treat it. YOU CAN'T KILL BRAIN CELLS WITHOUT TRADING OFF SOME VERY IMPORTANT BIO-FUNCTIONS.[49]

Areas of the brain affected by HIV include those controlling thought processes. This is a major reason for the high degree of mental and cognitive impairment in persons with HIV disease.[50] Analogous to an inoperable, malignant brain tumor, it is impossible to destroy or remove masses of HIV-infected tissue from vital areas of the brain without disastrous consequences. Brain cells which are latently infected maintain the presence of HIV infection.

Researchers from the University of San Diego note that even with prolonged AZT treatment, "dementia is a frequent, rather than a rare complication of AIDS."[51]

11. The nervous system is a conduit for HIV.

The AIDS virus targets nerve cells throughout the nervous system as well as the immune system.[52] This preference of the AIDS virus for infecting nerve cells is known as neurotropism (Greek, *neuron*, "nerve" and *trope*, "turning," "affinity for").[53] Productive HIV infection of the CNS is frequent in AIDS and can produce symptoms which resemble those of multiple sclerosis (MS).[54]

HIV destroys the spinal cord. The AIDS virus damages the spinal cord and nerves, leading to agonizingly painful burning sensations in the feet and difficulty walking.[55] Paresthesias (burning, prickling feelings sometimes accompanied by formication, a tactile sensation of insects crawling on the skin) and dysesthesias confined to the feet are common symptoms in patients in the pre-terminal stages of AIDS . . . [indicating] *a "dying back" process of the primary sensory axon.*[56]

The human nervous system serves as a deadly conveyor belt for transporting HIV disease throughout the body.

12. There is no way of eradicating HIV disease from nerve cells throughout the body.

It is impossible to eradicate the AIDS virus without destroying the infected nerve cells. AZT has been cited as causing inflammation of the peripheral nervous system, thus exacerbating the damaging effects of the virus.[57]

Damage to the autonomic nervous system may occur early in the course of HIV disease. In a study of patients with early HIV disease, 30% showed signs of autonomic neuropathy.[58]

13. The AIDS virus targets all vital organs.

In addition to the brain and nervous system, HIV infects and destroys vital organs throughout the body.

Heart: HIV disease causes deterioration of the heart muscle. This condition, known as cardiomyopathy, occurs in the absence of opportunistic infections such as toxoplasmosis.[59] Researchers from George Washington University, Washington, D.C. report "50% OF HIV-INFECTED PATIENTS HAVE UNSUSPECTED CARDIAC ABNORMALITIES. . . . The frequency of abnormalities is higher in patients with more advanced disease, but is not related to concurrent opportunistic infections . . . suggesting that HIV ITSELF IS A HEART PATHOGEN."[60] There is evidence that autoimmunity also has a significant role in HIV-associated cardiomyopathy.[61]

HIV disease causes inflammation of the muscle walls of the heart (myocarditis) and has been linked with fatal congestive cardiomyopathy and congestive heart failure in children.[62]

As drugs are used to treat some of the secondary diseases associated with immune deficiency, many AIDS patients who would have died earlier will face HIV-induced heart deterioration. "We feel that cardiac problems could emerge," says Constance Weinstein, Ph.D., chief of the cardiac diseases branch of the National Heart, Lung, and Blood Institute, Bethesda, Maryland.[63] Cardiac abnormalities are common in AIDS patients.[64]

The risk of cardiac disease should be taken into account by HIV-infected individuals and their physicians when considering any kind of exercise regimen or occupation requiring strenuous labor.[65] "Myocarditis is a frequent necropsy finding in patients dying with AIDS."[66] The fact that HIV causes heart disease makes it prudent for patients with known or suspected heart disease to be tested for AIDS infection.

Lungs Teem with HIV: The lungs have proven highly susceptible to AIDS-related pneumonias and tuberculosis. The lungs also provide a fertile breeding ground for growth of the AIDS virus. *Physicians have found a higher concentration of AIDS viruses in the lung secretions of AIDS patients than peripheral blood.*[67]

The AIDS virus infects cells in the lungs and directly causes a persistent inflammation of pulmonary tissue. This condition is known as chronic lymphoid interstitial pneumonitis (CLIP). HIV-induced lung disease (CLIP) can occur in the absence of or along with other lung ailments. Even when medications are used to alleviate the symptoms of other lung diseases such as *P. carinii* pneumonia, *the AIDS virus itself remains entrenched within the lungs and can directly induce disease.*

Researchers from the National Institutes of Health, the Armed Forces Institute of Pathology, Washington, D.C., and Beth Israel Medical Center in New York City, state that their study:

> . . . together with the knowledge that lymphocytic *pulmonary lesions may be caused by lentiviruses in humans and animals*, suggest that *HIV plays a significant role in the pathogenesis of both NIP* [Nonspecific Interstitial Pneumonitis] *and LIP* [Lymphocytic Interstitial Pneumonitis] *in adult HIV-infected patients.*[68]

Similar to maedi visna, a lentivirus disease of sheep, the AIDS virus itself induces lung disease. Since alveolar macrophages, a type of white blood cell found in the lungs, are long-lived cells, they may act as a reservoir for HIV infection, capable of transmitting the virus to other susceptible cells.[69] The CDC indicates that the lung secretions of AIDS patients expectorated into the air should be considered infectious.[70]

Kidneys: HIV can directly cause kidney disease, resulting in enlarged kidneys, weight loss and malnutrition.[71] Urinary albumin excretion is abnormal in patients with early HIV infection.[72]

A large percentage of AIDS patients have HIV infection of the kidneys. "Silent" HIV infection of the kidneys is frequent, approximately 50%.[73]

A rapidly progressive disorder of the kidneys may be the initial or the only sign of HIV disease.[74] Some AIDS researchers recommend that *all adult patients with signs of kidney disease be tested for HIV.*[75] Acute and chronic renal failure is a significant problem among AIDS patients and the survival rate is poor.[76]

Physicians from the New Orleans Health Department report:

Persons with HIV infections are at increased risk for heat-related illness during intense heat waves. Heat cramps developing in HIV-positive persons should be vigorously treated to prevent . . . *acute renal [kidney] failure*. Persons living with HIV infections in temperate zones who visit hot, humid areas should be cautioned about heat induced illness.[77]

Every precaution should be taken to avoid patient-to-patient spread of HIV in dialysis units treating AIDS patients.[78]

HIV has been detected in urine and should be considered an infectious body fluid in individuals with HIV disease.[79]

Liver: HIV infects the liver of the majority of AIDS patients.[80] HIV infection of the liver results in the dissemination of large numbers of viral particles throughout the body.[81] An enlarged liver is a common finding in AIDS patients. Infection with HIV-1 is the major determinant of liver enlargement (hepatomegaly) observed in various stages of HIV infection in hemophiliacs.[82] HIV infection in children can cause giant cell transformation of the liver.[83]

Liver lymphoma (cancer) is associated with HIV disease and can be a primary manifestation of AIDS. It has a poor prognosis.[84]

Spleen: Spleen enlargement has been reported in AIDS patients, and spontaneous rupture of the spleen has been reported in a patient with HIV disease.[85]

Pancreas: HIV disease causes devastating deterioration of the pancreas, the vital gland which produces insulin. In an analysis of the autopsies of 113 AIDS patients, about half were found to have pathological alterations of the pancreas. In some, the deterioration (necrosis) of the pancreas was so extensive that an examination of the organ could not be interpreted.[86] Researchers from the Johns Hopkins Medical Institutions report that "pancreatitis, [inflammation of the pancreas] is commonly found in AIDS patients."[87]

The fact that HIV disease causes pancreatitis should be taken into account when considering the usage of certain medications to treat AIDS patients. AIDS activist groups pushed for access to the experimental drug DDI (dideoxyinosine), but the drug has caused fatal inflammation of the pancreas in AIDS patients as well as painful nerve damage.[88]

AIDS Virus Causes Arthritis: HIV disease can result in acute and severe arthritis involving the ankles, knees, wrists, fingers and lower back.[89] HIV has been found in the synovial fluid, the lubricating fluid secreted by membranes in joints, cavities, sheaths of tendons and bursae.[90] Dr. Leonard Calabrese of the Cleveland Clinic Foundation in Ohio, states: "Articular disease appears to be relatively common in the setting of HIV infection."[91] According to

Italian researchers, "HIV is directly involved in relapsing and migrating arthrosinovitis."[92]

HIV infection has been associated with Reiter's syndrome (urethritis, conjunctivitis, and arthritis), dry eyes, and Raynaud's phenomenon, "intermittent bilateral attacks of ischemia [lack of blood flow] of the fingers or toes and sometimes of the ears and nose, marked by severe pallor, and often accompanied by paresthesia and pain."[93]

Bone Marrow: HIV infects the bone marrow at very early stages of HIV disease.[94] The bone marrow serves as a reservoir of HIV disease.[95] This has dire implications.[96]

> Even if viral replication could be suspended indefinitely, patients with AIDS will not be able to regain their health without reconstitution of their immune system. . . . Recent experience using bone marrow transplantation, even when cells from an uninfected twin were available, have been disappointing.[97]

Muscles: HIV has been associated with muscle inflammation (myositis).[98] "Neuromuscular involvement, mainly neuropathy, can be identified in up to 95% of patients with AIDS."[99]

Intestines: HIV can directly infect intestinal epithelial cells and cause disease within the colon and gastrointestinal (GI) tract. This is a major reason why male homosexuals have proven so extraordinarily susceptible to contracting HIV disease. HIV damage of the gut can result in chronic diarrhea. Canadian researchers report: "biological and ultrastructural abnormalities [of the intestines] are common in HIV positive patients, even in the absence of infectious pathogens."[100] Carcinomas (cancers) of the stomach and esophagus have also been reported in AIDS patients.[101]

> Cells of . . . the human small intestine and colon bearing lymphocyte or macrophage markers can be directly infected by and support the replication of HIV-1 and this may be important in the pathogenesis of HIV enteropathy [bowel inflammation].[102]

The GI tract is a major target site for HIV and the virus is present in high amounts at all sites.[103] The high amount of HIV in the GI tract indicates the fecal material (both solid waste and diarrhea) of AIDS patients should be considered infectious for HIV as well as for parasitic bowel diseases.

Skin, Nose and Mouth: *The AIDS virus directly infects Langerhans cells located in the skin and mucous membranes.*[104] In addition to skin, Langerhans cells are inside of the nose, mouth and the genital tract. Contrary to the reassurances given medical personnel,

HIV can be transmitted across intact skin *in the absence of* sores, cuts, lesions, or open wounds.[105]

Seborrehic dermatitis (a dandruff-like condition of the scalp and forehead) is a common symptom of HIV infection and can be accompanied by widespread skin lesions, Yellow Nail Syndrome, and severe psoriasis.[106]

Researchers from the Department of Virology at the renowned Robert Koch Institute in Berlin, along with researchers from Norway, have demonstrated:

> Epidermal Langerhans cells [in the skin] from symptom-free HIV-positive individuals may be latently infected. In ARC/AIDS patients, HIV HAS BEEN DEMONSTRATED IN THE EPIDERMIS OF THE SKIN, and we have previously demonstrated that epidermal Langerhans cells can be infected in vitro with HIV, and that they produce and release HIV into the culture medium.[107]

The skin teems with HIV. Researchers from the Laboratory of Tumor Cell Biology, NCI, NIH, Bethesda, Maryland, and the Department of Dermatology, University of Vienna Medical School, Vienna, Austria, have determined:

> . . . ACTIVE VIRUS CAN BE RESCUED FROM THE SKIN OF HIV-INFECTED INDIVIDUALS. Our findings conclusively confirm that (I) Langerhans cells are an actual target for HIV infection and production, supporting the view that besides T cells, cells of the monocyte/macrophage lineage are a major target population of this virus and (II) THE SKIN MAY SERVE AS A VIRAL RESERVOIR DURING THE COURSE OF HIV INFECTION.[108]

HIV infection has been associated with an increased susceptibility to skin rashes, psoriasis, and skin cancer (basal cell carcinoma).[109]

Exposure to ultraviolet light triggers a dramatic growth of HIV. In a study reported in the British scientific journal *Nature*, exposing HIV-infected cells in a test tube to ultraviolet light caused the virus to multiply 150 fold. Martin Rosenberg, a member of the team of Smith-Klein and French researchers who conducted the study, has stated, "We call these stress responses caused by UV light." This result raises the possibility that the virus can be activated by direct sun exposure.[110] A report from the United Nations Environment Program based in Nairobi, Kenya, indicates: "It is becoming clear that activation of HIV-1 by UV rays is a cause for concern. Increased exposure to ultraviolet rays can "result in increased severity of the disease or a more rapid course of infection."[111]

HIV Causes Blindness

Eyes: The AIDS virus directly infects the tissue and nerves of the eye causing lesions and impaired vision (e.g., cotton wool spots). HIV-induced eye damage and visual impairment occurs in the absence of and in addition to retinitis caused by cytomegalovirus (CMV). Blindness is one of the most dreaded aspects of HIV infection.[112]

Between 50%-70% or more of adult AIDS patients have ocular lesions.[113] Personnel performing eye examinations should be certain to thoroughly disinfect instruments having any direct contact with the eye.[114]

HIV Infects Sites in the Throat

Lymphoid Tissues: The lymph nodes, tonsils and adenoids are major reservoirs of HIV disease. There are higher concentrations of HIV-infected cells in the lymphoid tissues than in peripheral blood.[115] In addition, HIV disease can result in swelling of tissue (hypertrophy) in the nose and pharynx. An ear, nose, and throat examination is mandatory for all patients with known or suspected HIV disease.[116]

Testes and Prostate Gland: HIV infects and apparently causes disease within the testes and prostate gland. This is consistent with research demonstrating the presence of HIV in seminal fluid.[117] Physicians may consider it prudent to order an AIDS test for patients with prostate problems.

Bladder: HIV disease has also been associated with bladder problems, including painful frequent urination and blood in the urine in the absence of any other demonstrable urinary tract infection.[118]

14. HIV-infected cells can act as virtual cluster bombs for releasing massive amounts of virus.

If an HIV-infected cell is locked in a compartment of the body with no direct access to infectible cells and therefore no chance for fusing, the virus programs the cell to produce hundreds of viral particles, which can rapidly diffuse in extracellular fluids or in the bloodstream.

> The RNA genomes and viral proteins assemble into infectious [HIV] virus particles which, in some instances, massively bud from the cell surface, thereby destroying the cell. MASSIVE VIRAL REPLICATION MAY OCCUR. . . . *A SINGLE INFECTED CELL MAY PRODUCE 500 TO 1000 OF THESE.*[119]

DAUNTING OBSTACLES TO AN AIDS "VACCINE"

1. The body's natural defenses are incapable of combatting the AIDS virus. With other diseases, the immune system produces antibodies which attack and kill invading organisms. Vaccines are utilized to raise antibody levels in the bloodstream high enough to kill invading pathogens. In the case of HIV infection, the antibodies which develop have little or no capacity to neutralize. Injecting HIV into a human subject would be a death sentence.

2. The AIDS virus is constantly mutating within the body of each infected individual. HIV mutates (changes) with such ferocious rapidity, that *antibodies which have formed in response to the initial strain (form) of the virus do not recognize the new mutations.* This process is known as *antigenic drift,* a term previously coined for the mutation found among influenza viruses. Researchers from the University of Miami and the Laboratory of Tumor Cell Biology, NCI, Bethesda, Maryland, note:

> The AIDS virus, HIV, has been shown to exhibit striking genomic variation when isolates obtained from different individuals are compared. Extensive genetic variation is generated *in vivo* [in the body]. The degree of viral heterogeneity has been heretofore underestimated and MANY DIFFERENT VIRAL FORMS EXIST IN PERSISTENTLY INFECTED INDIVIDUALS, and thus "ISOLATES" OBTAINED FROM SUCH PERSONS for use in the study of HIV biology and immunology, unless cloned, ARE ACTUALLY COMPLEX MIXTURES OF GENETICALLY-DISTINCT VIRUSES.[120]

Scientists are not dealing with merely one viral entity. Each of the millions of individuals infected with HIV harbors numerous mutant forms of the virus.[121] Attempting to develop a "vaccine" for AIDS is like trying to hit countless moving targets simultaneously. Researchers from Washington, D.C., and elsewhere report:

> *More than 100 HIV-1 isolates from ten countries on four continents have been studied by PCR* [DNA "fingerprinting"]. Isolates from one country in Africa are genetically similar to each other by the PCR technique. . . . These isolates differ by sequence from both Zairean and North American/European isolates. Isolates from North America are relatively homogeneous and similar to known prototypes. In Asia and South America, disparate patterns were observed in different locales. One Asian country exhibited isolates principally of the North American/European type while another exhibited broad genetic diversity of HIV-1.
> *THE GENETIC DIVERSITY OF HIV-1 IN AFRICA AND SPECIFIC REGIONS OF ASIA AND SOUTH AMERICA MAY BE MORE EXTENSIVE THAN PREVIOUSLY APPRECIATED. If the first vaccines are incompletely protective against some HIV-1 variants, a profile of genetic diversity in different countries may be needed for effective vaccine development.*[122]

Even if there was a way of developing a vaccine against one particular mutant of the virus in one infected individual, it would not be effective against the countless other HIV mutants which already exist, and the new ones which are constantly arising.

3. Antibodies produced by a vaccine could further the spread of HIV disease within the body.[123] HIV disease is an immunological nightmare. Non- or poorly neutralizing antibodies which form in response to HIV infection can actually serve to spread AIDS viruses to other cells in the body. *These antibodies perpetuate rather than eliminate HIV infection.* Antibodies and killer T8 lymphocytes in AIDS patients are capable of attacking their own normal, uninfected T4 cells.[124]

Dr. Jay Levy of the University of San Francisco School of Medicine states:

> In many individuals and in HIV-infected animal model systems, THE VIRUS HAS ALSO BEEN SHOWN TO INDUCE ANTIBODIES THAT do not neutralize but rather *ENHANCE* VIRUS INFECTION. THESE ANTIBODIES COULD POTENTIALLY INCREASE THE SPREAD OF HIV IN THE INFECTED INDIVIDUAL and contribute to pathogenicity by expanding the host range of some viruses....[125]

Even if scientists were able to able to inoculate an individual with a non-infective killed virus or portion of the virus, *the antibodies which form could expedite rather than hinder the spread of HIV infection in the body when the person is subsequently exposed to the virus.* If the person is already infected with HIV, *enhancing antibodies produced by a vaccine would accelerate the destructive course of the disease.*[126]

4. A vaccine would not prevent infection. Dr. Peter Nara, D.V.M., Ph.D., chief of the Virus Biology Section, Laboratory of Tumor Cell Biology at the National Cancer Institute, explains:

> Given our current understanding of lentiviral infections, it appears that CONVENTIONAL VACCINE STRATEGIES ARE UNSUITABLE TO THE PREVENTION OF LENTIVIRAL DISEASES [SUCH AS AIDS]. Since the time of Jenner and Pasteur, all successful human and animal antiviral vaccines have been made either from virus attenuated in tissue cultures (called modified "live" virus particles), or from a part or parts (termed subunit) of the virus that activates the immune system. The vaccines confer immunity by eliciting what is termed an *anamnestic response*, which basically means to "not forget."
>
> On subsequent introduction of wild-type virus (other than lentiviruses) into the body, infection occurs, but the immune system, previously sensitized through vaccination, responds and eliminates the viral invader. The success of these vaccines was due primarily to the nature of the viruses involved. *Viruses successfully blocked by vaccine-induced protection generally do not*

integrate themselves into the host's genome and do not exclusively parasitize the immune system of the body....

A KEY POINT WITH REGARD TO AIDS IS THE FACT THAT THE IMMUNE RESPONSE GENERATED BY OUR CURRENT VI-RAL-BASED VACCINES DOES NOT ALWAYS PREVENT THE INI-TIAL INFECTION. Since HIV is capable of integrating itself into the genetic material of infected cells, *a vaccine would have to produce a constant state of immune protection, which could totally block the initial infection of the host cells at all times. Such complete and constant protection has never before been accomplished and works in direct opposition to the normal immune suppressor network, which dampens or turns down, specific immune responses.* A state of perpetual immune activation may have as yet undefined detrimental consequences to the host.[127]

5. An AIDS vaccine could cause autoimmune disease. HIV can induce autoantibodies resulting in autoimmune disease.[128] A vaccine utilizing a "killed" virus or portion of the virus could produce autoantibodies resulting in autoimmune disorders.

Canadian researchers from the University of British Columbia have cautioned: "Vaccines consisting of gp120, gp160, and anti-CD4 *may cause AIDS* in individuals belonging to high risk groups."[129]

6. The AIDS virus changes its genetic code more rapidly than any other known virus. Findings at the Los Alamos National Laboratory show that HIV is altering its genetic code as much as five times as fast as the influenza virus, which was previously thought to be the fastest in mutating. *The flu virus has taken 50 years to change as much as the AIDS virus has in ten years.* Dr. Gerald Myers, a molecular geneticist who participated in the research, states:

> The AIDS viruses now manifest themselves as a complex family tree, sprouting new genetic branches — and apparently quickly at that.[130]

7. The AIDS virus is transmitted through AIDS-infected cells in body fluids. Dr. Albert Sabin, an internationally renowned scientist and developer of the oral polio vaccine, doubts that a vaccine can be found to halt the spread of the AIDS virus. Writing in the *Proceedings of the National Academy of Sciences*, Dr. Sabin said he is pessimistic because the AIDS virus is transmitted differently than polio, measles or other diseases whose spread is prevented by vaccine. These other infections are prevented by vaccines which induce antibodies that attack invading viruses rather than cells. By being transported via infected cells, the AIDS virus is shielded from detection by antibodies. This creates a biological Trojan Horse mechanism.[131]

SUMMARY OF OBSTACLES TO FINDING AN AIDS "CURE"

1. The human lentivirus disease called "AIDS" destroys the very system designed to ward off invading organisms. HIV uses cells which normally protect the body to spread disease. This is analogous to a country using its defensive weapon system to bomb its own population.

2. It is impossible to eradicate the virus without destroying the cells it infects. The AIDS virus incubates within the skin, eyes, brain, spinal cord, nervous system, bone marrow, heart, lungs, muscles, liver, pancreas, kidneys and other vital organs. There is no way of destroying the virus throughout the body without killing the patient. Even if all the blood within an HIV-infected person was replaced with clean, "immune-boosted" healthy blood, HIV would remain fatally ensconced in vital organs throughout the body.

3. There is no way of reconstituting the human immune system. This assures that opportunistic disease(s) will continue to occur. AIDS patients who live somewhat longer are falling prey to a new variety of infections, cancers, nervous system disease and striking levels of wasting. According to Dr. Samuel Broder of the National Cancer Institute in Bethesda, Maryland, "*AIDS-related cancers are being seen in record numbers. Cancer is emerging as the biggest new challenge in the treatment of AIDS.*"[132]

4. The AIDS virus targets and destroys cells in the brain and other vital organs. HIV is not a "harmless microbe." Even if there was a way of maintaining or improving immune function for a prolonged period of time, the virus would continue to cause death directly through destruction of various major organs.

5. AIDS appears to induce autoimmune disease. Suppressing the multiplication of AIDS viruses would not stop the formation of destructive autoantibodies.

"AIDS" IS A MISNOMER

Acquired Immune Deficiency Syndrome (AIDS) was originally called the Gay Related Immune Deficiency (GRID). The name was changed in deference to homosexual groups who complained that the term GRID was "stigmatizing." As pointed out in the *Journal of the Royal Society of Medicine*, the term "AIDS" is in itself misleading because it diverts attention away from the disease's direct attack on the brain and lungs.[133] "AIDS" is actually a *human lentivirus disease* which directly attacks and destroys the body through a variety of means even in the absence of immune deficiency.

BLOOD ON WHOSE HANDS?

Homosexual and AIDS advocacy demonstrators have a penchant for holding up their hands wearing white gloves smeared with red paint. They do this to luridly illustrate their charge that the government has "blood on its hands" for not spending enough money on AIDS. In light of financial and scientific realities, their claim is unfounded.

In truth, the harder scientists have worked to combat HIV disease, the tougher and more pernicious the virus has become. Mutant versions of the AIDS virus–often a whole new colony–emerge which resist any drug treatment. The virus churns out millions of copies of itself, and no two are alike.[134]

THE BRICK WALL OF BIOLOGICAL REALITY

In confronting AIDS, all the human pathos, grief, rage, and rational arguments for greater efforts to find a cure or vaccine have collided head-on with the brick wall of unyielding biological reality. No amount of hysteria, sloganeering, guerilla street theater, bitter accusations or politicizing can change the extraordinarily complex and virulent nature of the AIDS virus itself.

Vast sums of money have been invested and countless intense hours of research conducted by a legion of international scientific experts. These monumental efforts have met with dismal results. Progress toward developing an effective treatment or vaccine for the human lentivirus disease called AIDS has been less than negligible. It is dreadfully clear that there is not even a remote expectation of a cure or vaccine anytime in the foreseeable future.[135]

When attempting to cope with a plague which could annihilate substantial portions of mankind, it is imperative that public policy be based on medical reality rather than political chauvinism, hysteria, or Pollyanna-like idealism. If it is not, the consequences will be catastrophic.

CHAPTER TWO

THE DEVASTATING IMPACT
OF HIV BRAIN DETERIORATION

The patient told the psychiatrist in a vague and convoluted manner that for the past two weeks he had become increasingly short of breath and had been tortured at night by the voice of a college psychology professor telling him that he was going crazy and should prepare "to kill or be killed."
- From a case study of a 24-year-old homosexual prostitute with AIDS dementia[1]

The idea of an epidemic of dementing illness amongst young people in our community is not a nice one. We regard this as a frightening complication of AIDS.
- Dr. Johnathan Weber, British AIDS Specialist[2]

Every time he forgot a phone number or left a pot on the stove, Aladar Marberger worried that he was losing his mind. In an interview, the 40-year-old New York art dealer haltingly recalled that one time he had started to tell some friends about his favorite hotel in Venice, but he stopped in mid-sentence, unable to recall its name. "Oh no," he thought with consternation, "it's happening." The "it" he feared was the dementing illness brought on by the AIDS virus. Similar in its effects to Alzheimer's disease, AIDS dementia leaves the minds of those affected a patchwork of confusion and forgetfulness. It is the insidious affliction that many HIV carriers dread more than AIDS-related tuberculosis or cancer. "I'm not frightened of death," said Marberger. "But the thought of losing one's mind—well that frightens me terribly."[3] Marberger has since succumbed to the ravages of the disease.

Studies indicate that the vast majority of persons with HIV disease will experience mental deterioration.[4]

Dr. Burton C. Einspruch, M.D., of the University of Texas Southwestern Medical Center, states:

Since the extensive neurological complications of this disease may affect not only the brain, but also the spinal cord, meninges, peripheral nerves, and muscles, it is obvious that THIS ILLNESS HAS AN ENORMOUS

CAPACITY TO CREATE BEHAVIORAL CHANGES of an organic and functional basis IN A SUBSTANTIAL PERCENTAGE OF HIV-POSI-TIVE PATIENTS.[5]

A major report in the *New England Journal of Medicine* on the abnormalities found in the "asymptomatic" stage of HIV disease states:

Destruction of the brain is one of the most fearsome consequences of infection with human immunodeficiency virus (HIV). *Many patients with the acquired immunodeficiency syndrome become demented,* and at autopsy more than 90% have abnormalities of the nervous system.[6]

Neurological complications are the second most frequent cause of death in AIDS patients.[7]

THE BEST KEPT SECRET OF THE AIDS EPIDEMIC

For almost a decade, leading national and international scientists have demonstrated that the AIDS virus invades the central nervous system producing dementia and death.[8] Media coverage of the mental impairment and psychiatric disorders caused by the virus has been remarkably sparse. Although it has received extensive coverage in the medical literature, HIV brain deterioration is a critical aspect of the AIDS epidemic about which the public has not been well informed. According to Dr. John Ward, medical epidemiologist for the Centers for Disease Control (CDC):

The existence of the neurological complications of AIDS infection has been one of the best kept secrets of the AIDS epidemic.[9]

Since 1987, the CDC has officially acknowledged that HIV causes dementia.[10] When describing the effects of HIV, however, most of the media mention immune deficiency but almost invariably omit the fact that brain deterioration is a very prominent feature of AIDS. Notwithstanding the lack of media emphasis on the subject, medical experts from around the world concur that dementia is a pervasive aspect of HIV disease. According to physicians from the Departments of Neurology and Pathology, Memorial Sloan-Kettering Cancer Center in New York City:

The AIDS dementia complex *commonly complicates* the course of HIV infection and AIDS. It is now clear that CNS infection and injury are not simply another complication of HIV infection, but *a principle aspect of its biology.*[11]

According to a report in the *Annals of Neurology:*

A progressive dementing illness, the AIDS dementia complex (ADC) is the most frequent neurological complication of the acquired immunodeficiency syndrome.[12]

The AIDS Clinic at the University of California San Francisco reports:

> *Neuropsychiatric problems have assumed an increasingly prominent role in HIV-infected individuals.* Disease occurs at all levels of the central and peripheral nervous systems by a variety of mechanisms. *The AIDS dementia complex is the prototypical example of the "direct" effects of HIV on the neuraxis [central nervous system],* while infections such as toxoplasmosis and cryptococcal meningitis are complications of HIV-induced immunosuppression.[13]

Physicians from Northwestern University Medical School, Chicago, Illinois, state:

> *The nervous system is profoundly affected by acquired immunodeficiency syndrome. . . .* Human immunodeficiency virus can directly infect the brain, producing a dementia.[14]

Many AIDS patients develop a variety of neurological manifestations which cause great distress to their loved ones.[15] The World Health Organization's Division of Mental Health/Global Programme on AIDS reports that there is a broad spectrum of mental and psychiatric disorders associated with HIV disease.[16] Dementia and other nervous system complications are so pervasive in HIV disease that a 410-page medical textbook has been exclusively devoted to the subject.[17]

AIDS DEMENTIA DEFINED

The word dementia is derived from the Latin, *dementare*, meaning "to undo the mind."[18] Dementia is an organic disorder listed in the *Diagnostic and Statistical Manual of Mental Disorders* and characterized by:

> . . . a general loss of intellectual abilities involving impairment of memory, judgement, and abstract thinking as well as changes in personality.[19]

Dementia may be caused by a number of conditions. Certain types of cancer and brain tumors cause dementia. The personality disintegration caused by Huntington's and Alzheimer's diseases are familiar examples of organic dementia. In some cases, "the recognition of HIV infection followed the clinical diagnosis of probable/possible Alzheimer diagnosis. *A serological screening for HIV should be included in the diagnostic program of organic brain syndromes* and dementias with presenile/senile onset."[20]

DEMENTIA CAN BE CAUSED BY SECONDARY DISEASES

When the human immunodeficiency virus (HIV) cripples the immune system, it makes the body susceptible to a variety of cancers and diseases. These are called *opportunistic* diseases because they seize the opportunity provided by the weakened immune system to attack and devastate the body. This is known as the *indirect* means of AIDS death. In addition to brain deterioration caused by HIV itself, secondary diseases such as toxoplasmosis, cytomegalovirus (CMV) and herpes simplex also devastate the brain causing dementia and death.[21]

EARLY CASE STUDY OF AIDS-RELATED DEMENTIA

Brain deterioration was seen early in the course of the AIDS epidemic, as illustrated by the following 1983 report from the National Institutes of Health (NIH). Note that, at the time, the virus causing AIDS had not yet been identified:

Acquired Immune Deficiency Syndrome (AIDS) is a newly described, highly virulent disease of unknown etiology [cause] which primarily affects previously healthy, promiscuous homosexual males. *Dementia and delirium due to infection and/or disseminated lymphoma may frequently occur in these patients, especially as the illness progresses.*

A previously healthy, highly promiscuous white homosexual male in his early thirties had become ill after a trip to Haiti. He was transferred to NIH after approximately seven months of unsuccessful inpatient treatment at another hospital for *pneumocystis carinii* pneumonia, persistent perianal herpes simplex, and ocular CMV infection. . . . Before this initial hospitalization the patient was reported to have episodes of *confusion, depressed mood, lack of energy and a loss of interest in his appearance and hygiene. . . .*

After transfer to NIH, yet another psychiatric consultation was obtained because *the patient was exposing himself to the nurses and giving away his food.*

One month later, a neurological consultant noted frontal lobe release signs. . . . EEG and CT scan showed diffuse slowing and cortical atrophy [brain wasting], respectively. . . .

On examination, the patient appeared as an emaciated, chronically ill man. He showed markedly blunted affect, motor retardation, and striking impoverishment of verbal output: the patient simply would stop speaking after a few words, although he could be prompted to continue. Even though the patient was oriented to date and name of hospital, he either confabulated[22] or was unable to provide accurate details of his previous life, hospital stay, and medical history. While some findings were quite subtle, *tasks of attention, concentration, calculation, abstraction, and recent remote memory showed impairment.*

The patient was notably unconcerned when his difficulties were called to his attention [indicative of a psychiatric disorder known as "denial"]. . . .

During this time the consulting psychiatrist also worked with the medical and nursing staff to help them understand the implications of organic and frontal lobe syndromes and *the limitations which such disorders can place on a patient's ability to respond cooperatively, consistently, and coherently to his environment.*

After a steadily downhill course, the patient died. ON AUTOPSY, THE BRAIN LITERALLY WAS POURED FROM THE CRANIUM; THE LARGEST BRAIN FRAGMENT WAS ONLY EIGHT CENTIMETERS.

Only CMV virus could be isolated from brain tissues. Tissue degradation prevented more complete analysis of the brain pathology.[23]

BACKGROUND OF AIDS DEMENTIA

The fact that the AIDS virus directly destroys cells in the brain apart from immune suppression has been medically established since the mid-1980s.[24]

It was realized early in the course of the AIDS epidemic that central nervous system (CNS) complications were common features of the disease.[25] At the time attention was focussed on the secondary AIDS-related brain diseases such as cytomegalovirus (CMV), toxoplasmosis, cryptococcosis and others.

In the January 11, 1985 issue of *Science*, researchers from the National Cancer Institute, Cornell Medical School and elsewhere presented a report which described the high prevalence of the AIDS virus in the brains of adults and children with encephalopathy [brain disease].

The researchers found:

> *The abundance of HTLV-III [now called HIV] in these brain samples was generally equivalent to and sometimes higher than, that found in other tissues including peripheral blood,* lymph node, spleen, and bone marrow of other ARC and AIDS patients.
>
> Our results indicate that *HTLV-III, in addition to its role in causing the immune deficiency of AIDS may also have a role in the pathogenesis of AIDS encephalopathy* [development of AIDS brain disease].

Shortly thereafter, researchers from the Department of Medicine and Cancer Research, University of California School of Medicine, reported that the AIDS virus had been isolated from the cerebrospinal fluid and brain of homosexual men presenting with neurological symptoms:

> The data strongly suggest that *AIDS-related viruses can infect and replicate in cells in the brain and give rise to neurological symptoms.* In this regard, *they resemble the lentivirus subfamily* of retroviruses. These observations emphasize the potential difficulty in eliminating the virus from the host; *it could remain latent in the brain as well as other cells in the body.*[26]

The December 12, 1985 issue of *New England Journal of Medicine* presented two major studies indicating the AIDS virus was directly causing brain deterioration. In the first study, researchers concluded:

> [The AIDS virus] . . . is neurotropic [has a preference for nerve cells], is capable of causing acute meningitis [inflammation of the membranes around the brain and spinal cord], is responsible for AIDS-related chronic meningitis and dementia and may be the cause of the spinal cord degeneration and peripheral neuropathy [disease of the nervous system]. . . .

... THE BRAIN IS THE MOST HEAVILY INFECTED TISSUE, as compared with spleen, lymph node, liver and lung.

We believe that HTLV-III [HIV] is directly involved in the pathogenesis of subacute encephalitis [brain inflammation] associated with AIDS and AIDS related complex [ARC].

In the second study, researchers reported:

In addition to the variety of complications resulting from the underlying immune dysfunction caused by the AIDS virus, central nervous system dysfunction occurs frequently in patients with AIDS. Spinal cord disease . . . afflicts approximately 20 percent of patients with AIDS.
HTLV-III [HIV] INFECTION OF NEUROLOGIC TISSUE OCCURS IN THE MAJORITY OF PATIENTS WITH AIDS OR ARC.[27]

These studies demonstrated that the AIDS virus has a marked preference for infecting cells in the brain and nervous system as well as the immune system. In technical terms, this is known as neurotropism (Greek, neuron, nerve and trope, toward). Numerous medical studies since then have confirmed that HIV infection of the brain is a central aspect of HIV disease.[28] Dr. Anthony Fauci, director of the National Institute of Allergies and Infectious Disease, has stated: "HIV also has a tropism [preference] for the brain, leading to neuropsychiatric abnormalities."[29]

DEMENTIA OCCURS PRIOR TO IMMUNE DEFICIENCY

Dr. Alexandra Beckett of Harvard Medical School is one of the nation's leading experts regarding the neuropsychiatric manifestations of HIV infection. The most common neurologic disorder, she states, is HIV dementia complex, characterized by cognitive, behavioral, and motor problems. The complex once was thought to strike only in the end stage of AIDS but, she notes, it has proved problematic in patients who are otherwise asymptomatic.[30]

Dr. Joseph Berger of the Department of Neurology, University of Miami Medical School, states:

Human immunodeficiency virus can produce an array of neurologic manifestations. . . . NEUROLOGIC DISEASE FREQUENTLY PRECEDES CLINICAL EVIDENCE OF IMMUNODEFICIENCY IN HIV-SEROPOSITIVE PERSONS AND IS OFTEN THE MOST OVERWHELMING COMPLICATION OF THE INFECTION.[31]

Physicians from the Department of Radiology, NYU Medical Center/Bellevue Hospital Center in New York report:

It has become apparent that the HIV itself is responsible for a significant percentage of neurological disease in the HIV-seropositive individual. The onset may be subtle and may occur before the onset of frank immunosuppression ["AIDS"].[32]

A study in the *Archives of General Psychiatry* states:

> . . . *asymptomatic subjects with human immunodeficiency virus may be neuropsychologically impaired early in the course of the disease.*[33]

Later, researchers from the Department of Psychiatry at Cornell Medical University Medical College delineated in greater depth the complications of AIDS infection of the brain:

> . . . recent evidence indicates that HTLV-III, THE VIRUS THAT CAUSES AIDS, DIRECTLY INFECTS THE CNS [central nervous system] AND MAY CAUSE PSYCHIATRIC SYMPTOMS *BEFORE* SIGNS OF IMMUNODEFICIENCY, cognitive impairment or neurological symptoms emerge. AIDS-related organic mental syndromes may mimic functional disorders such as chronic mild depression and *acute psychosis*.

In their study of the course of HIV infection of patients having AIDS or AIDS-related disease they found:

> THERE WAS A SUBTLE AND INSIDIOUS COGNITIVE [MENTAL] DECLINE IN MANY PATIENTS THAT SOMETIMES *PREDATED BY MANY MONTHS* ANY EVIDENCE OF IMMUNODEFICIENCY. The answer to this puzzle now appears to lie in compelling new scientific data indicating that neurological symptoms may also result from direct effect on the central nervous system of HTLV-III.
>
> The history of many patients with AIDS or AIDS related complex revealed that for weeks, months, or even years before developing prodromal symptoms of immunodeficiency, e.g., fever, night sweats, and lymphadenopathy, *these patients suffered* lethargy, apathy, withdrawal, and other unexplained, often *subtle psychiatric symptoms*.
>
> Second, *even considering the stress of having AIDS or ARC, the incidence of severe psychiatric disturbances in these patients seemed unusually high.* Moreover, the disturbances themselves – depression, mania [a mood disorder characterized by agitation and hyperexcitability], personality change, and psychotic disorganization–often had atypical features and occurred in individuals who before acquiring AIDS or ARC were reasonably well adjusted.
>
> . . . *HTLV-III, in addition to its deleterious effects on lymphocytes, can also directly infect and replicate in brain cells, giving rise to pervasive neuropathological changes.* . . . It has been noted that visna virus, a [lenti-] retrovirus that infects sheep and is similar to the AIDS virus, infects both brain and lymphocytes, has pronounced cytopathic [cell-killing] activity, and causes chronic degenerative CNS disease.[34]

The AIDS virus directly infects and destroys cells in the brain causing progressive mental deterioration. HIV destruction of the brain can occur in the absence of immunosuppression, as well as in tandem with secondary dementing illnesses.[35]

HIV RAPIDLY ATTACKS THE BRAIN

Physicians from the Institute of Clinical Psychology, University of Copenhagen, Denmark, state:

... not only patients with AIDS but also *asymptomatic subjects with HIV may be neuropsychologically impaired early in the course of the disease.*[36]

German researchers have reported that their study of the psychiatric status of a group of 76 patients at various stages of HIV infection found:

- 75% of the patients had some form of psychopathology.
- 50% of the patients suffered from chronic psychoorganic disorders (34% organic personality disorders, 16% dementia).
- 9% suffered from an acute psychosis.
- 9% demonstrated psychoreactive disturbances (anxiety and reactive depression).[37]

Physicians from the Mount Sinai Medical Center in Miami Beach, Florida state: The AIDS virus penetrates the blood-brain barrier *early in the course of infection* and "CNS dysfunction *occurs frequently* in patients with HIV."[38]

German AIDS researchers who examined HIV-infected patients found:

- 46% of apparently healthy "asymptomatic" HIV-antibody positive patients had indication of a very early HIV infection of the central nervous system.
- 70% of patients with ARC and 65% of AIDS patients showed evidence of HIV-encephalitis (brain inflammation).[39]

At autopsy, evidence of subacute encephalitis [brain inflammation] is found in *90% of AIDS patients,* according to researchers from the Department of Neurology, Massachusetts General Hospital in Boston.[40]

It is apparent that *HIV infection of the brain occurs very early in the clinical course of AIDS* and frequently is a survival-limiting factor.[41]

In order to determine the characteristics and prevalence of cognitive deficit (mental impairment) in HIV infection, researchers at the San Diego Veterans Administration Medical Center and the UCSD School of Medicine performed neuropsychological assessments of four groups of homosexual men. Neuropsychological abnormality was detected in:

- 87% of subjects diagnosed with AIDS.
- 54% of subjects with ARC.
- 44% of "asymptomatic" HIV positive subjects.
- 9% of homosexual men who were negative for AIDS antibodies.[42]

Slowed information processing was the most common finding, followed by impaired abstract thinking ability and defects in learning and remembering. The researchers concluded, "*cognitive impairment occurs early in the course of HIV infection and may be detected even in those who do not qualify for a diagnosis of AIDS or ARC.*"[43]

EARLY SYMPTOMS OF HIV MENTAL IMPAIRMENT

The onset of mental and cognitive problems among HIV carriers can occur gradually or abruptly, without warning signs.

Brain aberrations can occur in the early stages of HIV disease.[44] The AIDS dementia complex may be the earliest, and at times the *only* evidence of HIV disease.[45] Researchers from San Diego Veterans Administration Medical Center in California report that HIV causes disturbances in mood, thought, and behavior. Symptoms range from memory loss, impaired judgement and mental confusion to outbursts of rage, hallucinations and firesetting.[46]

Early HIV disease of the brain causes a variety of mental problems such as:

- memory loss
- mental confusion
- impaired judgment
- proneness to accidents
- irrational behavior
- paranoia[47]

BRAIN AND NERVOUS DISORDERS ARE COMMON IN AIDS

Central nervous system disease caused by HIV is an overwhelming consequence of HIV infection which has been described by both national and international AIDS experts. London psychiatrists working with AIDS patients state: "Neurological, neuropsychological and psychiatric manifestations are an *integral part* of HIV disease."[48] Reports from around the world demonstrate that dementia is a major complication of AIDS.*[49]

HIV CAUSES PSYCHOTIC BEHAVIOR

The potential for HIV to induce psychotic behavior was illustrated early in the course of the AIDS epidemic.

In August of 1985, doctors from the Department of Psychological Medicine, King's College Hospital, London, England, reported:

> We describe here a 22-year-old homosexual man who presented with lymphadenopathy [swollen lymph glands] and *psychiatric disturbance* and was later discovered to be HTVL-III positive.
>
> Three months after the lymphadenopathy was recognized, HE HAD A PARANOID PSYCHOSIS. HE BELIEVED THAT HE WAS IN GREAT DANGER OF COMING TO HARM AND THAT HE HAD SUPER-

---

*For further documentation of the high prevalence of dementia in HIV carriers, see Appendix A.

HUMAN POWERS GIVEN TO HIM BY GOD. HIS BEHAVIOR WAS BIZARRE, at times childlike and attention seeking, at other times withdrawn. . . .

A year later he became ill again and *tried to throw himself in front of two passing vehicles.* He was mute and negativistic [resistant to advice, suggestions or commands] and was admitted to a hospital. . . .

After five days his behavior became more bizarre–he picked up objects with his mouth, refused to communicate and HAD OCCASIONAL OUTBURSTS OF AGGRESSION.

After treatment [with medication] he said he felt guilty and depressed. . . . HE ALSO ADMITTED TO THIRD-PARTY AUDITORY HALLUCINATIONS [hearing voices] several days earlier. He was fully oriented but had some difficulty concentrating. . . . No opportunistic disease was found [indicating the dementia was due to the AIDS virus itself].[50]

Sometime later, physicians from the University of Wales College of Medicine described a case of schizophrenia in a patient with HIV disease:

A 27-year-old man known to have antibodies to HIV but who was otherwise healthy was admitted with a suspected diagnosis of *Pneumocystis carinii* pneumonia. . . . He was noted to be disoriented in time; *he sat staring at other patients and COMPLAINED OF HEARING VOICES* and being too frightened to sleep. The following day he was fully oriented, but *continued to complain of auditory hallucinations, of birds flying under his bed and of fellow patients trying to harm him. . . . HIS SPEECH WAS INTERRUPTED BY THOUGHT-BLOCKING, INTERPRETED AS THOUGHTS BEING WITHDRAWN FROM HIS HEAD BY AN ALIEN FORCE.* He believed that people could read his thoughts, and that they were being passed by telepathy to television, and broadcast so that everyone would know he had AIDS. He misidentified the female psychiatrist either as an old friend of his or as Barbara Streisand. HE EXPERIENCED A FEELING AS OF AN ELECTRIC CURRENT PASSING THROUGH HALF HIS BODY, SO THAT ONE HALF WAS GOOD AND THE OTHER BAD.

The presumptive diagnosis was acute schizophrenia. . . . The next day his mental state was worse, with marked suspicion, perplexity and commanding voices, and he was transferred to a psychiatric hospital. . . . He refused medication and wanted to leave the hospital; he was compulsorily detained.

The patient's father confirmed that his son had been hearing voices for two months before this admission. . . .

Could there be a link between this man's acute schizophrenic illness and HIV carrier status, without symptoms of AIDS?. . . In one series of 70 fatal AIDS cases, two-thirds of the patients had progressive dementia, and it was suggested that EARLY DEMENTIA MIGHT BE THE FIRST OR ONLY SIGN OF OVERT AIDS in up to one-quarter of patients, and may, in an early stage, be masked by a more obvious mental disorder. NEUROLOGICAL ILLNESS MAY DEVELOP BEFORE, OR IN THE ABSENCE OF HIV-RELATED IMMUNODEFICIENCY.[51]

MENTAL DISORDERS COMMON IN HIV DISEASE

According to Dr. Alexandra Beckett, "In addition to physical and psychological effects, *HIV infection can produce neuropsychiatric signs and symptoms.* Clinicians working with HIV-infected patients should be familiar with the multiple pathological changes with which it can be associated."[52]

Canadian physicians from Montreal who reviewed the medical charts of a group of AIDS patients over a four-year period found, "Neuropsychiatric complications in AIDS patients are common."[53] Mental changes are common in patients with AIDS.[54]

Physicians from the Division of Behavioral Medicine and Consultation Psychiatry, Mount Sinai School of Medicine, in New York City state:

> *Mental symptoms are common in patients with AIDS.* Optimal management involves the identification and treatment of underlying mental disorders rather than symptomatic treatment alone. ORGANIC MENTAL DISORDERS ARE VERY FREQUENT IN AIDS....[55]

HIV CAUSES SUICIDAL AND HOMICIDAL BEHAVIOR

The mental disorders affecting individuals with HIV disease can be severe. American military psychiatrists who analyzed the records of 573 HIV-infected soldiers found a significantly higher incidence of *psychosis, organic mental disorders, and adjustment disorders* than in an uninfected control group.[56]

Researchers from the HIV Center for Clinical and Behavioral Studies at Columbia University in New York describe the spectrum of mental problems which beset people with HIV dementia:

> Confusion, memory loss, disorientation, and lethargy were prevalent among the demented. PSYCHIATRIC SYMPTOMS INCLUDED BIZARRE BEHAVIOR, DEPRESSION, *SUICIDAL OR HOMICIDAL BEHAVIOR,* borderline personality, adjustment disorder, mutism, hallucinations (auditory, visual or tactile), paranoia, and conversion symptoms.[57]

HOMICIDAL DENTISTS?

A homosexual friend of the late dentist Dr. David Acer says he suspects Dr. Acer intentionally infected at least two of his patients with the AIDS virus. In an interview with the *Palm Beach Post,* Edward Parsons, 35, an AIDS-infected male nurse, said he based his "uncomfortable conclusion" on 1988 conversations he and Dr. Acer had about AIDS. Parsons alleges the dentist said, "*When it [AIDS] starts affecting grandmothers and younger people, then you'll see something done.*"

Parsons said that Dr. Acer may have selected Kimberly Bergalis, a 21-year-old college coed who later died of AIDS, and Mrs. Barbara Webb, a 64-year-old grandmother, to make his deadly point.

Mrs. Webb said she considered the homosexual nurse's revenge theory a possibility. "In a weird way, it makes some kind of sense," she said.[58] The ailing former schoolteacher traveled from Florida to Albany, New York, in order to urge lawmakers to enact legislation protecting patients from AIDS-infected medical workers. "There are many more Dr. Acers in this world," she warned.

EARLY INDICATORS OF HIV-INDUCED MENTAL DETERIORATION

Though not in themselves diagnostic, the following symptoms may be early indications of an AIDS-related dementia:

- apathy
- fatigue
- sleep changes (including both insomnia and excessive sleeping)
- anorexia, weight loss
- imbalance
- enuresis [involuntary discharge of urine]
- withdrawal
- impaired judgement
- erratic and impulsive behavior
- suspiciousness
- avoidance of complex tasks
- shortened attention span and concentration
- forgetfulness
- proneness to accidents
- rigidity of defenses
- obsessive ruminations [the constant preoccupation with certain thoughts with inability to dismiss them from the mind[59]]
- denial
- breakdown of defenses [such as uncharacteristic spending or risk-taking]
- distractibility
- change of speech patterns
- increased sensitivity to alcohol and prescribed medications[60]

The Cornell researchers continue:

Despite vigorous efforts to confirm an organic diagnosis, sometimes only time will tell. For this reason, *even in the absence of cognitive deficits, patients in high risk groups who present with psychiatric symptoms should undergo neurological and neuropsychological assessment every few months, more often if the clinical situation changes inexplicably.*

SYMPTOMS OF MODERATE AND ACUTE HIV DEMENTIA

The second cluster of AIDS-related organic mental syndromes is characterized by *psychotic features* whose onset is generally more acute than that of the depressive symptom cluster.[61] Syndromes in this category include:

SCHIZOPHRENIA: Personality disintegration, insanity.

ACUTE PARANOID DISORDER: The word paranoia is derived from a Greek word meaning "madness, delirium, a mind beside itself." A psychotic disorder marked by persistent delusions of persecution or delusional jealousy, and such behavior as suspiciousness, mistrust, and combativeness.

BRIEF REACTIVE PSYCHOSIS: Marked by frequent incoherence, associated features include: extreme social withdrawal, grimacing, mannerisms, mirror gazing, inappropriate giggling, and other bizarre behavior.[62]

PSYCHOTIC PHASES OF HIV DEMENTIA

HIV disease of the brain can induce psychosis.[63] Psychosis is a severe mental disorder characterized by gross impairment in an individual's ability to differentiate between reality and distorted imaginations. The psychotic patient is not aware of the irrational nature of his thinking and behavior.[64] Signs of HIV-related psychosis include:

GRANDIOSITY: An exaggerated belief or claims of one's importance or identity, often manifested by delusions of great wealth, power or fame.[65]

DELUSIONAL THINKING: Irrational, unfounded thoughts of persecution (paranoia), belief that strangers are conspiring against the patient or can read his mind.

HALLUCINATIONS: Visual or auditory impressions of objects, events or people which the individual believes are real but have no objective basis in reality.

PSYCHOMOTOR AGITATION: Can include rapid pacing back and forth, inability to sit still, repeated abnormal hand motions.

RAMBLING AND REPETITIVE SPEECH: Marked impairment of verbal fluency, inability to connect sentences and thoughts, frequent repetition of statements without an awareness that they are being repeated.

CONFUSION AND BLUNTED AFFECT: Inability to comprehend or cope with circumstances, emotional indifference.

CASE STUDY OF HIV-RELATED PSYCHOSIS

As an example of acute AIDS-induced psychosis, researchers cite the case of a 24-year-old male prostitute who was also an IV-drug abuser. He was initially brought to the hospital after being found in the street in a stuporous state.

> During treatment, he was diagnosed with Pneumocystis carinii pneumonia and AIDS. During his third day in the hospital, while the social worker continued to try to reach his friends or relatives, *the patient ripped out the intravenous tube and demanded his clothes so he could leave the hospital.* An emergency consultation was requested.

The patient told the psychiatrist in a vague and convoluted manner that for the past two weeks he had become increasingly short of breath and had been tortured at night by the voice of a college psychology professor telling him that he was going crazy and should prepare to "kill or be killed."

After medical treatment the "voice" no longer was apparent. Three weeks after the initial admission, treatment of the patient's pneumonia was completed and he began to press for discharge. . . . He left the hospital against medical advice, only to return two months later with fulminating [severe] pneumonia and marked dementia. He died five days later. *Autopsy revealed cerebral atrophy* [wasting of the brain]. . . .[66]

MANIA

HIV brain disease can also induce an acute manic syndrome.[67] Mania (Greek, meaning literally, "madness") is a mood disturbance characterized by abnormal hyperexcitability which causes marked impairment in occupational functioning and interpersonal relationships. It can be severe enough to necessitate hospitalization to prevent harm to self or others.[68]

CASE STUDY OF HIV-RELATED MANIA

A 33-year-old AIDS-infected lawyer became acutely manic three weeks after his regular homosexual partner died of AIDS:

After psychiatric hospitalization, he paced up and down the ward night and day screaming that he had discovered a cure for cancer through telepathic messages from his deceased partner. [After receiving medications] he fell into a profound depression and required constant attention because of suicidal intent. . . .

In the tenth week of hospitalization, *he developed thrush and severe diarrhea*, which are consistent with AIDS, necessitating his transfer to the infectious disease service. There, despite rigorous antibiotics and palliative therapy, he rapidly declined and died four weeks later. His distraught and shocked parents refused postmortem examination of their son.[69]

MENTAL DISTURBANCES CAUSED BY HIV – NOT STRESS

Deanne Walcott of the University of California at Los Angeles, Neuropsychiatric Institute, studied the medical histories of more than 200 deceased AIDS patients. It was found that severe depression, suicidal tendencies and paranoia often are the first signs that an AIDS patient is suffering with a life-threatening brain disorder:

Patients experiencing stress due to [other] life-threatening illnesses may have similar symptoms, but they are much less severe and not serious enough to be classified as psychiatric disorders. *"Physicians who assume all mental symptoms* [among AIDS patients] are *due to stress are making a tragic mistake."*[70]

HIV CAN WORSEN PRIOR PSYCHIATRIC PROBLEMS

Pre-existing psychogenic disturbances may be substantially worsened by HIV brain disease.[71]

A chilling example of how AIDS may exacerbate prior emotional problems was illustrated by a case involving an HIV carrier who allegedly bludgeoned his mother to death with a clawhammer. The man's mother had flown from California to New York City in order to assist him in returning with her so she could care for him at her home.

Police identified the suspect as Earl Imbert, 39. The body of his mother, Leona Imbert, 63, was discovered in Imbert's apartment after police got a call from another son in Van Nuys, California, who said he was concerned because he had not heard from her. The brother described him as an AIDS sufferer with a history of emotional problems.

When officers arrived at the apartment late Thursday, Earl Lambert greeted them in an incoherent state and blood spattered clothes. Inside, the officers found the body of Mrs. Imbert propped up in a chair and wrapped in a blanket, a scene reminiscent of the shocker ending in the classic Alfred Hitchcock film, "Psycho." The psychopathic protagonist in the film, played by Anthony Perkins, kept the skeletal remains of his deceased mother in a rocking chair in the basement.

Imbert's mother was apparently asleep when she was bludgeoned repeatedly on the head with a clawhammer and a wooden statue, said NYPD Sgt. Alfred King.

"He just killed her and he wanted to kill himself," King said. *"He definitely incriminated himself. There was no rhyme or reason."* Police said there was blood all over the apartment walls. The woman appeared to have been dead for three days.

Imbert had second and third degree burns over his body. He told officers that after killing his mother he tried to set himself on fire but changed his mind and doused the blaze by wrapping himself in a shower curtain.

According to Joseph Imbert, his mother had come to New York only recently to look after her sick son and to arrange to take him to California so she could nurse him at home. Two one-way airline tickets for a flight to California were found in the apartment, police said.[72]

AIDS DEMENTIA IS PROGRESSIVE

HIV disease of the brain is a relentlessly progressive condition. The following case example illustrates how HIV brain deterioration intensifies over time.

A homosexual artist in his mid-fifties had been receiving medical and psychiatric treatment for a generalized weakness, changes in sense of taste and smell (which caused many foods to have a vile vinegar-like quality) and emotional difficulties. Sometime apparently prior to the start of treatment, he had been infected with AIDS. He had been engaging in anonymous homosexual promiscuity at bathhouses and had semi-regular encounters with a younger homosexual.

> During the course of treatment, *the patient developed loss of memory. He had difficulties in drawing a clock, in calculating and remembering.* A CAT scan revealed significant cerebral atrophy [wasting of brain matter]. A Western Blot test was positive for AIDS antibodies.
> This occurred over a three year period. In the fourth year, the patient's increasingly severe dementia was accompanied by fever, night sweats swollen lymph glands and impaired immunity. EVENTUAL NURSING HOME OPTIONS WERE DISCUSSED.[73]

The above case indicates that mental deterioration can occur *several years prior* to developing what is called "Classic AIDS"–severe immune deficiency accompanied by opportunistic disease.[74] It also raises the specter of millions of HIV-infected young adults requiring nursing home care as they become mentally and physically incapacitated.

HIV CAN CAUSE IMPAIRED SENSE OF SMELL

The distorted sense of smell/taste cited in the previous case appears to be one of the peculiar signs of early HIV invasion of the central nervous system. Researchers from the Department of Psychiatry, New York University School of Medicine and the New York VA Medical Center did a study of 42 HIV seropositive asymptomatic patients compared with a control group of 37 non-infected patients and found that the HIV-infected group scored significantly lower on Smell Identification Tests than the control group. They concluded:

> Impaired odor identification is described in a number of CNS disorders. . . . Clinically, impaired olfaction [sense of smell] might serve as a marker of early CNS HIV involvement.[75]

HIV-RELATED HEADACHE

Severe recurrent headaches are a frequent symptom among HIV-infected patients. These are probably due to chronic recurrent aseptic meningitis (an inflammation of the membranes around the brain) which often occurs during seroconversion (the process in which antibodies develop in response to infection with the AIDS virus). Australian immunologists have reported: "Headache may be a prominent feature in HIV-infected patients. . . . This is a distinct entity and we have termed it HIV-related headache.[76]

According to the San Francisco Headache Clinic:

Because the acquired immunodeficiency syndrome (AIDS) virus is neurotropic, physicians will continue to see a rise in the number of neurologic complications of this syndrome. Much of this increase will be accompanied by headache, not only as a primary symptom of HIV infection or opportunistic disease but also as a result of diagnostic tests and therapeutic efforts. Complete understanding of the ramifications of headache in AIDS will be important in the 1990s as we continue to treat a younger population, usually affected by benign vascular and muscle contraction-type headache.[77]

German neurologists report: "Headache represents a frequent symptom in HIV-infected patients."[78]

HIV-RELATED HEARING LOSS

HIV disease causes marked sensorineural hearing loss in a substantial percentage of infected persons. Physicians from the United States Air Force Medical Center at Lackland Air Force Base in Texas conclude:

HIV infection produces clinically and statistically significant sensorineural hearing loss. Audiometry [hearing tests] should be added to testing battery on detection of positive HIV serology.[79]

HIV DISEASE CAN INDUCE BELL'S PALSY

Loss of control of the muscles of the face with resultant twitching and facial distortion is frequent in ARC patients and in HIV positive, otherwise apparently healthy patients. This condition is known as Bell's Palsy.[80]

SKIN AND MUSCLE ABNORMALITIES

The lower legs may develop hair loss and thinning of the skin. In severe cases, there may be a dark reddening of the skin and large swelling of the feet. More advanced cases are marked by muscle weakness and loss of sensation in the toes. As this loss of sensation rises to mid-calf, loss of sensation is also noted in the fingers.[81]

HIV RAPIDLY INVADES THE NERVOUS SYSTEM

In addition to destroying the brain, HIV disease attacks the nervous system. Nervous disorders can occur within 2 to 3 weeks after acute HIV infection.[82]

HIV DISEASE ATTACKS THE SPINAL CORD
The AIDS virus also attacks the spinal cord causing painful tremors and paralysis. This is known as the "dying back" process as major nerves degenerate due to HIV disease.[83]

The nerves in the spinal column help control movement and sensation in various areas of the body. When these nerves are damaged, it causes pain and the inability to coordinate movement in the affected areas.[84]

Common symptoms of HIV spinal cord degeneration include:
- weakness in legs
- partial paralysis of legs
- uncontrollable muscle spasms
- shooting pains in legs
- lack of ability to coordinate muscle movements[85]

FECAL AND URINARY INCONTINENCE
In some AIDS patients, progressive disease of the nervous system causes early impairment of bladder and rectal sphincter control resulting in involuntary discharge of urine and fecal matter. Loss of sensation in the lower back also occurs. CMV has also been implicated as causing this disorder.[86]

ABNORMAL SENSATIONS IN THE HANDS AND FEET
Most patients with HIV disease of the nerves initially notice numbness or tingling in the toes that gradually spreads to the fingers.[87] The symptoms are insidious and develop over weeks to months. Burning or sharp shooting pains develop, most noticeably in the feet.

Dr. David Cornblath of Johns Hopkins Department of Neurology reports many patients have complained of their feet being so sensitive and sore they were unable to walk on them:

> Indeed, *several of our patients arrived for consultation walking only on their heels, unable to bear the discomfort of placing their soles on the ground. With time the symptoms progressed to involve the entire foot.*[88]

ABNORMAL HEART RATE AND BLOOD PRESSURE
HIV disease can affect the autonomic nervous system, the portion of the nervous system which regulates the activity of the cardiac muscle, smooth muscle and glands.

Physicians from the Department of Medicine, Middlesex Hospital, London, England, report seeing a 53-year-old homosexual male who had AIDS and autonomic neuropathy in association with dementing illness and Parkinsonism.

There was evidence of dementia, with loss of short-term memory and disorientation of time and space. Formal autonomic nervous system tests REVEALED SERIOUS ABNORMALITIES IN ALL THREE HEART RATE AND BOTH BLOOD PRESSURE TESTS, indicative of severe sympathetic and parasympathetic nervous system damage. . . . The patient deteriorated and nocturnal diarrhea developed before death.[89]

PHYSICIANS EXPRESS CONCERN

Physicians working with AIDS patients regard the growing problem of dementia with deep concern. Dr. Jonathan Weber, a British AIDS expert states, "The idea of an epidemic of dementing illness amongst young people in our community is not a nice one. We regard this as a frightening complication of AIDS."[90] An article in the *British Journal of Neurosurgery* warned brain surgeons to expect increasing numbers of patients with AIDS since "Most, if not all, patients with AIDS will develop neurological manifestations."[91]

Dr. Paul Volberding, head of AIDS services at San Francisco General Hospital has stated:

It is reasonable to consider that *everyone who is seropositive [infected with the virus] will develop central nervous system complications*. We are seeing an increasing number of signs of this on our ward. They take the form of varying degrees of dementia.[92]

German researchers have reported:

The central nervous system of *virtually every HIV-positive patient* becomes affected by the AIDS virus itself or by one of the associated diseases during the course of the illness.[93]

SIGNS FOR HEALTH PROFESSIONALS TO WATCH FOR

Because its signs and symptoms can be subtle, nurses and other health professionals may not recognize HIV dementia complex, especially in its early stages. Dr. Alexandra Beckett recommends looking for the following:

Cognitive: Forgetfulness, confusion, mental slowness, and inability to sustain a conversation. The patient may have trouble following a television program or finishing a book.

Behavioral: Apathy, agitation, social withdrawal, or inappropriate behavior. In more severe cases, psychiatric disturbances, including hallucinations and paranoia, may result.

Motor: Ataxia [failure of muscular coordination], dysarthia [confused or garbled speech], or tremors. The patient may feel unsteady on his feet. Or, his handwriting may deteriorate.

Unfortunately, HIV dementia complex doesn't follow a predictable course. Some patients may have trouble with only memory and concentration. . . . But in other patients, the complex progresses rapidly. In just a few weeks or months, patients develop noticeable psychomotor slowing, apathy, motor abnormalities, spasticity, incontinence, and seizures. . . .

When HIV dementia complex is suspected, a thorough evaluation—including computed tomography or magnetic resonance imaging scan, electroencephalogram, lumbar puncture, and neuropsychiatric testing—helps confirm the diagnosis.[94]

HIV DEMENTIA AND MILITARY POLICY

The onset of HIV brain deterioration may be acute or gradual. Associated deficits range from subtle to incapacitating.[95] The U.S. Armed Forces views the actual or potential manifestation of such impairments as sufficient grounds for restricting "asymptomatic" HIV-infected personnel from sensitive occupations. In their view, it would not be safe to permit individuals subject to impaired judgement, erratic and impulsive behavior, forgetfulness, proneness to accidents and other mental problems to participate as a crew member on a plane or tank or to handle heavy weaponry.[96]

The United States Navy has established the policy of permanently grounding all flyers who test HIV positive, including those who have not yet been diagnosed as having end-stage AIDS. A study in *Aviation Space and Environmental Medicine* underscores the harmful effects of HIV on the brain and nervous system early in the course of the disease as the basis for the policy.[97]

PUBLIC POLICY IMPLICATIONS
OF HIV DEMENTIA

> **CAUTION:** The recommendations contained in this book do *not* in any way represent a legal or medical opinion as to their legality under federal, state or local laws. Public and private employers, businesses and schools MUST OBTAIN PROFESSIONAL LEGAL ADVICE PRIOR TO ESTABLISHING ANY POLICY with regard to mentally and/or physically impaired employees, job applicants, customers, clients, visitors and students. Concerned parties should read the important disclaimer on page v regarding the Americans with Disabilities Act (ADA).

1. It would be compassionate and prudent to implement HIV screening for occupations in which HIV-induced mental and cognitive disruption could pose a threat to public health and safety.

Most of the controversy surrounding the hazard of AIDS in the workplace has focused solely on the risk of disease transmission. While the transmissibility of HIV is an important issue, *it is critical to evaluate the hazard of AIDS in the workplace with regard to the mental, cognitive and psychiatric disruptions triggered by HIV.*

HIV-infected individuals are at high risk of impaired judgement, memory loss, mental confusion, slowed reaction time, proneness to accidents and other mental problems. etc. Any of these or other impairments can occur subtly and precipitously at any time during the course of HIV disease, including persons who have no overt symptoms of physical disease ("asymptomatic" HIV carriers).

Legal Expert Urges Compulsory AIDS Testing

The high incidence of mental deterioration among HIV carriers has sparked increasing concerns regarding public safety. Prominent legal and medical experts have called for mandatory HIV screening in occupations where HIV-induced mental dysfunction could pose a serious danger.

Writing in the *Preventive Law Reporter* published by the University of Denver's National Center for Preventive Law, Professor Edward P. Richards, a public health attorney, contends that employers should transfer individuals with HIV disease out of "physically risky" jobs. Otherwise, companies could be liable in case of an accident caused by HIV dementia.

> An employee who is unfit for hazardous activity endangers himself and other employees. In jobs such as driving a truck or providing professional services, an impaired employee may also endanger customers and the general public.

Richards recommends that employers routinely screen employees and job applicants for evidence of HIV infection, particularly in occupations where mental impairment caused by HIV could endanger the infected individual(s) and others.[98]

Dr. Eric S. Berger, M.D., then Medical Director of the prestigious American Council on Science and Health in New York City, has urged that the policy of the U.S. Armed Forces restricting HIV-infected personnel from sensitive occupations be adopted in the private sector.

HIV Mental Dysfunction and Public Safety
By Eric S. Berger, M.D.

> One of the most significant AIDS-related stories of the year has received scant coverage from the media. It's the Defense Department's removal of "asymptomatic" AIDS infected personnel from sensitive jobs.
>
> The rationale for the action was simple: to protect the integrity of the U.S. military. The need was equally straightforward: the AIDS virus frequently causes impaired mental functioning. Thus, its victims pose too great a risk.
>
> In a substantial number of cases, neurologic symptoms are the first indication of AIDS infection. Writing in the *Annals of Internal Medicine*, researchers showed impaired or unusual mental abilities and behavior,

commonly called dementia. In addition, the research showed that 44% of the individuals who tested positive for HIV but exhibited no symptoms of the disease, had the same functional disorders as the AIDS patients. The test measured intelligence, short-term and visual memory, mental processing and cognitive abilities. Dr. Edmund C. Tramont of the Walter Reed Medical Center in Washington [D.C.] explained the Pentagon's action:

> IF A PERSON'S BRAIN IS NOT FUNCTIONING CORRECTLY, YOU DO NOT WANT HIM FLYING HIGH-PERFORMANCE AIRCRAFT . . . OR DRIVING TANKS.

While the military seems to have read the data properly, others in government appear unconcerned, and continue to oppose more general testing of individuals in sensitive occupations.

But DON'T WE HAVE REASON TO BE CONCERNED IF AN AIRLINE PILOT OR AIR TRAFFIC CONTROLLER, A PUBLIC TRANSIT BUS DRIVER OR THE SURGEON WHO PLANS TO OPERATE ON US IS INFECTED WITH THE AIDS VIRUS AND MAY BE MENTALLY IMPAIRED? DON'T WE CARE WHETHER THE DAY-CARE WORKER GUARDING OUR CHILDREN SUFFERS FROM AIDS DEMENTIA? ISN'T THEIR BEHAVIOR A POTENTIALLY LIFE-AND-DEATH MATTER TO US?

An estimated 1.5 million Americans are infected with HIV [CDC figures], but show no physical symptoms. According to the *Annals of Internal Medicine*, 600,000 of these infected but symptom-free individuals might be neurologically impaired. I raise this issue neither to incite terror and not to unnecessarily complicate anyone's life, but rather because it is an agonizing problem that begs a rational solution. Ignoring it will not make it go away. . . .

While there is no question that AIDS patients deserve compassion and adequate medical care, IT IS ALSO TIME TO STOP BURYING OUR HEADS IN THE SAND. THE PUBLIC DESERVES COMPASSION TOO.

The Pentagon has crafted a medically and morally sound policy for dealing with personnel infected with HIV.

The rest of America must also now do the same.[99]

2. HIV-infected individuals can have nervous system abnormalities without obvious symptoms. The neuropsychological dysfunction may be too subtle to be detected by conventional methods, giving further weight to the necessity of using HIV seropositivity per se as grounds for excluding HIV-infected individuals from certain sensitive occupations.[100]

3. There are a number of occupations in which HIV-induced mental dysfunction could adversely impact public health and safety.

THE HAZARD OF HIV-INDUCED BRAIN DYSFUNCTION IN VARIOUS OCCUPATIONS

COMMERCIAL AND PRIVATE PILOTS AND FLIGHT CREW MEMBERS; AIR TRAFFIC CONTROLLERS:

DANGERS TO PUBLIC SAFETY: HIV-related mental and nervous system dysfunction would interfere with a pilot's ability to fly and navigate safely. Mentally impaired flight crew members, including flight attendants, would be unable to respond appropriately in case of emergency situations. Mentally impaired air traffic controllers could cause massive loss of life.

RECOMMENDATIONS: Implementation of restrictions imposed by the U.S. Navy. Universal mandatory HIV screening of commercial and private pilots and flight crew members, including flight attendants. Permanent grounding without waiver of all seropositive personnel, including individuals with "asymptomatic" HIV disease. Mandatory HIV screening of air traffic controllers; exclusion of those testing positive from directing air traffic.

DENTISTS, PHYSICIANS, NURSES AND PARAMEDICS:

DANGER TO PUBLIC SAFETY: HIV-related mental/CNS impairments would pose a serious threat to the health and safety of patients. Areas of liability include: inability to respond appropriately in a medical emergency, misdiagnosis of disease or medical conditions, errors during medical/surgical/dental procedures, prescribing the wrong medications, forgetting to prescribe the correct medication, administering incorrect amounts or types of drugs or anesthesia.

RECOMMENDATIONS: Universal mandatory HIV screening of professional medical, dental and nursing personnel involved in direct patient care or medical management of patients. MANDATORY HIV SCREENING SHOULD BE A PREREQUISITE FOR OBTAINING OR RENEWING OCCUPATIONAL LIABILITY INSURANCE.
(1) Require HIV-infected personnel to obtain written informed consent from patients prior to performing treatment. This does not necessarily absolve the hospital, physician, dentist or nurse from legal liability in the event of injury due to dementia or accidental infection of patients. (2) Termination of operating room privileges and barring of HIV-infected personnel from direct patient care. *Possible Option:* Transfer HIV-infected personnel to other areas of service not involved with direct care and medical management of patients, e.g., administrative and office positions.

LAW ENFORCEMENT PERSONNEL:

DANGER TO PUBLIC SAFETY: HIV brain and nervous system impairment would render law enforcement personnel unable to respond appropriately in hazardous situations. Slowed reaction time, mental confusion, inability to recall how to perform essential job tasks, such as the proper and accurate use of firearms, would endanger the HIV-infected personnel involved, the lives of other law enforcement officers and civilians. Paranoia, confused thoughts, emotional instability, homicidal and suicidal behavior, outbursts of rage and other HIV-induced psychiatric problems could have a serious adverse impact on a police officer's ability to respond rationally and safely in working situations.

RECOMMENDATIONS: (1) Universal mandatory HIV screening of federal, state and local law enforcement personnel and armed security personnel. (2) Restrict HIV-infected personnel from sensitive job tasks, particularly those involving potential use of firearms and other weapons. *Possible Option:* Transfer HIV-infected personnel to other areas of service not necessitating direct participation in sensitive situations, e.g., administrative and office positions.

FIRE DEPARTMENT PERSONNEL:

DANGER TO PUBLIC SAFETY: High risk firefighting situations can involve navigating through heavy smoke and burning buildings, climbing ladders, removing trapped and injured civilians or fellow firemen and maneuvering hoses and other firefighting equipment. These situations involve intense emotional and physical stress and can be disorienting per se. HIV brain dysfunction and psychiatric disorders would pose extreme danger to the infected personnel, other firemen and civilians.

RECOMMENDATIONS: (1) Routine mandatory HIV screening of fire department personnel. (2) Restrict HIV-infected personnel from job tasks involving firefighting or emergency medical situations. *Possible Option:* Transfer HIV-infected personnel to other areas of service not necessitating direct participation in firefighting or provision of medical treatment.

HEAVY EQUIPMENT OPERATORS/CONSTRUCTION WORKERS:

DANGER TO PUBLIC SAFETY: Workers with HIV-induced cognitive impairments and/or psychiatric disorders who operate cranes, bulldozers, pneumatic drills, logging machines, etc., would be highly susceptible to accidents threatening their own safety as well as the lives of other workers and the public. Construction workers with HIV-induced memory loss, mental confusion, imbalance, proneness to accidents, etc., would also pose a serious workplace hazard.

RECOMMENDATIONS: (1) Routine mandatory HIV screening of heavy equipment operators and construction workers. (2) Restrict HIV-infected personnel from job tasks involving the operation of heavy equipment or high-rise construction work or other risky situations. *Possible Option*: Transfer HIV-infected personnel to other areas of service not necessitating direct control of heavy equipment or dangerous job tasks.

PUBLIC TRANSPORT WORKERS, TRAIN AND SUBWAY ENGINEERS, SWITCHMEN, BUS DRIVERS:

DANGER TO PUBLIC SAFETY: HIV-induced avoidance of complex tasks, mental confusion, and/or psychiatric disorders would result in the inability to properly and safely conduct public means of conveyance or manage mass transit equipment.

RECOMMENDATIONS: (1) Routine mandatory HIV screening of public transport workers, train and subway engineers, switchmen and bus drivers. (2) Restrict HIV-infected personnel from job tasks involving the operation of public means of conveyance or mass transit. (3) *Possible Option:* Transfer HIV-infected personnel to other areas of service not necessitating direct control of heavy equipment or dangerous job tasks, e.g., administrative and office positions.

In New York City, a mentally impaired subway engineer driving an estimated 50 mph on a curve caused his train to plow into steel posts, resulting in one of the worst fatal accidents in the city's history. Several people were killed and over a dozen seriously injured. This tragic case underscores the imminent danger to public safety posed by mentally impaired public transport workers.

QUESTIONS AND ANSWERS

Q. *Instead of testing for HIV, why not run tests for a spectrum of cognitive/mental impairments and psychiatric disorders on every job applicant and employee?*

A. The cost of running a comprehensive battery of neuropsychiatric tests on every job applicant or employee would be excessively time-consuming and cost prohibitive. In addition, some of the more subtle HIV-induced cognitive impairments may remain undetected except by more complex, time consuming and costly testing. Even if the individual with HIV disease initially were to pass these tests he or she would be at high risk of developing brain dysfunction at any time. While there are other causes of mental impairment, HIV disease per se indicates a high probability of cognitive dysfunction. Forty-four to 67% of HIV-infected males who had not yet developed ARC or AIDS have been shown to manifest varying degrees of cognitive impairment.[101] Mental deterioration and psychiatric problems are rampant among patients with ARC or full-blown AIDS.[102] HIV disease poses an intrinsic risk of mental, cognitive and psychiatric impairments.

Q. *Instead of excluding individuals with HIV disease from certain occupations on the basis of their being seropositive, why not wait until they manifest symptoms which obviously endanger the safety of others?*

A. That would be tantamount to not excluding someone with a positive test for drugs or alcohol until they have an accident. The idea is to prevent accidents occurring in the first place, not try to cope with the loss of human life and injuries after the event. Furthermore, an individual infected with HIV disease has a condition which will inexorably grow worse over time. HIV-induced cognitive or neuropsychiatric impairments can occur almost imperceptibly to the person with the disease. In point, one of the psychiatric disorders associated with HIV disease is denial, a blithe apathy toward or inability to comprehend the gravity of one's impaired condition.

SUMMARY OF HIV DEMENTIA

1. The AIDS virus *directly* infects and destroys critical areas of the brain causing psychiatric disturbances and loss of thinking and reasoning abilities. This condition is known as AIDS dementia or AIDS dementia complex (ADC).

2. HIV also attacks the spinal cord and nervous system leading to painful tremors and paralysis which can mimic the symptoms of Multiple Sclerosis (MS) and Parkinson's disease. HIV damage to the nerves of the eye results in loss of vision.

3. Brain and spinal cord deterioration can commence in the absence of severe immunodeficiency due to HIV's preference for attacking nerve cells (neurotropism).

4. AIDS dementia is an integral aspect of HIV disease. Most – probably all – persons infected with HIV will experience progressive mental and intellectual decline.

5. Symptoms of HIV brain and nerve degeneration can include: severe recurrent headaches, hearing loss, loss of or changes in the senses of smell and taste, memory loss, mental confusion, depression, incontinence, paranoia, rage, violent impulses, psychotic behavior, and auditory hallucinations ("hearing voices"). In its final stages AIDS dementia leads to personality disintegration and death.

6. Mental deterioration caused by the AIDS virus can emerge early in the course of HIV infection, among individuals who are otherwise asymptomatic. Over time, everyone infected with the AIDS virus can expect to develop dementia. Mental, cognitive and physical impairments can appear abruptly or gradually.

7. HIV infection of the central nervous system (CNS) poses formidable obstacles to treatment.

> *The prospects of an epidemic of AIDS-related dementia are ominous, particularly as antiviral therapy alone is unlikely to either eradicate the virus or restore brain function.*[103]

CHAPTER THREE

HETEROSEXUAL AIDS: GAINING MOMENTUM

The AIDS pandemic not only remains volatile, dynamic and unstable, but it is gaining momentum and its major impact in all countries is yet to come. Regardless of which groups in a community are infected first, the maturing epidemic will tend to spread within and throughout society. It is reasonable to assume that HIV will reach most, if not all, communities.
- Dr. Johnathan Mann, director of the International AIDS Center at Harvard School of Public Health[1]

I'm afraid the worst is yet to come.
- Dr Michael Merson, director of the World Health Organization's Global Program on AIDS[2]

The widely publicized cases of famous entertainers and athletes with AIDS have intensified public awareness about the spread of the disease. Millions of callers have flooded AIDS hotlines across the United States with anxious inquiries. As the epidemic has grown, the general public has come to the stark realization that AIDS is indeed no longer merely someone else's problem. U.S. Surgeon General Antonia Novello, M.D., has warned:

AIDS cases attributed to heterosexual transmission are increasing faster than any other exposure category.[3]

LENGTHY INCUBATION PERIOD OVERLOOKED
For a period of time, many people were lulled into believing that AIDS would remain confined to certain "high risk groups." There was a general sense of security because the United States had not yet witnessed the explosion of AIDS among heterosexuals that had taken place in many other areas of the world.

What was largely overlooked is that AIDS is a lentivirus disease with a lengthy (lenti=slow) incubation period. Most AIDS cases reported in the 1990s reflect individuals who were infected several years previously. The incubation period or lag time between infection with the AIDS virus and development of "full-blown" disease can be quite lengthy.[4] Researchers from the Robert Koch Institute in Berlin state:

> HIV is, to our knowledge, the first lentivirus to ever infect mankind. THE LONG INCUBATION PERIOD OF UP TO 19 YEARS AND MORE (with an average of 10 years) results in unusual phenomena such as . . . *a general delay of various dynamic effects.* The increasing potential of infectivity in recently infected young virus carriers is considerably postponed.[5]

CURRENT CASES ARE THE "TIP OF THE ICEBERG"

The long "slow" incubation period of HIV disease masks the true extent of its spread into the population. The mean incubation period for transfusion acquired AIDS can be up to 12 years or longer.[6] The number of AIDS cases published by the Centers for Disease Control (CDC) only represents individuals who have reached the end stage of disease. Individuals in the initial or middle stage (ARC) of HIV disease are not reported. Consequently, the official count of AIDS cases is merely the tip of the iceberg in terms of the number of people actually carrying HIV.

AIDS cases "continue to reflect infection acquired in the past," according to Dr. Johnathan Mann, director of the International AIDS Center at Harvard School of Public Health.

HIV SILENTLY SEEDED AMONG HETEROSEXUALS

While the focus of public attention was diverted by the explosion of AIDS cases among male homosexuals, HIV was silently being seeded in the heterosexual population.

In the United States overall, AIDS is now the second leading cause of death in young men ages 15-44 and the fifth leading cause of death in young women. Those rates are higher in some urban areas. The early 1990s saw a substantial growth in the number of AIDS cases among heterosexuals.[7]

Newly reported cases among heterosexuals actually represent people who have been carrying the disease for up to 12 years or longer. Though outwardly appearing to be healthy, HIV carriers remain infectious during this prolonged incubation period. The individuals whom they infected have in turn been passing along the disease to others. This is the vicious silent cycle of HIV seeding waves which, barring effective disease control measures, advances in an ever-expanding circle of death. After the highest risk group, e.g., homosexual males, is saturated (most of its members are infected) a saturation wave of HIV infection proceeds to lower risk groups.[8]

WHY HETEROSEXUAL AIDS IS GAINING MOMENTUM

1. HIV disease is transmitted through normal heterosexual relations from men to women and women to men.[9]

There is a vast group of people at risk for acquiring HIV disease through heterosexual relations.[10]

HIV is contained in semen and incorporated in sperm.[11] Male HIV carriers secrete ("shed") infective virions in semen at all stages of disease.[12] HIV targets cells in the testicles and epididymis.[13] HIV is found in seminal plasma, indicating that pre-ejaculate fluid can transmit disease.[14]

According to researchers from the Department of Microbiology and Immunology, UCLA School of Medicine, Los Angeles, California and the Pasteur Institute, HIV binds to sperm and can be transported to host cells thereby.[15]

In females who carry HIV disease, the virus is found in cervical and vaginal secretions.[16] Researchers from the Pasteur Institute report:

> The relatively high incidence of HIV isolation from vaginal secretions confirms the risk of HIV contamination from women to men.[17]

Cells in the female reproductive tract may host and transmit HIV.[18] The presence of vaginitis (vaginal inflammation) enhances risk of HIV transmission as does the practice of anal copulation.[19] The presence of HIV-infected blood cells increases the danger of female-to-male transmission when sexual contact takes place during a woman's menstrual period.[20]

It should be underscored, however, that *HIV disease can be effectively transmitted through normal penile-vaginal intercourse* in couples who do not practice sodomy, do not engage in sexual relations during menses, and in the absence of venereal disease or genital inflammation.

One of the reasons why homosexual males have been so susceptible to acquiring HIV disease is the fact that the practice of rectal sodomy circumvents mucosal defenses against infectious agents.[21] The AIDS virus directly infects epithelial cells which line the internal surface of the colon (large intestine).[22] HIV replicates in the gastrointestinal (GI) tract providing a "reservoir" which persistently releases virus.[23] "Evidence of HIV in rectal mucosa is common" in this group.[24] Sperm deposited in the rectum of the passive sodomy partner results in immune suppression – even in the absence of HIV infection.[25]

In contrast to the rectum, which is designed for the expulsion of feces, the lining of the vaginal mucosa has multiple layers of cells capable of protecting against abrasion.[26]

Notwithstanding the difference in anatomical design, it has been established that the AIDS virus can directly infect tissue in the genital tract via Langerhans cells. This type of transmission has been described in the British medical journal *Lancet*:

> *Langerhans cells occur in skin and mucous membranes, including oral, vaginal and cervical epithelium.* We therefore conclude that *the accessory cells (target cells) for HIV are within these barriers themselves.*
>
> The assumption that HIV infection occurs exclusively by the entry of virus through wounds in skin and mucous membranes into the blood can no longer be considered valid. Our results suggest that the *Langerhans cells in the skin and mucous membranes are the primary targets* for sexually transmitted HIV infection.[27]

HIV targets Langerhans cells located in the outer skin and urethra (the inner tube through which urine and semen is discharged) of the penis as well as inside the vagina.[28]

"Safe sex" guidelines which advise visually inspecting the genitals of prospective paramours for venereal lesions or sores are superficial. Males and females with "asymptomatic" HIV disease, though outwardly appearing to be healthy, are able to transmit the fatal disease to others.[29]

Males and females are both at risk of acquiring HIV disease through heterosexual relations.[30] Researchers from the Centers for Disease Control state: "The role of heterosexual transmission in the HIV epidemic in U.S. women is increasing."[31] HIV/AIDS has emerged as a leading cause of death in women of reproductive age. [32]

Dr. Renslow Sherer of the Cook County Hospital in Chicago, Illinois, writes in the *Journal of the American Medical Association*:

> Here in the United States there was a 36% increase in heterosexually transmitted AIDS in a one year period; this ranks with perinatally [mother to infant] transmitted HIV (38% increase) as the fastest growing categories of transmission. Furthermore, 25% of women in the United States acquired the disease heterosexually; for these individuals, *HETEROSEXUAL AIDS IS NO MYTH....*
>
> In high prevalence areas, *HIV PREVALENCE AMONG HETEROSEXUALS AT SEXUALLY TRANSMITTED DISEASE CLINICS IS AS HIGH AS 9.0%.*
>
> Physicians who adopt the sanguine view that the AIDS virus "almost exclusively" infects homosexually active men and injectable drug users do so at their peril, and more important, at the peril of their heterosexual patients.[33]

2.   Evidence from around the world indicates that heterosexual relations are an effective means of transmitting HIV disease.[34]

The vast majority of AIDS cases worldwide have occurred through heterosexual relations.[35] Internationally, AIDS has become a disease profoundly affecting the heterosexual population.[36]

The Specter of Heterosexual AIDS in Africa: A Portent of Things to Come Elsewhere

The incidence of HIV disease has reached catastrophic proportions among heterosexuals in many areas of the continent of Africa.[37] The disease has cut a lethal swath across social, cultural and geographic boundaries.

Dr. Richard W. Goodgame, a physician from the Baylor College of Medicine in Houston, Texas, who has worked extensively with AIDS sufferers and their families in the east central African nation of Uganda, states:

> Uganda can be seen as a microcosm of the African AIDS situation. . . . *Of a population of approximately 17 million people, it is estimated that 1 million adults are HIV-seropositive,* and AIDS is already the most common cause of admission and death among hospitalized adults in many parts of the country.
>
> In 1986, serologic surveys indicated that 67% of the barmaids and 32% of truck drivers were infected with HIV. By 1989, the HIV infection rates among pregnant women and unselected blood donors in Kampala, the capital of Uganda, exceeded 20%. The national serologic survey conducted by the AIDS control program in 1988 showed rural HIV-seropositivity rates of 7 to 12 percent and urban rates of 8 to 30 percent. *Because of the high prevalence rates in the general population, knowing a patient's social history rarely helps in making a diagnosis of HIV infection.*
>
> *Old and young, men and women, rich and poor, rural and urban, married and single are all commonly infected.* Similarly, members of all ethnic groups, religions, and professions are at risk.[38]

The Ugandan Ministry of Health has reported that there are currently twice as many AIDS cases among girls 15 to 19 years old as among boys in the same age group. This reflects a trend among HIV-infected older men, worried about high rates of AIDS infection among women their age, who are having sex with teenagers and younger women.[39]

At a sexually transmitted disease clinic at Mulago Hospital in Uganda, an appalling 42.5% of the men and 62.5% of the women, most of whom were in their early twenties, have been found to be carriers of HIV disease. "The magnitude of HIV seroprevalence among young, non-prostitute females has enormous implications for design of HIV control strategies."[40] The rate of HIV disease among women in 8 different districts of Uganda ranged from 4.6% to 21.8%.[41]

A Ghastly Nightmare

In an article in the *New York Times Magazine* entitled "Scenes from a Nightmare," journalist Kathleen Hunt writes:

> In Uganda, no district has remained untouched. But the affliction is heaviest in the capital, where *about one in five adults has the virus*, and in the southwestern districts along Lake Victoria, where IN SOME OF THE TRADING CENTERS AS MANY AS HALF OF THE WOMEN BETWEEN 20 AND 29 YEARS OF AGE ARE INFECTED....
>
> ... One of the senior residents in charge when I visited the [AIDS] ward was 32-year-old Dr. David Serwadda. His deep resonant voice was showing signs of strain. "The number of patients is so overwhelming," he said....
>
> ... As Serwadda stooped over a 40-year-old man with HIV symptoms–fever, cough and oral thrush–two men arrived to transfer a patient with raging AIDS-related diarrhea, whose corner bed stood in a fulvous pool. Arms stiffened and faces rigid with terror, they hoisted the mattress like a sagging stretcher. The sick man slid down into the soiled center as they staggered out the door.
>
> Like a surrealistic backdrop, this scene went on noiselessly behind Serwadda, who was listening with his stethoscope as his patient stared blankly, sucking short breaths through his mouth. Holding a chest X-ray up to the window, Serwadda instructed his junior resident to run tests for tuberculosis.[42]

Religious leaders in Uganda are urging young people and adults to refrain from sex relations outside of marriage and recommending couples to have themselves tested for AIDS before getting married.[43]

Malawi: In this country of 4.5 million inhabitants located just above South Africa, an analysis of 1482 pregnant women undergoing prenatal care at a large urban hospital found 1 out of 5 women were HIV-1 positive. Promiscuity and a history of genital warts (HPV) were the major risk factors.[44]

AIDS Causing Cemeteries to Run Out of Space

Zimbabwe: Although poverty has been cited as a contributing factor in the growth of the AIDS epidemic in Africa, in a number of areas AIDS has become a disease of the middle and upper classes. In the southern nation of Zimbabwe, Health Minister Timothy Stamps states that AIDS is draining the nation of badly needed professional and skilled classes. An estimated one million people, a staggering 10 per cent of the population, are estimated to be carriers of HIV disease. Most of those presently infected will be dead or dying of the disease by the year 2000. Fifty-eight percent of those succumbing to the disease are in professional or skilled groups. "This is having a crippling effect on our nation's social and economic development," Stamp said.[45]

Speaking at a press conference in Harare, after the recall from the market of 30,000 defective condoms, Stamps remarked that "we are going to see an escalation in deaths from AIDS even if we don't have one more infection." The Health Minister argued that even the best-made condoms are no guarantee against contracting AIDS. He therefore urged people to adhere to one sexual partnership. "Only a mutually faithful lifelong partnership will not put people at risk of getting AIDS," Stamps said.

The number of people dying of AIDS has become so immense that authorities in Zimbabwe's capital, Harare, say they will have to insist that the corpses of AIDS sufferers be cremated rather than buried, because of the shortage of cemetery space.

A spokesman for the city has reported that the city's four cemeteries will run out of space by 1995. "With the AIDS epidemic, we foresee the city council passing a law asking that all those who die of a certain disease to be cremated," said Myles Zata, a spokesman for the city.

The country's largest private medical aid society states that by the year 2000, it will be paying out $100 million annually for medical care for AIDS sufferers, a monumental sum for this developing nation.

According to John Viljoen, managing director of a firm of undertakers, "*the demand for coffins would create a severe strain on the nation's timber industry.*"[46]

Tanzania: Heterosexual transmission is the predominant mode of spread in this nation. One million people in Tanzania are HIV carriers. One out of every seven infected are teenagers. This number is expected to triple by the end of the century.[47]

Rwanda: A survey of pregnant women in this east central Africa nation of 3.5 million people found an average of 10.2% of the women carrying HIV disease. Rates of HIV disease ranged from 5% in rural areas to 14% in an urban health center. Promiscuity and early age of first intercourse (age 17 or earlier) were significant factors.[48] Another study found 1 out of 3 women were HIV positive. Researchers concluded:

THE EPIDEMIC OF AIDS IN RWANDA HAS SPREAD BEYOND HIGH-RISK GROUPS TO THE GENERAL POPULATION OF WOMEN WITHOUT KNOWN RISK FACTORS. For most of these women, a steady male partner is the source of their HIV risk. . . . A SIMILAR PATTERN MAY EMERGE IN THE UNITED STATES, where an increasing number of women without known risk factors may acquire the infection from high-risk partners.[49]

Ivory Coast: A largely French speaking nation in West Africa, the Ivory Coast ranks fourth in Africa in reported number of AIDS cases. In the early 1980s, there were very few reported cases of AIDS here. In 1986, the ratio of male:female AIDS cases was 7:1; that ratio decreased to 4:1 in 1989. The number of infected females has grown substantially over the past several years.[50]

Zaire: A study of 90 employees at a large bank in Kinshasa, the capital of the central African nation of Zaire, found an HIV infection rate of 6.3%. Over a two-year period, AIDS was the leading cause of death among employees. Fifty-three percent of deaths at the bank were caused by AIDS.[51]

Researchers from the National Institutes of Health in Bethesda, Maryland, and the Department of Public Health, Kinshasa, Zaire, report:

> We conclude that HETEROSEXUAL PROMISCUITY AND THE RESULTANT RISK OF ACQUIRING A SEXUALLY TRANSMITTED DISEASE HAS PLAYED AN IMPORTANT ROLE IN PROMOTING HIV-1 TRANSMISSION in this large Kinshasa population.[52]

Jacques Baudnoy of the World Bank, Africa Department, reports that the majority of those infected in Zaire are women in their twenties and men in their forties. Those who contracted the fatal disease usually came from the well-educated middle class and were in occupations such as business executives or government employees which are essential for the nation's economic progress. HIV disease will cause a 20% rise in infant mortality and a skyrocketing death rate among young adults. *"AIDS threatens to bring economic development to a halt in Zaire and other African nations,"* he warned.[53]

Burkina Faso: In the West African nation of Burkina Faso, the rate of HIV infection among a cohort of 1400 pregnant women who were screened at Banfora Hospital more than doubled between 1987 and 1989 from 2.3% to 5.1% (1 out of 20 mothers).[54]

Zambia: Physicians from the Departments of Surgery and Immunology at the University of Zambia in Lusaka conducted HIV screening of 243 patients of both sexes age 15 years or older who were admitted to urban or rural hospitals in Zambia in 1989. The mean level of HIV disease in patients was 23%, the male:female ratio being 1.5:1. *"HIV infection is present in nearly one quarter of unselected patients in Zambia."*[55]

AIDS Terrorism

Kenya: By 1985, 62% of the prostitutes tested in Nairobi were infected with HIV disease.[56] The AIDS crisis in this nation of 12 million has escalated to such an extent that Kenyan President Daniel Arap Moi has called for the isolation of AIDS patients to curb the spread of the disease. President Moi has directed the Health Ministry to "identify and isolate" AIDS carriers from the rest of society to help check the spread of the deadly disease. The President stated:

> ... a number of AIDS carriers have vowed not to die alone but to take along scores of others with them to the grave.[57]

Nigeria: After a long delay that may have lulled Nigerians into a false sense of security, AIDS has begun to creep into the population of over 120 million, prompting warnings that the disease may soon reach the epidemic levels reported elsewhere in sub-Saharan Africa. "There is a great deal of denial and apathy here," said Pearl Nwashili, director of Stop AIDS, an information program based in Lagos and financed by the Ford Foundation. *"When the AIDS epidemic finally hits – and it will, believe me – what we've seen in other parts of Africa will be small compared to the devastation here."*[58] In Lagos, out of 546 prostitutes tested, a total of 72 (13.2%) were positive for HIV-1, HIV-2 or both.[59]

AIDS Threatens to Shred the Fabric of South Africa's Economy

We are talking about over 45%, up to half the adult population, being AIDS carriers by the turn of the century.
– Theo Hartwig, Chief Actuary of Old Mutual Assurance Company

By the year 2000, AIDS will be ravaging the economy of South Africa, according to reports by three of this nation's major financial institutions. Two major banks, Nedcor Ltd. and Volskas Group Ltd. and the Old Mutual Assurance Company warned respectively of the impact of the AIDS epidemic on South African health care, housing, education, employment, productivity, export markets and population growth.

The Volskas company report said that by 1995 the medical costs for treating AIDS patients could rise to 14 billion rand and by the year 2000 could rise to 90 billion rand ($35 billion U.S.). There is *"no dispute about the inevitability of a major catastrophe. There will be radical changes* to cost structures, mechanization trends, consumer demand patterns and markets." The report by Nedcor Bank stated:

As the numbers of sick and dying soar, the entire nature of the labor market will change drastically. . . . It will be difficult if not impossible, to attract skilled immigrants to a country that is seriously threatened by AIDS.

The institution's report also said "the effects of AIDS in the rest of southern Africa could collapse South Africa's regional export market."

Old Mutual Assurance also mentioned the dampening effect of AIDS on the tourism industry, which had been seen as a major area of growth.[60] Scientists from the Institute for Biostatistics, South African Medical Research Council state, "It is unlikely that peak infection levels among the sexually active population will exceed 30%-40%. However, especially in urban populations, *it cannot be ruled out that infection levels of 30% [1 out of 3 people] will be reached in the next 10-15 years.*[61]

Massive Depopulation Expected

In the paper "How Bad Will It Be? Modelling the AIDS Epidemic in Eastern Africa," researchers from the Center for International Research U.S. Bureau of the Census state:

HIV infection levels are increasing rapidly in many regions, especially in urban areas. . . . Mortality levels will substantially increase, especially among newborns and adults under age 50. This mortality will remove many productive members from the economy, while HIV-related illness will reduce the productivity of the infected population. Health care facilities will be severely strained to bear the increases in hospitalized populations. . . .

By the year 2015 in terms of the entire sub-Saharan Africa region. . . . THE TOTAL POPULATION OF THE REGION COULD BE REDUCED AS MUCH AS 50 MILLION BY THE AIDS EPIDEMIC [and many millions more people who remain alive will be carrying HIV disease].[62]

Unless there is a radical alteration in cultural and behavioral mores, much of the continent of Africa will face depopulation over the coming decades. This will leave many nations susceptible to political and economic upheaval and explosive social unrest.

By the year 2000, AIDS will lower life expectancy in Africa 10 years and will hit 25 per cent of the farming families, spreading famine, other diseases and social disorder.[63]

Asia: "Like a Volcano Ready to Explode"

Asia will be ravaged by AIDS at a rate surpassing the depopulation of sub-Saharan Africa, according to the World Health Organization (WHO). By the mid-to-late 1990s, the WHO predicts that more people in Asia will contract HIV disease annually than persons in Africa.

Thailand: In Thailand, health officials estimate that over 500,000 people carry HIV disease and expect the number of carriers to soar into the millions by the year 2000. Early in the course of the AIDS outbreak in Asia, AIDS was largely confined to homosexuals and drug abusers. Homosexual magazines and tabloids have regularly run advertisements for tours to Thailand along with pictures of young Thai males. Bangkok's first identified case of AIDS was a Thai homosexual who had resided in the United States. As the AIDS epidemic progressed among the primary risk groups, it spilled over into the heterosexual population through the extensive prostitution network in Thailand.

Thailand is notorious for its commercial sex industry. There are an estimated 20,000 brothels and massage parlors in Thailand. At least 25% of the nation's estimated 1 million prostitutes are believed to be carrying HIV disease. *Health experts estimate that close to one half million men, both local and foreign, visit brothels every evening throughout Thailand,* generating an estimated $4 billion annually in revenue. Heterosexual contact with prostitutes greatly facilitates the spread of HIV and other virulent diseases.[64]

Noy, a 23-year-old Thai prostitute who says she has spoken at international AIDS conferences on the problem of combatting AIDS among prostitutes, says that while insisting clients use prophylactics might help prevent transmission of AIDS it interferes with business.

"If I tell a customer to use a condom and he refuses, I lose money. We bar girls need money and it is very difficult to say no. Too difficult." A typical prostitute in Bangkok earns 80 *cents* ($US) per customer and needs to sell her body to at least 10 men an evening to make a living. "The condom is the enemy of these prostitutes because it prolongs ejaculation and wastes the prostitutes valuable time which she could be using to sell her body to more men," said an AIDS activist there.[65]

India: The increasing rate of HIV disease has deeply alarmed health officials in this nation of over 800 million inhabitants. Physicians from the Institute of Immunohaematology in Bombay report an "exponential increase" in the rate of HIV disease among paid blood donors.[66]

According to Sriram Tripathy of the Indian Council for Medical Research in Delhi, up to a third of prostitutes in Bombay may be carrying HIV disease.[67] Physicians treating these women say that "If not checked . . . this alarming rise in HIV infection in promiscuous females will be a threat to India."[68]

HIV disease in India is predominantly heterosexually transmitted.[69]

Foreigners with high risk activity have constituted a sizeable proportion of the seropositive population in India. A diplomat from the U.S. embassy was asked to leave the country after it was learned he had AIDS. State Department officials did not reveal how he contracted the disease.[70] The rate of HIV disease among national residents is growing.[71] HIV-2 has been reported mostly among indigenous residents who have never traveled outside of India.[72]

Although pre-marital relations are taboo in India, physicians from the Medical University of Madras who conducted HIV testing of Indian women attending a prenatal/infertility clinic over a three-year period, say their study has revealed an "ominous trend" in HIV disease:

> ... THERE IS A SUDDEN SURGE OF INFECTION OF HIV AMONG WOMEN from the general low risk population WHICH IS INDICATIVE OF ONLY THE TIP OF THE ICEBERG in a group that has previously not shown any infectivity.[73]

AIDS is spreading through India's prostitute population with frightening speed.[74]

Researchers from the Stanley Medical College in Madras state that HIV disease has taken root in India and will intensify in coming years.[75]

Singapore: Researchers from the Communicable Disease Center in Singapore report that "the pattern of risk groups seems to be changing from predominantly homosexuals to one in which heterosexual transmission is becoming more evident. This trend has potentially ominous implications for the future of HIV infection in Singapore."[76]

Japan: Several years ago the Japanese government enacted tough health measures to control the spread of AIDS. All individuals who test HIV positive must be reported by name to the government and their contacts followed up and tested for AIDS. Individuals who are found to knowingly expose others to the disease are subject to criminal prosecution and imprisonment. Diametrically opposite to the United States, doctors who *fail* to report cases of HIV infection to health authorities are subject to heavy penalties. As a result of its tough mandatory reporting and contact tracing laws, the number of AIDS cases in Japan is extremely low. Only a few hundred AIDS cases have been reported here and a mere 3,500 people are estimated to be HIV positive.[79]

Communist China: This nation of approximately one billion inhabitants has reported a growing number of AIDS cases mostly among foreigners.[78] Several hundred million Chinese have been exposed to hepatitis B virus (HBV). Since the routes of spread of HIV and HBV are highly similar, the potential for the growth of HIV disease in China is enormous. In an effort to head off a major AIDS crisis, the government has instituted a policy of mandatory blood donation by citizens. The blood is tested for the presence of AIDS. Strict quarantine measures are likely to be instituted for those found to be infected.

The Communist party newspaper *People's Daily* has reported that the government has launched a nationwide crackdown on pornography and will impose tough penalties on dealers. "Money motivated people engaged in illegal publishing activities are trying every means to sell this spiritual opium, which poisons teenagers and the social environment as well," the paper said.

Taiwan (Free China): There have only been a handful of reported AIDS cases in Taiwan, with almost half of them occurring among foreigners. Taiwan has passed a tough package of laws to combat AIDS, including a measure which mandates up to seven years in prison for people who knowingly transmit the deadly virus to others through sexual contact or donating infected blood or organs.

A spokesman for parliament, which passed the laws, said health officials have been given the power to quarantine carriers of HIV disease and require them to receive publicly-funded treatment.

Health officials are empowered to ask foreigners resident in Taiwan for more than three months to take an AIDS test. Those who test positive or who refuse to be tested will be deported.

Viet Nam: A number of AIDS cases have been reported, mostly due to IV drug abuse. It appears likely that government will impose strict measures, such as compulsory HIV screening and isolation of carriers in an effort to keep the epidemic under control.

Malaysia: Malaysia is located on the southern border of Thailand. Malaysia's Health Ministry has reported over 1200 carriers of HIV disease since 1985 and health officials are taking stringent steps to prevent further dissemination of the deadly virus.

The Malaysian government has proposed a program of isolating convicts with HIV disease in prison camps on remote islands in the South China Sea. In the past, convicts with AIDS were kept in separate cells from uninfected prisoners within the same prisons. Other carriers of the deadly virus will be required to carry health identification cards and may also be isolated if they put others at risk.

Health Minister Datuk Lee Kim Sai, said the policy is planned out of compassion for the uninfected, "so that those infected will be prevented from infecting them."

Most physicians and health care workers in the country support the government's policy. Dr. S. Salmah, a Malaysian physician who backs the proposed policy, asserts:

> AIDS is a killer disease and if left unchecked it is worse than cancer, it can be worse than going to war. . . . *Face the facts, doctors around the world are desperately trying to find a cure for AIDS, but nothing is forthcoming and the disease is spreading like wildfire.* Soon millions and millions of people will die–perhaps wiping most of the human race from this earth. Tell me what do we do?

Researchers from the Philippines report:

> The potential for widespread HIV dissemination in Asia is evident. Urbanization, prostitution and changing moral values . . . supported by growing entertainment and tourism industries make Asia vulnerable for AIDS spread.[79]

According to Krishna Singh, Deputy Administrator of the United Nations Development Program (UNDP), the AIDS epidemic in Asia is *"like a volcano waiting to explode"* and the region must act rapidly to contain the disease. "There is enormous reluctance on the part of countries to acknowledge the threat but I believe that is changing," Singh said. UNDP officials estimate that tens of millions of people in Asia may contract HIV disease by the year 2000. Singh likened the potential for the explosion of AIDS in Asia to that of Africa, where many communities have been depopulated of adults who would have been working in agriculture, factories and skilled occupations.[80]

Middle East: Islamic cultural and religious prohibitions regarding homosexuality and pre-marital relations will likely help constrain significant spread of the disease in this region. Pre-marital virginity, particularly among women, is normative. Saudi Arabia demands AIDS tests of all foreigners prior to being allowed into the country.[81]

Turkey: Between 1985 and 1990 only 100 cases of AIDS were reported. "HIV-1 infection in Turkey is introduced by incoming foreign tourists, workers coming back from abroad and imported but unchecked blood products. HIV-1 is not an indigenous, but an imported, virus in Instanbul, Turkey."[82]

Heterosexual AIDS Spreading in Latin America and the Caribbean

The World Health Organization classifies areas where AIDS has predominated among homosexual males and intravenous drug abusers as Pattern I type of HIV transmission. Extensive spread of HIV began in these areas in the late 1970s/early 1980s. This pattern has been seen in North America, Western Europe and Oceania (Australia, New Zealand and Pacific islands).

Countries in which AIDS is found predominantly among heterosexuals are classified as Pattern II areas. Extensive spread of HIV probably began in these areas in the mid-to-late 1970s. Pattern II areas are sub-Saharan Africa and some parts of the Caribbean.[83]

There is mounting evidence that a number of countries in Latin America and the Caribbean are undergoing a transition from the Pattern I to Pattern II. Many Latin American countries were initially classified as belonging to Pattern I. However, by the mid-to-late 1980s, sexual transmission among heterosexuals had increased to such an extent in this region that Latin America is now classified as Pattern I/II.[84]

Brazil: Health officials estimate that this South American country of 150 million people has hundreds of thousands people who are infectious carriers of HIV disease.[85]

Researchers from the School of Medicine, Federal University of Rio De Janeiro and the University of California Los Angeles (UCLA), report that bisexual males are a major bridge for the spread of retrovirus disease into the heterosexual population.[86]

The Pan American Health Organization has reported that Brazil and Honduras are undergoing transition from Pattern I to Pattern II, in which extensive HIV spread occurs among heterosexuals.[87]

Heterosexual contact has become the greatest risk factor for HIV disease among women in Rio de Janeiro.[88]

Health Minister Alceni Guerra predicts that by the year 2000, one million Brazilians will have developed end-stage AIDS and an additional three million persons could be carrying HIV disease.

Argentina: Researchers from the Department of Microbiology, School of Medicine, STD Section, University Hospital, Argentina, found 13.8% of heterosexuals attending a venereal disease clinic in Buenos Aires were carrying HIV disease. *None of those tested suspected they were HIV positive.*[89] There is an increase in the incidence of AIDS in children in Buenos Aires.[90]

Physicians in Argentina have reported an outbreak of AIDS at dialysis centers.

[Contamination occurred] through a transfusion and was propagated through tubulations and contaminated filters. . . . We conclude that, as we have shown, transmission of HIV may occur in dialysis if disposable material is not used.[91]

Researchers from the University of Miami and Abbot Laboratories in Chicago have reported that "In addition to HIV-1, the prevalence of HTLV-1 is high (4.6%) in U.S. urban dialysis centers. Blood transfusion might be a way of contamination."[92]

Costa Rica: Physicians in Costa Rica forecast an increase in AIDS among women due to the high prevalence of HIV disease among bisexual males.[93]

Trinidad: This lush Caribbean nation located off the coast of Venezuela provides a striking example of how sexual transmission of HIV can shift from homosexual to heterosexual. In 1983-1984 the risk group for AIDS was exclusively homosexual/bisexual males. By 1989, 43% of AIDS cases were reported among heterosexuals, making them the largest risk group. The male:female ratio of AIDS cases shifted drastically from 19:0 in 1984 to 3:1 by 1989.[94] Researchers from the National Cancer Institute assert that since intravenous drug abuse is not practiced in Trinidad, the upswing in reported cases among heterosexuals "provides a model for sexual transition from homosexual/bisexual to heterosexual AIDS."[95]

Dominican Republic: AIDS has progressed in waves from homosexuals to heterosexuals. In 1983 the male:female ratio of AIDS cases was 9:0. By 1985 this ratio decreased to 3.6:1, and by 1988 the ratio was 2.2:1.[96]

Cuba: Cuba has conducted mandatory AIDS screening of the general population for several years. HIV carriers are required to live in designated housing units where they receive free food and medical care. Individuals infected with HIV are prohibited from engaging in conduct which can spread the disease. As a result of its strict policy of disease control, Cuba has one of the lowest AIDS rates in the Western Hemisphere.

Mexico: Mexico, with a population of more than 85 million inhabitants, borders the states of Texas, New Mexico, Arizona and California. The Department of Epidemiology of the Ministry of Health has estimated close to 100,000 people in Mexico are already infected with HIV. The Department predicts there will be an astronomical jump in the number of reported AIDS cases over the next several years. The male:female ratio of AIDS cases is 4:1.[97]

The National Health department surveyed 2195 AIDS cases among persons older than 12 years of age and found that heterosexual transmission of HIV is on the increase: 17.9% of those in the upper classes contracted the disease through heterosexual relations; 28.4% of heterosexual AIDS cases occurred among persons in the poorer classes.

Heterosexual transmission of HIV is occurring among all economic classes in Mexican society. Mexican health officials conclude that "extension of HIV/AIDS to persons in lower socioeconomic strata will contribute in the near future to an increasing demand for public medical care as well as having a negative impact on the productive infrastructure."[98] There is a high rate of HIV disease among Mexican blood donors.[99]

Epidemiologists from the Mexican Ministry of Health and the U.S. Centers for Disease Control have reported a mass outbreak of HIV contamination among plasma *donors* in Mexico City.

> The rate of HIV seropositive donors increased from 6% to 54% [over a nine-month period] at which time the center was closed. Of 281 HIV seropositive donors identified, 58 (21%) had documented seroconversion during this period. HIV seropositive donors were more likely than seronegative donors to have four or more donations per month. . . . The data suggest that MANY OF THESE DONORS BECAME INFECTED WITH HIV IN THIS PLASMA CENTER.[100]

Homosexual and bisexual males in Mexico are spreading AIDS to their male and female partners. A survey conducted by the General Directorate of Epidemiology in Mexico City of 5040 homosexual and bisexual males in Mexico between the ages of 16 and 44 years of age revealed high levels of hazardous conduct:

- 73% passive anal sodomy
- 57% fellatio (oral-genital copulation)
- 26% passive "fisting" or "handballing"
- 40% rectal douches (giving and receiving enemas)

On average, members of the groups surveyed had 45 male partners *and* 49 female partners. HIV prevalence is growing among homosexual/bisexual males in Mexico. These males provide a conduit for the spread of AIDS to the general female population who in turn can pass the disease on to their children and subsequent male partners.[101]

Russia and Eastern Europe

"Patient Zero" Russian Style

In the United States, a promiscuous homosexual Canadian flight attendant has been dubbed "Patient Zero."[102] He was one of the earliest AIDS "super-spreaders" identified as having seeded the disease in countless partners across the country. Researchers from the Central Institute of Epidemiology in Moscow have described Russia's own version of "Patient Zero":

> The penetration and spread of HIV has been detected in the USSR. The infection was brought by a homosexual man who got infected in East Africa

in 1982. *In the USSR he infected 5 of his 22 bisexual partners [and] gave the virus to 2 of 6 female partners and to 5 of 6 recipients of his blood.*[103]

Physicians from the AIDS Reference and Research Laboratory in Leningrad report that the HIV seroprevalence is "extremely low" and the majority of HIV positive Soviet citizens have had multiple sexual contacts with foreigners.[104]

HIV disease is in its relatively nascent stages in Russia and the countries of Eastern Europe.[105]

Authorities in Russia have conducted large-scale mandatory AIDS testing of the population. Only a very small number of individuals have been found to be infected. Known HIV carriers are prohibited from placing others at risk.

Health officials in Hungary have instituted mandatory HIV testing of STD patients. HIV positive patients are reported to health authorities and their contacts are notified and required to be tested.

England, Wales and Northern Islands: AIDS and known HIV-1 infections in women in these areas are increasing. Among women known to be HIV positive, the proportion infected through sexual intercourse is rising.[106]

3. Infected homosexual/bisexual males are transmitting HIV disease to their female partners: girlfriends, wives and prostitutes.

In the United States and other Pattern I countries, male homosexuals were initially the segment of the population primarily affected by HIV. The ferocity of HIV spread among male homosexuals was not a biological anomaly or mere happenstance. The practice of anal sodomy, analingus (oral/anal/fecal contact), fisting (insertion of the fist and forearm into the rectum and colon), and other unhealthy acts combined with hyperpromiscuity (scores to hundreds of partners) provided ideal conditions for the rapid dissemination of a novel blood-borne viral disease.[107]

The national and international infrastructure of homosexual bars, sex-shops, and bathhouses, which promote *en masse*, anonymous encounters, provides an open conduit for the spread of mass contagion.[108]

Physicians from the Faculty of Medicine, University of Toronto, Canada state their analysis of homosexual males with AIDS or ARC found:

> ... activities involving or potentially causing anorectal mucosa injury such as rectal douching [enemas are used to evacuate the bowel prior to fisting], perianal bleeding, receipt of object in rectum [e.g., dildoes] and receptive fisting were strongly associated with HIV seropositivity.[109]

Written prior to the discovery of the AIDS virus, a national case study found:

> Blood from rectal mucosal lesions [which] *are known to be common in homosexual males* who engage in rectal intercourse [sodomy] could contain the infectious agent . . . [causing AIDS].[110]

In the classic medical textbook, *Sexually Transmitted Diseases in Homosexual Men*, Dr. David G. Ostrow noted that prior to the onset of AIDS, the extremely high levels of promiscuous anal sodomy among male homosexuals had resulted in pandemic levels of hepatitis B and other infections:

> . . . *90% of homosexually active men* demonstrate chronic or recurrent viral infections with herpesvirus, cytomegalovirus (CMV) and hepatitis B. . . .[111]

The unsanitary practices and hyperpromiscuity endemic within the homosexual subculture provided an optimal "hothouse" for the astronomical growth of a host of virulent diseases including AIDS.[112] Homosexual practices involving fecal contamination resulted in a pandemic incidence of intestinal diseases normally considered "tropical." Amebiasis, giardiasis, shigellosis, salmonellosis, etc., became so prevalent among male homosexuals that physicians coined the term "gay bowel syndrome" to describe them.[113] Amebiasis, a parasitic bowel disease, apparently acts as a co-factor in the triggering of severe HIV disease among male homosexuals.[114]

By 1985, 48.5% of male homosexuals in San Francisco were infected with AIDS. For those reporting more than 50 partners, the rate of infection was 71%.[115] From this group AIDS spread via homosexual IV drug abusers to heterosexual drug abusers.

Psychiatrists who interviewed and conducted HIV testing of male prostitutes in New Orleans, Louisiana, found many have wives or girlfriends. The male prostitutes perceived a majority of their customers to be heterosexual or bisexual, many (39%) of whom were thought to be married.

> Results from the study support the argument that male prostitutes serve as a bridge of HIV infection into populations with currently low infection rates through contact with both non-customer sexual partners and customers, and thus indirectly to spouses and sexual partners of these individuals.[116]

A majority of homosexual males report having sexual relations with girls and women and many have been or are married.[117] Australian investigators interviewed 176 bisexual males, many of whom frequented "beats" (public toilets, parks and isolated roads where homosexuals meet for anonymous encounters). Forty-six percent (46%) of the bisexual men admitted engaging in hazardous sexual practices with at least one man and one woman. Several of the men knew they were carriers of HIV.[118]

Despite millions of dollars spent on so-called "safe-sex" education, a survey of self-avowed, young (18-25 years of age) homosexual males found 43% *admitted* having engaged in anal sodomy without a condom during the six months prior to the interview.[119] As a consequence of this type of recalcitrant conduct, a substantial percentage of young males in their teens and twenties who identify themselves as homosexual/bisexual have contracted HIV disease.[120] Younger and older bisexual males who engage in relations with females pose an ongoing risk of HIV transmission.[121] The females they infect are at risk of passing the disease along to their subsequent male partners.

Men Who Lead Deadly Double Lives

There are a number of males who, though professing a preference for sodomy with other men, also engage in relations with women.[122] They often express a peculiar penchant for copulating anally with women they have relations with, but are capable of normal sexual intercourse as well. These males compose a worrisome reservoir of HIV disease. Australian researchers state:

> A significant proportion of homosexually active men also report heterosexual behavior. There is a great crossover in terms of risk.[123]

Clandestine homosexuals with HIV endanger the lives of their unsuspecting wives and girlfriends. The following is a chilling testimonial by the daughter of a woman infected by her husband who led a secret life as a homosexual:

> To me AIDS is not a statistic or someone else's problem. For you see, BOTH MY FATHER AND MY MOTHER ARE DYING FROM AIDS.
>
> I grew up in the most ideal all-American family. My father was a successful senior partner in a thriving business. My mother took care of seven of us at home. We went to church each Sunday and were sent to the finest private schools money could buy. We belonged to country clubs. My parents were outstanding civic and conservative political leaders in our community and our well-adjusted family was the envy of all.
>
> BUT FOR THE LAST TWO DECADES MY FATHER LED A VERY SECRET LIFE AS A HOMOSEXUAL. He discreetly received pornography and letters from his homosexual partners through a private post office box. HE FREQUENTED HOMOSEXUAL BARS AND BATHHOUSES. He courted boys my youngest brother's age and hosted them in the penthouse suites of the finest hotels. He squandered away the family's savings account. We now know that over the years he contracted herpes, lice, rectal lesions, gonorrhea of the throat, among other diseases, as a direct result of homosexual encounters. [The family physician prescribed medication for the venereal disease the mother contracted from her husband but told her it was for an ordinary "female infection."]
>
> Last October my father underwent open-heart surgery, one of the bloodiest surgical procedures, *with over twenty vulnerable health care profes-*

sionals in attendance. At Christmas he appeared so frail and weak that he was readmitted into the hospital for a series of diagnostic tests, including an HIV blood test. His doctors diagnosed histoplasmosis, then *pneumocystis carinii* pneumonia (Pcp) and when the blood test came back, AIDS was confirmed. But MY FATHER FELT NO OBLIGATION TO SHARE THE FINAL DIAGNOSIS WITH MY MOTHER. AND THE DOCTOR WAS LEGALLY PROHIBITED FROM INFORMING MY MOTHER OF THE DIAGNOSIS WITHOUT MY FATHER'S CONSENT. It was days later, when my mother called in a rare disease specialist in an effort to ensure my father's good health that she was told that my father had AIDS and that she was at risk.

MY MOTHER IS IN THE ARC STAGE NOW AND SHE'S BEEN GIVEN ONE MONTH TO FIVE YEARS TO LIVE. . . . I think back nine months, during a happier time, when she stood beside me as I gave birth to my first child. If there had been any complications I would have asked her to give me blood. I would then have slept beside my husband and breastfed my newborn child. . . .

My mother's doctor, who specializes in AIDS treatment, has expressed concern that there are tens of thousands of unsuspecting wives now infected with the virus who have never engaged in high risk behavior other than sleeping with their own husbands.[124]

In a grim irony, the homosexual husband became a local AIDS victim celebrity, speaking at churches and religious seminars in which he angrily decried his family's lack of acceptance of his homosexual proclivities.

Congress Rejects Spousal Notification

The above letter was received by every member of the U.S. Congress. Despite its powerful heart-wrenching message, a majority of the House *rejected* a provision of an AIDS funding bill which mandated that States receiving federal monies require health officials to notify the *spouses* of HIV carriers. Billions of federal dollars have been poured into finding a "cure" for AIDS, while virtually *nothing* has been done to protect the unsuspecting spouses (and other partners) of those carrying the disease.

Bisexuals Spreading Disease in Central America

The rapid spread of HIV-1 disease in Central America, including Honduras (where the male to female ratio of AIDS cases is 1.3:1), Guatemala and Costa Rica is attributed to infected bisexual males.[125]

4.   Drug abusers are spreading HIV disease to unsuspecting heterosexuals.[126]

Physicians from Staten Island Hospital In New York have reported an outbreak of AIDS among middle class ($42,000 average income) white heterosexuals. "HIV spread is occurring among the middle class, with the predominant sources being intravenous drug abusers who do not fit the stereotype of being minorities and lower class.[127]

AIDS researchers from Belgium, report:

Heterosexual bi-directional (from males to females and vice versa) is now clearly proved. IN WESTERN COUNTRIES THE EXISTENCE OF CLUSTERS OF HETEROSEXUAL TRANSMISSION DEMON-STRATES THAT, AS IN CENTRAL AFRICA, THE EPIDEMIC COULD SPREAD AMONG HETEROSEXUALS. Sexual contacts with partners who belong to different high risk groups for HIV may introduce the virus in the general population. This is mainly true with bisexual men, IV drug abusers or people originating from endemic areas.[128]

5.   Middle class heterosexual men who patronize female prostitutes are in danger of contracting HIV disease and passing it to their girlfriends and wives.

Female prostitutes are at risk of contracting a variety of venereal diseases including AIDS.[129] The Rand Corporation, a major think tank located in Santa Monica, California, drew information from a 1982 survey of 80,434 readers of *Playboy* magazine and examined data on 52,527 exclusively heterosexual men age 18 and older who answered a question about having sex with a prostitute in the last five years. Their analysis found that *one out of five of the men admitted using prostitutes.* The average annual income of the men was at least $40,000. Thirty-four percent of the men reported having 25 or more lifetime partners. The researchers concluded:

Men who use prostitutes appear to have stronger sexual appetites and more sex partners than men who do not. Certain specialized tastes [e.g., anal sex] are also associated with usage of prostitutes. As a group, *men who use prostitutes are likely to engage in other behaviors that place them at elevated risk of acquiring HIV infection.*[130]

6.   The epidemics of sexually transmitted disease (STD) sweeping the United States and other countries are priming the bodies of millions of heterosexuals for the acceleration of the AIDS epidemic.

The astronomical worldwide incidence of sexually transmitted diseases (STDs) indicate that vast numbers of heterosexuals are engaging in behaviors which can transmit HIV. *At least 250 million cases of STDs occur annually worldwide.* The rampant growth of venereal infections is creating "a public health nightmare," warns Dr. Hiroshi Nakajima, Director General of the World Health Organization.

Young adults comprise the largest share of the mammoth 250,000,000 infections, with the highest incidence reported among people ages 20 through 24. Dr. Nakajima warns:

Sexually transmitted diseases have reached epidemic proportions globally. If sexual behavior is not modified and effective new prevention and control programs are not implemented immediately, the resulting disease and mortality rates will be even more staggering.

These diseases can cause serious health problems such as sterility, blindness, brain damage, cancer and death.

In addition, Nakajima said there is evidence that the sores and inflammation caused by sexually transmitted diseases enhance the risk of contracting the deadly AIDS virus during sex.[131]

The Connection Between STD and HIV

In simpler times, the common term for sexually transmitted disease was venereal disease (Latin, *venereus, venus,* love, lust; Venus was the mythological Roman goddess of love and beauty) or VD. Syphilis and gonorrhea were the ailments most people thought of as venereal diseases. Over the past several decades, physicians have witnessed the emergence of an extraordinary array of diverse sexually transmitted disorders. Currently, at least 20 organisms and 25 diseases are recognized as being sexually transmitted.[132] Sexually transmitted diseases have been linked with a number of devastating, sometimes lethal complications in those infected and in babies born to those affected.

In the United States, *a colossal 12-14 million cases of STD occur annually,* mostly among heterosexuals. Among others, these include:

- 1.5 million cases of gonorrhea
- 110,000 cases of syphilis
- 4 million cases of chlamydia
- 500,000-1 million cases of human papillomavirus (venereal wart virus)
- 200,000-500,000 cases of genital herpes
- 3 million cases of trichomoniasis
- 200,000 cases of hepatitis B[133]

The mammoth levels of STD among heterosexuals has critical implications for the present and future health of millions of Americans of all ages. STDs have been linked with cancer of the cervix, vulvar carcinoma (cancer of the external vagina), cervical intraepithelial neoplasia, cancer of the penis, mouth, rectum, liver cancer and vascular cancer.[134]

STD causes the vast majority of cases of pelvic inflammatory disease (PID) in the 1-1.2 million American women who develop the disorder each year. The high rate of PID results in 150,000-200,000 adolescent and young adult females rendered sterile each year. The number of ectopic pregnancies, which result in spontaneous or therapeutic abortions, skyrocketed to over 88,000 cases in 1987.[135]

How STD Facilitates HIV Transmission

A comprehensive analysis in the journal *Fertility and Sterility*, underscores several reasons why STDs are associated with an increased danger of HIV transmission:

> *One,* because STD often results in the increased presence of white blood cells in the reproductive fluids of both men and women (semen, vaginal and cervical secretions), STD can enhance HIV transmission. Genital tract infection is accompanied by dramatic increases in CD4 positive lymphocytes and macrophages, which are the primary targets for HIV.
>
> *Two,* STD causes apparent and inapparent lesions and/or inflammation of the lining of the infected areas including male and female genitalia, rectum and mouth. This increases susceptibility to HIV by providing a portal for entry and exit of the virus. The disruption of the genital epithelium [breaks or lesions of the outer skin surface and/or internal genital tissue] by STD permitting HIV penetration can facilitate HIV infection. The breaks in the lining of internal genitalia frequently are not readily discernible by visual inspection. . . . The exudate [secretions] from venereal lesions have been found to contain HIV.
>
> *A third* relationship between STD and HIV is the direct effects of the STD. The transient immunosuppression during various STDs can alter host defenses to HIV.[136]

Individuals with HIV disease have an increased vulnerability to STD. STD increases the giving off ("shedding") of infective viruses in the genital tract thereby amplifying the effect of STD on the transmission dynamics of HIV.[137] *The impaired immune response caused by HIV disease can facilitate spread of STD by permitting the proliferation of infectious viruses and organisms.*[138]

Public focus on the AIDS epidemic has obscured the dangerous undercurrent of a host of virulent other STDs. These STDs expedite the transmission of HIV and serve as markers for behaviors which can transmit AIDS.

7.   Individuals who carry HIV disease become more infectious over time thereby increasing the danger of transmission to their heterosexual partners.[139]

According to George Rutherford, Medical Director of the AIDS Office, San Francisco Public Health Department, *"AIDS is spread more easily the longer a person is infected."*[140]

This increasing contagiousness has critical implications for the growth of the AIDS epidemic among heterosexuals.[141]

Physicians from the Institute of Tropical Medicine, Antwerp, Belgium report that 58% of the heterosexual female partners of HIV-infected males became infected with HIV. The study found that persons in the more advanced stages of AIDS were more able to transmit the lethal virus to others.

This study confirms a high transmission rate of HIV infection among female heterosexual partners from European and African descent. *A more advanced clinical stage* and a low concentration of OKT4+ lymphocytes appear to *markedly enhance the infectiousness through sexual intercourse of HIV-infected persons.* This was independent of the duration of exposure or the number of sex acts.[142]

Over the coming decade, millions of persons in whose bodies the AIDS virus is presently incubating along with those newly infected, will progress to the middle and latter stages of HIV disease. Many of these individuals will not have readily apparent outward signs of disease. They will nevertheless become progressively more infectious and place others at increased risk of acquiring HIV. Dr. William Haseltine, a prominent investigator at Harvard's Dana-Farber Cancer Institute notes:

THIS SYSTEM IS VERY POTENT IN PERMITTING VIRUSES TO REPLICATE AT A FEROCIOUS RATE. It's one of the reasons this is such a devastating disease. It's one of the reasons this virus can be transmitted so easily from person to person.[143]

According to Dr. Jay A. Levy of the University of California, San Francisco:

Individuals who progress to severe disease have HIV that emerge with properties suggesting increased virulence [ability to cause disease]. These isolates replicate [multiply] rapidly in *a wide variety* of human cells.[144]

The increasing contagiousness of AIDS carriers in the latter stages of disease appears to be driving a slower epidemic of HIV disease among the Western heterosexual drug-free population. Leading researchers from the Los Alamos Institute have postulated that among the high risk population (e.g., male homosexuals) the disease spreads most during the short, initial, highly infectious period, whereas among the low-risk population, the disease spreads most during the five to ten years of increasing infectivity in the later stages of the disease.[145] They suggest that *this mode of slower spread may be the strategy adapted by the virus to survive among human hosts for an indefinite period of time.*

Rather than being rapidly "burned out" of existence, which would occur if those infected died shortly afterward (effectively halting further spread of the disease), the virus incubates for years, during which time it is silently being seeded within the bodies of countless other people. By the time those currently infected reach the terminal stage of HIV disease and die, vast numbers of other people will have become infected. The long, slow incubation period ensures the continued survival of the virus in other human hosts.

A lower rate of AIDS among Western heterosexuals does not mean that the disease is not spreading in this population. German statisticians report:

> ... if the actual growth [of HIV disease] inside the heterosexual population is slower than expected from the early growth pattern amongst homosexuals, this might be due to slower transport into this group, while it may not necessarily be taken as a sign of significantly slower transmission rate or of low penetration depth of HIV-infection into the heterosexual population.[146]

The research team at Los Alamos indicates that after the highest risk group is saturated with HIV, a saturation wave of infection gradually proceeds to lower risk-groups producing further growth of the epidemic.[147] They state:

> ... lower risk populations will have a significantly higher probability of becoming infected from contacts with people in the later more infectious stages of the disease. Thus the future danger is still alarming.[148]

According to Scandinavian researchers:

> ... heterosexual HIV transmission is likely to be followed by a relatively long latency period, which in turn suggests that the rate currently observed for heterosexual transmission of HIV will probably change accordingly. WITH THE PASSAGE OF TIME, NEW HIV CARRIERS WILL NECESSARILY ENTER THE STAGES OF INCREASED INFECTIOUSNESS AND THUS ACCELERATE THE FURTHER SPREAD OF HIV IN A PREDICTABLE WAY.[149]

8. Different strains of the AIDS virus may be more readily transmissible through heterosexual relations.

Some scientists have speculated that some variants of HIV are more infectious than others.[150] Researchers from the Los Alamos Institute have suggested that mutant forms of HIV may be more easily transmitted:

> ... the very rapid spread of infection in the Kagera region of Tanzania, from only a few seropositive persons in 1984 to 43% of urban adults in 1988, may indicate that a more virulent strain has emerged.[151]

The Pasteur Institute in France and Cetus Corporation in Emoryville, California, have found: ". . . some infected cells harbor *as many as seven genetic variants* [mutant forms of HIV]." Their findings underscore the phenomenal ability of the virus to mutate in the bodies of those infected.[152]

The British Newspaper, the *Daily Mirror*, reports:

"Super AIDS" Worry for Doctors
A new drug-resistant super-strain of AIDS is sweeping through the Third
World. Scientists say it is even more deadly than the original version. And
they fear it could soon reach Britain – passed on by normal sexual inter-
course. . . .
  Health officials say HIV-2 mainly affects heterosexuals in Africa.
  Now they fear the same pattern could be repeated here.
  Six million Africans are already infected with one of the two AIDS
strains, according to the World Health Organization (WHO) estimates.
  That figure is expected to rise to ten million by 1995.[153]

There are types of HIV-2 which have a marked preference for
cells present in the genital tract, increasing the risk of heterosexual
transmission.[154]

In the United States, 5% of 19,369 blood samples from patients
attending STD clinics between 1988 and 1990 were positive for
HIV-1 and 5.8% were positive for the variant of the AIDS virus,
HIV-2.[155]

HIV is a human lentivirus which is incessantly mutating.[156] This
rapid mutation can increase the contagiousness of the virus by developing a preference for infecting different types of cells in the
body (such as cells in the genital tract or the lungs).[157]

There are strains of HIV which are highly destructive to brain
cells but do not do much apparent damage to the immune system.[158] Likewise there appear to be strains of HIV which are
highly specific in attacking vulnerable cells in the female and male
genital tracts.

There are types of the AIDS virus capable of inducing full-blown
AIDS within a matter of months.[159] These potent strains of HIV
may also be more easily transmissible through heterosexual relations.

Cases of what are known as "super-spreaders" of HIV have been
cited – individuals who are highly infectious and readily transmit
the disease to almost every one of their partners.[160]

**9.   The widespread usage of steroidal birth control drugs ("The
Pill") has heightened the susceptibility of millions of women to
contracting HIV disease.**

Usage of the pill has been linked with an increased hazard of
acquiring STDs including chlamydia, HPV, gonorrhea, genital
herpes and others.[161] The presence of STD exacerbates heterosexual (both male to female and female to male) transmission of
HIV.

Physicians from the Division of Adolescent Medicine, University
of Alabama at Birmingham tested specimens from the lower genital tract of 102 urban adolescent females who had been engaging
in premarital sex for the common sexually transmitted diseases

(STDs). Forty-one percent of the girls were infected with the agent for one or more STDs including chlamydia, trichomoniasis, gonorrhea, venereal warts (HPV) and herpes. The physicians concluded:

> *Oral contraceptive use of more than six months appears to be a risk factor for an STD. No other factors, including the number of sexual partners, were significantly correlated with the presence of an STD.*[162]

The Pill does not prevent exposure to venereal pathogens and can act as a biological and behavioral co-factor in expediting heterosexual STD/HIV transmission.[163]

Dr. J. Neil Simonsen of the Department of Molecular Biology and Microbiology, Case Western Reserve University, and other researchers have suggested several major reasons why birth control pills may enhance a woman's risk of acquiring HIV disease:

> *First*, is A DIRECT BIOLOGIC ROLE OF ORAL CONTRACEPTIVES IN INCREASING THE SUSCEPTIBILITY OF THE FEMALE GENITAL TRACT TO HIV INFECTION. Oral contraceptives are well known to increase the frequency and size of cervical ectopy, which might provide easier access of HIV to susceptible cell types. [Ectopy results in a red-appearing cervix and may result in increased production of a vaginal discharge.[164]]
>
> *Second*, ORAL CONTRACEPTIVES MIGHT ACT INDEPENDENTLY TO INCREASE THE RISK OF HIV INFECTION. Oral contraceptives increase the risk of *C. trachomitis* cervicitis [inflammation of the cervix induced by chlamydia] and *Candida albicans* vaginitis [vaginal yeast infection]. Such infection could result in recruitment of immunologically competent cells to the genital tract, thereby increasing the population of cells susceptible to HIV infection.
>
> *Third*, is A DIRECT IMMUNOSUPPRESSIVE EFFECT OF ORAL CONTRACEPTION, making women systemically more susceptible to HIV.[165]

In addition to increasing a female's susceptibility to STD, the Pill can cause other medical complications. In the manual *Managing Contraceptive Pill Patients*, Dr. Richard P. Dickey, M.D, Ph.D., Clinical Associate Professor, Department of Obstetrics and Gynecology, Tulane University, documents a variety of the dangerous side-effects linked with oral contraceptives: increased risk of cerebral hemorrhage (stroke), cardiovascular disease, liver tumors, blood clots, and other disorders. The increased risk of stroke can persist for years after a woman has stopped using the Pill. An increased incidence of Crohn's disease, a devastating inflammatory disease of the intestines (similar to ulcerative colitis), has been reported in women who have been on the Pill:

> In a study of patients attending clinics for bowel disease, a significant excess (63%) of women with Crohn's disease confined to the colon had taken OCs [oral contraceptives] during the year before developing symptoms.[166]

California gynecologist Dr. James Caillouette contends there is a serious connection between the increased incidence of ovarian cysts and multiphasic birth control pills which have been generally prescribed for women since 1987. The gynecologist, who has been in practice for over 30 years, said he was horrified by what he was seeing among his patients on the pill:

> *It absolutely blew my mind. I thought something awful was happening to me. Every time I went into an examining room, I had a patient with ovarian cysts.*

Dr. Caillouette was instrumental in getting the FDA to intensify their studies of the triphasic pills.[167]

Long term oral contraceptive usage has been cited as increasing the risk of cervical cancer.[168]

Women who smoke cigarettes and use birth control pills have a 400% to 1100% increased risk of heart attack over those who do not use the Pill.[169] Smoking per se appears to increase susceptibility to HIV disease either directly through effects on the cervix or indirectly by increasing the risk of other infections that disrupt cervical epithelium (the surface of the cervix).[170]

The use of Norplant in which flexible rods releasing progestin are placed under the skin of the arm, does not prevent STD/HIV transmission and may, like the Pill, increase a woman's suscepti-bility to STD/HIV. Furthermore, by facilitating high-risk sexual behaviors in adolescent and adult females, Norplant may indirectly contribute to increased exposure to STD/HIV. The abortifacient so-called "morning after" pill does nothing to prevent acquisition of HIV disease.

For decades, population control groups have been promoting the Pill as allowing spontaneous sexual relations without the risk of undesired births. More than 50 million adolescent and adult fe-males worldwide use birth control pills.[171] These women are at in-creased vulnerability of acquiring STD and AIDS. *So-called family planning agencies, school-based clinics, parents, et al., which encour-age usage of the Pill and Norplant are aiding and abetting a chemi-cally-induced AIDS holocaust.**

10. The usage of condoms, diaphragms, IUDs and spermicide can cause contact dermatitis increasing risk of HIV transmission.

---

*Studies indicate that the Pill does not always prevent conception; rather it pre-vents the lining of the uterus from permitting the development of the baby after conception has taken place.[172] This post-conception abortifacient mechanism is also the way intrauterine devices and Norplant can function. Technically, this would classify the Pill, Norplant and IUDs as abortifacients rather than contra-ceptives (which prevent conception from taking place).[173]

Researchers from the Reproductive Health Center in South Carolina and the World Federation of Health warn:

CONTRACEPTIVE COPPER IUDS, CONTRACEPTIVE DI-APHRAGMS, RUBBER CONDOMS, AND SPERMICIDES MAY PRODUCE ALLERGIC CONTACT DERMATITIS [inflammation of the skin] in sensitized persons. Rubber chemicals may cause condom dermatitis/diaphragm balanitis [inflammation of the head of the penis] in rubber sensitive men and vulvitis/vaginitis [inflammation of the external and internal vagina] in rubber sensitive women. Dermatitis may be due to sensitizers [irritants] in contraceptive spermicides. . . .

Increased blood flow to the uterus and increased cellularity [greater number of cells] associated with IUDs enhances HIV heterosexual transmission. IUDs cause local damage of endometrial lining, which is a potential entry point for HIV, or a site from which it is transmitted.

Co-factors which enhance HIV heterosexual transmission include increased menstrual bleeding, adherence to IUD's tails by bacteria, viruses, cervical mucus, and fragmentation of copper spirals of copper IUDs. The infectivity rate of seropositive women wearing IUDs is aggravated further by absorption, by IUD tail, of HIV virions and infected cellular elements in semen. These adverse responses are protected from publication by certain wealthy pharmaceutical companies [and various "family-planning" agencies].[174]

The use of IUDs has been associated with an increased risk of HIV transmission.[175]

Use of a diaphragm with spermicidal jelly or use of a spermicidal foam with a condom markedly alters the environment of the vagina and strongly predisposes users to the development of urinary tract infections.[176] Vaginal and urinary tract infections cause inflammation of the affected areas as well as an increase of white blood cells which are targets of HIV.[177]

Dr. Howard I. Maibach, Professor and Vice Chairman of Dermatology at the University of California, San Francisco School of Medicine, has reported that San Francisco is currently experiencing an epidemic of allergic contact dermatitis (raw, scaling skin) among frequent condom users.[178] *Raw chapped skin can facilitate direct access by HIV to the bloodstream and susceptible cells.* "Natural" condoms made of processed sheep intestines are more porous and vulnerable to viral transmission.[179]

In addition to causing contact dermatitis, condoms are rejected by many people because they reduce tactile sensitivity, interfere with spontaneity and are seen as artificial barriers to natural eroticism.[180]

The risk of condom failure during rectal sodomy is so high that a U.S. Public Health Service task force issued a warning that the practice should be entirely avoided – with condoms or without.[181]

The inefficacy of condoms as a panacea for heterosexual AIDS is demonstrated by the massive levels of STDs in the heterosexual population. Although condoms are readily available through commercial outlets and cheaply or freely distributed through private and public health clinics, an estimated 14 million (14,000,000) cases of STD occur annually in the United States.

In an ironic twist, New York City health officials "recalled" *750,000* condoms for excessive pinhole leaks on the eve of a condom giveaway program in the city's public schools. The condoms had already been distributed to family planning agencies.*

11. HIV disease can be transmitted by oral-genital acts including fellatio and cunnilingus.

In 1988, physicians from the Claude Bernard Hospital in Paris identified five cases of homosexual males who became HIV positive for whom their only admitted risk behavior was fellatio (oral-penile sex). Two of the patients identified their only risk factors as "passive" participation indicating that *saliva can be a vector when in contact with genital mucosa.*[182] In 1990, Warren Winkelstein, professor of epidemiology at the University of California at Berkeley School of Public Health, reported a study of 82 male homosexuals testing positive for HIV in which 17% reported engaging exclusively in fellatio.[183] The usage of "dental dams" during these practices has not and probably will not gain widespread acceptance. Manual-genital contact or "heavy petting" could transmit HIV through skin contact with infective vaginal secretions or semen.

12. Kissing involving the exchange of saliva can transmit HIV disease.

In 1987, Dr. L.A. Kay of the Royal Infirmary in Sunderland, England, wrote in the *British Journal of Medicine*:

> The high risk rate of intravenous drug abusers suggests that fairly small amounts of blood, such as might contaminate used needles, may carry infective doses of HIV.
>
> During open-mouthed kissing, the juxtaposition of teeth and delicate vascular oral and glossal mucous membranes carries the risk of mucosal injury and bleeding for both partners. In addition, *oral lesions, such as herpes labialis [canker sores], apthous ulcers, gingivitis, and even toothbrush abrasions, must expose capillaries [tiny blood vessels] and are all very common. It therefore seems likely that OPEN-MOUTHED KISSING MAY TRANSMIT HIV,* but this is obscured by the fact that those who engage in such kissing also probably have sexual intercourse.[184]

---

*For a further analysis of condoms and HIV see "Now for a Little Condom Sense" in Appendix B.

Two years later, Italian researchers conducted a study which confirmed the presence of blood in saliva among couples who engaged in open-mouthed kissing. The researchers found *91% of the couples had detectable quantities of blood in saliva after kissing.*

> The presence or increase in the amount of blood in saliva after kissing is particularly important.
>
> DURING KISSING, two mucosae [mouth surfaces such as gums] come into close contact and BLOOD CAN PASS DIRECTLY FROM ONE SUBJECT TO ANOTHER. The intense rubbing that takes place during kissing favors this passage, and IF THE BLOOD OF ONE PARTNER IS INFECTIVE, HUMAN IMMUNODEFICIENCY VIRUS (HIV) CAN PASS INTO THE BLOOD STREAM OF THE OTHER PARTNER.
>
> [Brushing the teeth before kissing] is an activity that, as our results show, often causes intense bleeding.
>
> ... THE RESULTS OF THIS STUDY INDICATE THAT PASSIONATE KISSING CANNOT BE CONSIDERED PROTECTIVE ["safe"] SEX FOR THE TRANSMISSION OF HIV INFECTION.[185]

Contrary to popular misconception, the saliva of AIDS carriers is teeming with infective viruses.[186] Passionate kissing alone can result in AIDS transmission. Women using birth control pills have a greatly increased incidence of gingivitis [bleeding gums], tooth abscesses and mouth ulcers. These sores and lesions facilitate the entrance and emission of infective viruses.[187]

SUMMARY

A 1990 study found that a staggering 46% of college coeds who had engaged in pre-marital relations were infected with HPV, the incurable venereal wart virus which is the major cause of cervical cancer.[188] *Most of the young women were not aware that they had been infected.* The pandemic incidence of HPV and other STDs has horrific implications for the ongoing silent spread of HIV disease in the heterosexual population.

CHAPTER FOUR

AIDS TRANSMISSION THROUGH OTHER BODY FLUIDS

HIV has been isolated from blood, semen, saliva, tears, urine, cerebrospinal fluid, amniotic fluid, breast milk, cervical secretions, and tissue of infected humans and experimentally infected non-human primates.

. . . the skin (especially when scratches, cuts, abrasions, dermatitis, or other lesions are present) and mucous membranes of the eye, nose, mouth and possibly the respiratory tract [trachea, bronchi, lungs] should be considered as potential pathways for entry of the virus.
– U.S. Centers for Disease Control[1]

The AIDS virus can survive for hours or days outside the body.
– Dr. Harold Jaffe, Deputy Director for Science at the Centers for Disease Control[2]

HOW CONTAGIOUS IS HIV-INFECTED SALIVA?
AIDS INFECTS THE MOUTH

The mouth is an early target site of invasion by HIV disease.[3] Researchers from the National Institutes of Health in Bethesda, Maryland, state:

The oral cavity [mouth] is the site of numerous early signs of HIV infection.[4]

Individuals infected with HIV, including those who are asymptomatic, experience major alterations of the oral mucosa, the tissues lining the mouth.[5] HIV disease causes changes in the oral flora, the bacteria inhabiting the mouth.[6] These alterations produce the infiltration of AIDS viruses into saliva at a phenomenal rate.

AIDS-INFECTED CELLS FLOOD SALIVA

Canadian researchers from the Armand-Frappier Institute, the Dental Department of Jewish General Hospital, the Faculty of Dentistry, McGill University, and the Faculty of Medicine University of Montreal, have demonstrated that HIV-infected cells stream rapidly into saliva from the gingiva (gums) of individuals with HIV disease.

> After blood, saliva was the second body fluid from which HIV was isolated. The origin of salivary HIV is infected lymphocytes [white blood cells] from the gingiva [gums]. THESE CELLS EMIGRATE INTO THE SALIVA AT A RATE OF 10^6 [ONE MILLION] PER MINUTE. This emigration may increase up to 10-fold [ten million cells per minute] in oral diseases which are frequent in an immunocompromised host [such as an individual with HIV disease]. Recent immunocytochemical STUDIES SHOW A HIGHER INCIDENCE OF HIV IN SALIVARY LYMPHOCYTES THAN IN PERIPHERAL BLOOD LYMPHOCYTES OF DENTAL PATIENTS WITH AIDS. This suggests that the infected lymphocytes receive an antigenic and/or mitogenic stimulation by the oral flora [bacteria in the mouth] *resulting in a higher expression of the virus.* . . .
>
>   THE USE OF SALIVA FOR DETECTION OF HIV OFFERS THE FOLLOWING ADVANTAGES: a) collection of the specimens does not require medical competence b) quantity necessary for a test can be easily collected c) HIGH CONCENTRATION OF THE VIRUS ALLOWS EASY DETECTION OF INFECTION.[7]

Studies have demonstrated:

> . . . the presence of HIV-infected lymphocytes [white blood cells] in the gingiva [gums] of AIDS patients as well as *a higher incidence of HIV in salivary lymphocytes than in peripheral blood* of the same patients. HIV is brought into the saliva by infected blood lymphocytes which, following an infiltration of the gingiva, emigrate into saliva. This emigration is stimulated by oral diseases associated with AIDS. . . . This suggests that ORAL ENVIRONMENT MIGHT CONTRIBUTE TO A *HIGHER EXPRESSION OF THE VIRUS IN SALIVA.*[8]

These studies plainly demonstrate that the mouths of AIDS carriers are literally *teeming* with infective HIV. HIV-infected oral tissues emit up to ten *million* white blood cells *per minute* into saliva. As evinced by the high rate of AIDS among drug abusers who share needles, it only requires a minute amount of HIV, such as is contained in a contaminated syringe, to transmit AIDS.[9]

Ironically, many public health officials and the media continue to promulgate the false notion that HIV is scarcely present in saliva. "The virus is present in such small amount, it would take two quarts of saliva from someone with AIDS to transmit the virus by kissing" is one of the more popular illustrations used in sundry AIDS instruction lessons. Yet, as documented in the study above and others, there is a greater concentration of HIV-infective white blood cells in saliva than in blood. In fact, the researchers make a point of noting that there is a *higher* concentration of HIV in salivary lymphocytes than in peripheral blood (e.g., blood drawn from the arm).

Hopefully, no public health official would suggest that a half a gallon of HIV-infected blood is needed to transmit AIDS. Yet, the public is still being inculcated with the erroneous impression that it takes an ocean of HIV-contaminated saliva to transmit the disease.

SALIVA CAN TRANSMIT AIDS

Another contention of the AIDS establishment is that just because saliva and other body fluids contain HIV does not mean they can transmit AIDS.

Straightforward scientific studies reveal, however, that contaminated saliva *can* transmit HIV disease:

> The presence of HIV in saliva of infected individuals has been demonstrated before. Although transmission of HIV by saliva is difficult to prove, the transmission of HIV by oral route has recently been reported. *BODY FLUIDS (SALIVA OR OTHERS) WHICH CONTAIN INFECTIOUS AIDS VIRUS, when in contact with activated lymphocytes or other susceptible cells ...MAY EFFECT THE TRANSMISSION OF THE VIRUS to the susceptible host.*[10]

ORAL LESIONS ARE COMMON IN HIV CARRIERS

Individuals with HIV disease, including those who are "asymptomatic," commonly experience canker-like ulcers of the mouth called apthae, and oozing, "weeping" lesions, which permit the seepage of AIDS viruses into saliva.[11] These lesions occur in the roof of the mouth, on and under the tongue and inside the cheeks.*

Dutch AIDS researchers state, "Oral lesions *are common* in HIV-infected subjects and can be the *first sign* of HIV infection."[12] HIV-related oral lesions and inflammation of the gums seep copious amounts of infective HIV-infected cells into the saliva.[13]

BLEEDING GUMS DEVELOP EARLY IN HIV DISEASE

Gingivitis, a condition involving inflamed bleeding gums, and periodontal disease, a severe inflammation of the tissues and structure surrounding the teeth, are common in bisexual, homosexual, and heterosexual HIV carriers.[14] Both conditions expedite the seepage of HIV-contaminated blood into saliva. Researchers at the University of California School of Dentistry in San Francisco have determined that:

> ORAL LESIONS, such as hairy leukoplakia [which appears as a white cheesy substance on the sides of the tongue] and candidiasis, ARE NOW

---

*Oral lesions and other HIV-related conditions are graphically illustrated in *A Colour Atlas of AIDS* by C. F. Farthing et al., (London: Wolfe Medical Publications Ltd., 1986), available through medical bookstores.

AMONG THE FIRST CLINICAL SIGNS OF AIDS. . . . *An atypical gingivitis* [inflammation of and bleeding from the gums] *and a rapidly progressing periodontal disease* [inflammatory disease of the tissues and structure surrounding the teeth] may serve *as even earlier indicators of HIV infection.*

Atypical gingivitis is associated with general inflammation of the oral mucosa [which can give the inside of the mouth a "beet-red" appearance] and *does not appear to respond to conventional therapy.*

Rapidly progressing periodontal disease is often associated with significant pain, *bleeding*, and extremely rapid loss of periodontal bone.

. . . LESS THAN 25% OF THE PATIENTS WITH ATYPICAL GINGIVITIS WERE AWARE OF BEING SEROPOSITIVE [infected with HIV]. . . .

Our data suggests that rapidly progressive periodontal disease and atypical gingivitis [extensive inflammation of and bleeding from the gums] are intraoral diseases related to HIV infection and may have predictive value in identifying HIV-infected individuals. ATYPICAL GINGIVITIS APPEARS TO BE A VERY EARLY SIGN OF HIV INFECTION AND FREQUENTLY OCCURS IN THE ABSENCE OF OTHER HIV ASSOCIATED SIGNS AND SYMPTOMS.[15]

Physicians from the Albert Einstein College of Medicine in New York state:

Periodontal disease [inflammation of the tissues surrounding the teeth] *is common and severe in heterosexual patients with AIDS.*[16]

HIV disease is also associated with a tendency to incur oral warts containing a variety of types of HPV (human papilloma virus), including some novel forms of the virus.[17] HPV is frequently found in the oral mucosa of HIV carriers, indicating that HPV infection can be transmitted by oral-genital sex and deep kissing.[18]

MORE HIV FOUND IN SALIVA THAN BLOOD

The researchers from the School of Dental Medicine, University of Montreal have presented a study entitled, "Origin, Role and Infectivity of Salivary HIV" describing how HIV permeates the tissues of the mouth:

Human Immunodeficiency Virus (HIV) was searched for in peripheral blood lymphocytes [blood from the general circulation]; salivary lymphocytes, gingival [gum] biopsies; and subgingival plaque [plaque under the gums] from 94 patients at different stages of HIV infection.

. . . HIV particles and Ag were found in lymphocytes infiltrated in gingiva [gums] endothelial cells of crevicular origin [crevices and cracks in gums], epithelial cells and salivary lymphocytes, suggesting blood origin of HIV. THE INCIDENCE AND PERCENTAGE OF HIV IN SALIVARY LYMPHOCYTES WAS SIGNIFICANTLY HIGHER THAN IN PERIPHERAL BLOOD LYMPHOCYTES.

These findings suggest that virus-positive peripheral blood lymphocytes in gingiva receive antigenic and/or mitogenic stimulation by the oral flora [bacteria in the mouth] *resulting in greater expression of the virus* which is demonstrated by our current studies *in vitro.*

Presence of HIV in gingiva [gums] is associated with elimination of the local CD4+ cell mediated immunologic barrier and expression of pathogenicity of oral microorganisms, resulting in a high incidence and rapid progression of a variety of oral diseases. SALIVARY HIV IS INFECTIVE [able to transmit disease] as demonstrated in vitro.[19]

The mouth of an individual with HIV disease acts as a prolific viral incubator, fomenting the massive multiplication of infective AIDS viruses. HIV-infected cells have been found in "higher incidence and percentage" in saliva than blood, indicating that HIV-contaminated saliva is as infective, and possibly more infectious, than blood.

HIV INFECTS THE SALIVARY GLAND

Early in the course of AIDS in the United States, scientists from the Infectious Diseases Branch, National Institute of Neurological and Communicative Disorders and Stroke, identified AIDS-associated retrovirus-like particles in the salivary gland, prostate and testicles of AIDS patients. HIV disease of the salivary gland can generate infectious saliva:

These findings further suggest that *SALIVA* and semen *MAY TRANSMIT THE INFECTION* to susceptible individuals.[20]

SAIDS TRANSMITTED BY SALIVA AND URINE

Simian Acquired Immune Deficiency Syndrome or SAIDS (Latin, *simia,* ape) which is similar to AIDS in humans, can be transmitted by saliva and urine. Note that tissue from the parotid (saliva) gland was found to be "budding" viral particles:

Saliva and urine specimens from rhesus monkeys with SAIDS were found to contain a type D retrovirus related to Mason-Pfizer monkey virus (MPMV) which has been linked etiologically to SAIDS. Virus isolates from saliva and urine were shown to have the characteristics of the SAIDS agent. . . . *Electron micrographs of parotid [saliva gland] tissue from an animal with SAIDS also showed budding particles with type D retrovirus morphology.* A tissue culture grown virus isolate from urine of an animal with SAIDS, produced SAIDS when inoculated into two normal juvenile rhesus monkeys. SINCE SALIVA AND URINE OF MONKEYS WITH SAIDS CONTAIN INFECTIOUS SAIDS VIRUS, THEY ARE LIKELY SOURCES OF VIRUS BY WHICH THE DISEASE IS NATURALLY TRANSMITTED. Thus, care should be taken to avoid contact with normal and infected animals.[21]

Simian Immunodeficiency Virus (SIV) has been transmitted via conjunctival and oral mucosae (through the surface of the eyes and inside the mouth) in a newborn rhesus monkey.[22]

Simian Retrovirus Serotype 1 (SRV-1) commonly infects the gums and cheek pouches of rhesus monkeys inoculated with the virus intravenously, indicating that *the mouth is a target site for the virus.* "... SRV-1 commonly infects oral mucosal Langerhans cells in rhesus monkeys."[23]

SALIVA: AS ACCURATE AS BLOOD FOR AIDS TESTING

Scientists from the Department of Cancer Biology, Harvard School of Public Health determined as early as 1986 that a saliva test for AIDS antibodies could be feasible. Of 45 individuals with positive blood tests for AIDS antibodies, 100% were found to have detectable salivary antibodies to viral antigens. "The results showed that a Western Blot assay for salivary antibodies may be possible."[24]

Researchers from San Francisco General Hospital and Epitope Company in Portland, Oregon, have since reported:

Certain HIV antibodies in the oral cavity [mouth] can be detected by Western Blot analysis [using saliva] *with accuracy comparable to serum* [blood].[25]

SALIVA TEST SUITABLE FOR MASS SCREENING

Physicians from the Federal Centre for AIDS in Ottawa, Canada, report that there is a highly accurate saliva test for AIDS.* The Canadian health authorities recommend saliva as a suitable alternative to blood for large scale AIDS screening. The saliva test is painless and more acceptable to the public. Since it does not require drawing blood, there is no risk of needlestick injury to health care workers. Usage of the saliva test for AIDS testing on a mass scale would reveal how extensively the disease has spread in the population.[26]

Researchers from the Oral AIDS Center, University of California San Francisco, compared the presence of HIV in blood and saliva using a DNA probe and reported:

... detection of HIV in blood and gingival crevicular fluid (GCF) [saliva in the gums between the teeth] is approximately equal. .... The ease of sample collection and sample stability, may make examination of GCF an additional tool for epidemiologic surveys in large patient populations. ...[27]

---

*The saliva tests for AIDS have high sensitivity and specificity. *Sensitivity* is the probability that a test will accurately identify individuals who are disease carriers. *Specificity* is the likelihood that a test will give negative results for individuals who are not disease carriers.

PAPER TEST FOR AIDS IN SALIVA

The *Straits Times* of Singapore reports that Thailand's Chula-longhorn University has developed a special color-sensitive paper to test saliva for AIDS which can be used to check tourists entering the country.[28] Doctors in Thailand have been using a saliva test for AIDS since the late 1980s. Physicians report that the saliva test has advantages over conventional blood tests. According to a government hospital physician:

> Checking saliva is convenient, very quick and does not hurt. Just put about two teaspoons in a bottle and let the doctor check it. That's all.[29]

Physicians from Chulalonghorn University's Department of Medical Technology and Medicine and the Pasteur Institute, report:

> A commercial anti-HIV ELISA kit can be satisfactorily used to detect salivary anti-HIV.[30]

HOME AIDS TESTS DEVELOPED

American researchers have developed an inexpensive, over-the-counter saliva test for AIDS which will be available to people outside the country. Currently, the test is not being sold in drug stores in the United States.

Roger Clemmons, a professor at the University of Florida College of Veterinary Medicine, said the simple dipstick saliva test is also effective in detecting hepatitis B. Dr. Clemmons and his colleagues are in the process of expanding the test to detect other sexually transmitted diseases, including genital herpes, gonorrhea, chlamydia and syphilis.

"We now can simultaneously diagnose several diseases with one device," said Clemmons. He was granted a patent for the test in 1991.

DIPSTICK SALIVA TEST GIVES IMMEDIATE RESULTS

Similar to home pregnancy tests, *Clemmons' saliva test takes less than 8 minutes to detect HIV and less than 5 minutes to detect hepatitis B.*

In more than 2000 tests on hundreds of people, the test proved to be 100% sensitive in detecting HIV antibodies in saliva.

Easy to Use

The dipstick test is easy to perform. It merely requires placing a dipstick in a sample of saliva and reagent for one minute, washing the dipstick before and after a second chemical is added, and then applying a developer to see the results. If the circle on the end of the dipstick changes color, the results are positive.

Very Low Cost

"The tests will only cost about $5.00 each," said David Fowler, President of FutureTech Inc., of Gainesville, Florida. His company is marketing the test.

The test is being sold abroad, but cannot be sold in the United States until it is approved by the Food and Drug Administration.

The big advantage to the test, Clemmons said, is that it can be done almost instantaneously by anyone and does not require the handling of needles to withdraw blood. It also does not have to be sent to a laboratory.

> *If you could spit in a cup and do a very simple, very reliable, very inexpensive self-test for AIDS [and other STDs], wouldn't you want to?"* Fowler said. *"Conceivably, people could even bring it on a date and exchange tests before moving ahead in courtship.*

On the foreign market, the test will initially be used by doctors, dentists, emergency room personnel, the military, and possibly immigration officials to quickly determine if people are carrying AIDS. A home test version will be available very soon afterwards.

The test will be useful anywhere that access to central laboratories is limited such as rural areas and developing nations.[31]

SALIVA TEST MORE ACCURATE THAN BLOOD

The saliva test allows detection of a variety of normal and abnormal antibodies and antigens in body fluids, including HIV antigen, antibodies to HIV, hepatitis B surface antigen and antibodies against hepatitis B. The test can screen for both HIV-1 and HIV-2. Rapid HIV assays for testing urine and blood are also available. According to an informational report released by the FutureTech company:

> Current data suggest that the final configuration will offer sensitivity and specificity equal to or BETTER THAN THOSE OF CONVENTIONAL BLOOD TESTS.

The Epitope company in Oregon has also developed a rapid saliva test for AIDS. It uses the placement of a cotton pad placed inside the mouth between the gums and the cheek. The pad is then placed in a tube and sealed. The saliva-soaked pad can then be rapidly analyzed in the office or laboratory setting.

ANTIBODIES IN SALIVA DO NOT NEUTRALIZE HIV

Researchers from Harvard University and the University of Maryland in Baltimore analyzed the serum and saliva from people at various stages of HIV disease. They found specific antibodies to HIV-1 in the serum and saliva of all people tested. However, the antibodies in the saliva of those tested did *not* neutralize the virus.

> [These findings] suggest that the mucosal immune response in HIV-1 infected people is impaired long before any pathognomic symptoms [specific signs] of AIDS occur.[32]

THE MYTH OF THE "FRAIL" VIRUS

Public health officials have downplayed the risk of person-to-person transmission of HIV by body fluids other than blood. One of their chief arguments is that the AIDS virus is a weak, frail virus which "dies" shortly after leaving the body. Even if HIV is in saliva, blood, lung secretions etc., it is claimed that the virus is incapable of surviving outside the body for more than a few seconds. Though not widely publicized in the popular media, extensive analyses by respected French and American AIDS researchers reveal that HIV is actually a tough, hardy virus.

THE LENGTHY SURVIVAL OF HIV OUTSIDE THE BODY

Dr. James Slaff, former Medical Investigator at the National Institutes of Health, has reported:

> Unlike most other retroviruses, THE AIDS VIRUS CAN SURVIVE OUTSIDE THE BODY FOR HOURS TO DAYS.[33]

TOP VIROLOGISTS REPORT VIRUS IS UNUSUALLY HARDY

The September 28, 1985 issue of the British medical journal *Lancet* contained a study by a team of French researchers from the Viral Oncology Unit at the Pasteur Institute revealing that *the AIDS lentivirus can remain infectious outside the body for up to ten days.*

> LAV/HTLV-III [now called HIV], the agent causing AIDS, has been isolated from body fluids (blood, semen, saliva, tears). Its isolation in saliva prompted us to investigate the possibility of transmission by saliva, and we have studied the sensitivity of LAV/HTLV-III at room temperature....
>
> THE VIRUS used for the infectivity assay ... WAS LEFT AT ROOM TEMPERATURE FOR 0, 2, 4, OR 7 DAYS IN A SEALED TUBE OR ALLOWED TO DRY IN A PETRI DISH. After the times indicated in the figure the virus was used to infect stimulated T lymphocytes and viral production was determined in cell-free supernatant by testing for the reverse transcriptase activity twice a week. [THE DATA] SHOWS THE

UNUSUAL STABILITY OF THE AIDS VIRUS AT ROOM TEMPERA-TURE. No significant difference was found between 0, 2, or 4 days. Only a slight decrease is noted with a delay in the virus production indicating a loss of few infectious particles *after 7 days* at room temperature.

Two petri dishes containing 25,000 cpm equivalent reverse transcriptase of dry virus were kept at room temperature for 4 or 7 days and then resuspended in 0.220 ml water and used to measure the infectivity. Significant numbers of viral particles are then inactivated, but some infectious virus is still present since RELEASE OF VIRUS WAS SEEN ON DAY 10. This result indicates that THE VIRUS IS RESISTANT AT ROOM TEMPERA-TURE, EITHER IN DRY FORM OR LIQUID MEDIUM.

HARDINESS LINKED TO CASUAL TRANSMISSION

THE RESISTANCE OF LAV [THE AIDS VIRUS] AT ROOM TEM-PERATURE MAY EXPLAIN THE APPEARANCE OF SOME CASES OF AIDS IN NON-RISK GROUPS. To prevent possible contamination by viral particles in dry or liquid form, hygiene should be increased in the general population. Moreover, SOME MORE SAFETY PRECAUTIONS SHOULD BE TAKEN IN LABORATORIES AND IN HOSPITALS AND BY DENTISTS WHO USE A VACUUM PUMP FOR SALIVA ASPIRA-TION. Indeed, these data strongly support the use of disinfectants found to be effective against the AIDS agent.[34]

Worries over casual transmission have been dismissed as the product of ignorance, paranoia and "homophobia." The findings of the French researchers–specialists from the Pasteur Institute's elite Viral Oncology Unit–went unmentioned by major public health officials and were virtually blacked out by the media.

Two months after their findings were published in *Lancet*, the *Journal of the American Medical Association* commented in the Medical News section:

A recent report from the Pasteur Institute in Paris by the investigators who originally isolated the lymphadenopathy virus suggests that the AIDS virus might be pretty tough. The French study finds that THE VIRUS SUR-VIVES TEN DAYS AT ROOM TEMPERATURE EVEN WHEN DRIED OUT IN A PETRI DISH.[35]

DRIED OUT VIRUS REMAINS INFECTIOUS

Six months after the Pasteur Institute study was reported, researchers from the laboratory of Tumor Cell Biology, National Institutes of Health, reported their findings on the stability of the AIDS virus:

In view of the serious consequence of HTLV-III/LAV [now called HIV] infection, its stability under clinical and laboratory conditions and its inactivation by commonly utilized inactivating agents and disinfectants are of tremendous importance to health care workers and laboratory personnel.

Here, the results of testing the stability of HTLV-III/LAV under various experimental conditions are reported. . . .

To test the effect of some frequently encountered clinical and laboratory conditions on the infectivity of the HTLV-III(TM), virus diluted in media supplemented with 50% human plasma was dried and incubated at 23 to 27 degrees Centigrade [73 to 80 degrees Fahrenheit], or incubated in an aqueous state at one of several different temperatures; room temperature, 36 to 37 degrees Centigrade [up to 98.6 degrees F.], and 54 to 56 degrees Centigrade [133 DEGREES F.] for various periods of time. IN A DRIED STATE, COMPLETE INACTIVATION OF VIRUS REQUIRED BETWEEN THREE AND SEVEN DAYS. . . .

VIRUS REMAINS INFECTIVE FOR 15 DAYS

Exposing virus to different temperatures resulted in a reduction of infectious virus corresponding to increasing times of incubation and increasing temperatures. Complete inactivation . . . of infectious virus was seen between 11 and 15 days of exposure at 36 to 37 degrees Centigrade. INFECTIOUS VIRUS WAS STILL DETECTED AFTER 15 DAYS AT ROOM TEMPERATURE. . . .

RIGOROUS HEATING FAILS TO KILL VIRUS

Infectious cell-free virus could be recovered from dried material after up to three days at room temperature, and in an aqueous environment (e.g. water), infectious virus survived longer than 15 days at room temperature. EVEN UNDER THE MORE RIGOROUS HEATING CONDITIONS COMMONLY USED TO INACTIVATE COMPLEMENT (54 TO 56 DEGREES CENTIGRADE [133 DEGREES FAHRENHEIT]), INFECTIOUS VIRUS WAS DETECTED THREE HOURS AFTER EXPOSURE. . . . The stability of HTLV-III at 54 to 56 degrees Centigrade suggests that the inactivation of virus in blood products (e.g., antihemophilia factors) could require more extensive treatment, as has been suggested.[36]

VIRUS SURVIVES ON METAL STRIPS

Since those studies were performed, researchers from the Centers for Disease Control conducted their own analysis of the viability of HIV outside the body. Entitled, "Survival of the Human Immunodeficiency Virus [HIV] Under Controlled Drying Conditions," the CDC study documents that HIV is a tough, hardy virus which survives *for several days* after being dried out and placed on stainless steel strips in a desiccator jar at room temperature.[37]

HIV MULTIPLIES IN THE THROAT
CELLS IN THE ESOPHAGUS ARE A TARGET FOR HIV

HIV has been found in lesions of the esophagus among homosexual males who engaged in oral copulation. The esophagus, also called the gullet, is the passage from the pharynx to the stomach.[38]

THE TONSILS TEEM WITH INFECTIVE VIRUS

Researchers from the National Institutes of Health in Bethesda, Maryland, and St. Luke's Hospital in New York, have found that the *tonsils and adenoids of patients with HIV disease have a greater concentration of HIV-1-infected cells* (50 to 100 times higher) *than blood*. These glands, located in the back of the throat, serve as major reservoirs of HIV.[39]

Physicians from the Children's Hospital of Philadelphia have analyzed the distribution of HIV-1 disease in blood, throat and urine of infected children. The group was composed of 21 children aged 2 months to 15 years, who had clinical or past evidence of HIV infection.

HIV was isolated from the throat swabs of 9 of 19 (47%) children. The virus was usually, but not always present in small amount, and was both cell-free and cell-associated. Irradiation experiments confirmed that VIRUS IN THE THROAT WAS IN AN ACTIVE REPLICATING STATE. . . .[40]

The researchers stated their findings "do not yet have epidemiologic correlates, and their significance for virus spread is unknown." In other words, even though the virus is *actively replicating* in the throats of pediatric AIDS carriers, they adopted a "wait and see" attitude regarding person-to-person spread of the virus. It can be inferred from their findings, however, that infective AIDS viruses from the throat [and saliva in the mouth] would be expelled into the air through coughing or sneezing, thereby exposing other children and adults in close contact. Infants and young children frequently slobber or drool saliva on other children and toys, creating a further risk of exposure. The U.S. Centers for Disease Control has warned that *the skin and mucous membranes of the eye, nose, mouth and possibly the respiratory tract [trachea, bronchi, lungs] should be considered as potential pathways for entry of the virus.*[41]

CDC URGES WEARING PROTECTIVE GEAR

Blood, *saliva*, and gingival fluid from all dental patients *should be considered infective* [able to transmit disease]. . . . In addition to wearing gloves for contact with oral mucous membranes of all patients, *all dental workers should wear surgical masks and protective eyewear or chin-length plastic face shields during dental procedures in which splashing or spattering of blood, saliva or gingival fluids is likely.*[42]

The CDC warns outright against allowing blood *or saliva* to contact the skin of the hands and further cautions that plastic face shields, similar to welders' masks, be used to prevent infective blood or saliva from transmitting disease via the mucous membranes of the eyes, nose or mouth.[43]

The warnings of the CDC and other authorities make it abundantly clear that saliva is an "other body fluid" which can transmit AIDS.[44]

HIV-contaminated saliva that is dribbled, coughed, sneezed, spit or otherwise sprayed or spattered onto the skin or mucous membranes of the eyes, nose, mouth, or inhaled into the respiratory tract is a risk.

AIDS AND DAYCARE CENTERS

Until fairly recently, it was believed that hepatitis B (HBV) which is similar in epidemiology and modes of spread to HIV, could not be transmitted in daycare centers. Transmission of hepatitis B has now been documented in daycare settings. The March 1987 *American Journal of Epidemiology* presented a study of 269 children, ages one to three, attending five nursery schools in which there were children who were hepatitis B carriers. Fifteen of the children – 5.6% (other than those known to be carriers) – were found to have been exposed to hepatitis B. Ten of the children were thought to have been infected at the nursery school by hepatitis B carrier children and four became hepatitis B carriers themselves.

Researchers from the Hepatitis Branch of the CDC have reported in the December 1989 *Pediatric Infectious Disease Journal*:

> A 4-year-old boy who attended a daycare center developed acute hepatitis B; another child at the center who had a history of aggressive behavior (biting/scratching) was subsequently found to be a hepatitis B carrier. No other source of infection among family members and other contacts was identified. . . .

AIDS TRANSMITTED THROUGH BITING

A case involving transmission of HIV disease between two brothers through a bite has been reported. A little boy contracted AIDS from a contaminated blood transfusion traced back to a homosexual donor. Shortly after the child's death from AIDS, his brother, three years older, was found to have become infected with HIV. The physicians presenting the report state:

> One possible route of transmission was a bite on the older brother's forearm by the younger child about six months before he died. The mother had seen teeth imprints on the skin but no bleeding or haematoma. This observation suggests that EVEN MINOR BITES BY HIV-INFECTED CHILDREN MAY CARRY THE RISK OF VIRUS TRANSMISSION. Parents, teachers, and other people responsible for HIV-infected children should be aware of this possibility and try to prevent spread of the virus by this route.[45]

SOBERING RECOMMENDATIONS

The National Institute of Justice *AIDS Bulletin* has presented an eye-opening report entitled "Precautionary Measures and Protective Equipment: Developing a Reasonable Response," by Theodore M. Hammett, Ph.D.* While maintaining that "the risk of becoming infected with HIV in the course of Law Enforcement duties is extremely low," the report recommends:

GENERAL INFECTION CONTROL
Avoid smoking, eating, drinking, nailbiting, and all hand-to-mouth, hand-to-nose, and hand-to-eye actions while working in areas contaminated with blood and body fluids. . . .

LABORATORY ANALYSIS OF EVIDENCE
– all personnel who have direct or indirect contact with blood or body fluids should wear gloves
– gloved hands should not contact other items which may be touched by ungloved personnel
– face shields or protective eyeglasses and masks should be worn if there is potential for spattering of blood or body fluids
– fingers, pencils, and other objects should be kept out of mouths

HUMAN BITES
While the risk of infection through human bites is already very low, the following simple precautions will minimize the risk of HIV and other infection as well as promote basic hygiene:
– ENCOURAGE "BACKBLEEDING" by applying pressure and "milking the wound," AS WITH SNAKEBITE
– wash the area thoroughly with soap and hot water; and
– seek medical attention as soon as possible[46]

CHILDREN WITH AIDS PRONE TO BEHAVIOR PROBLEMS

Young children not infrequently drool, bite, scratch or engage in other activities involving the release of body fluids. Children with AIDS are very prone to neurological damage which can facilitate such behaviors.[47] Researchers from the Baylor Hospital of Medicine in Houston have reported that children with HIV disease can exhibit behavioral changes such as conduct disorders involving firesetting and deliberate destruction of other's property and physical abuse to people.[48] Developmental abnormalities may be the first sign of pediatric HIV disease.[49]

In light of their serious cognitive disabilities, it is in the best interests of children with HIV disease (as well as non-infected

*Points of view or opinions expressed in the *Bulletin* are those of the authors and do not necessarily represent the official position or policies of the U.S. Department of Justice.

children) to attend specialized education classes or receive personalized tutoring designed to best meet their unique learning and behavioral needs.[50]

CHILDREN WITH HIV SUSCEPTIBLE TO OTHER DISEASES

Due to their weakened immune systems, children with HIV disease/AIDS are especially vulnerable to contracting other infectious diseases. Routine childhood ailments can be life-threatening in immunocompromised children.

PEDIATRIC AIDS PATIENTS AND VACCINATIONS

Many children with HIV disease do not respond adequately to routine vaccinations against childhood diseases. Physicians from the State University of New York Health Science Center at Brooklyn and Temple University School of Medicine, St. Christopher's Hospital for Children in Philadelphia, found:

> A significant percentage of children with HIV infection had antibody levels to Diphtheria, Polio, Measles, Mumps and Rubella below indicated [protective] levels.[51]

Measles can be particularly virulent in children with AIDS.[52] Chickenpox, which is caused by the varicella-zoster virus, is a highly contagious disease spread by contact with infective lesions and the airborne route.[53] There is no effective vaccine to prevent chickenpox. Children who are immunocompromised are considered at high risk of varicella. Recurrent episodes of varicella-zoster virus has caused fatal stroke in HIV-infected infants.[54]

Contagious illnesses are readily spread in settings where large groups of children are in constant close contact with each other such as school classrooms and daycare centers. A host of communicable diseases and viral infections are endemic in daycare centers: hepatitis A, meningitis, influenza, cytomegalovirus, giardiasis, intestinal viruses and others.[55]

It is in the best interests of infants and children with AIDS to be shielded from environmental and social situations which could expose them to other infectious diseases.

HIV FOUND IN URINE

Researchers from New York University Medical Center state:

> The fact that HIV-1 RNA can be detected in urine pellets suggests that URINE MAY BE AN INFECTIOUS BODY FLUID IN SEROPOSITIVE INDIVIDUALS....[56]

Skin and mucous membrane contact with known or potentially infective urine should be avoided.

URINE SAFER FOR AIDS TESTING

Researchers from New York University and Calypte Biomedical Company in Berkeley, California, have reported that a dipstick test for detecting AIDS antibodies in urine provides highly accurate results:

> These data suggest that urine instead of blood can be used as a sample source for detection of HIV-1 antibodies. THERE IS A LOWER RISK TO HEALTH CARE WORKERS TESTING FOR HIV-1 IN URINE RATHER THAN BLOOD due to 1) substantially lower incidence of infectious HIV-1 virus in urine and 2) eliminating venipuncture and exposure to blood.[57]

URINE SUITABLE FOR LARGE SCALE AIDS TESTING

Based on their studies of urine tests demonstrating 99.7% and 99.9% accuracy in detecting AIDS antibodies, physicians from Middlesex Hospital in London conclude:

> Class-specific antibody tests . . . reliably detect anti-HIV in urine and *could provide HIV prevalence data that was previously unobtainable.*[58]

Scientists from the University of Toronto, the Federal Centre for AIDS in Ottawa, and the Ontario Ministry of Health, state:

> Detection of HIV Ab [antibodies] in URINE IS A SUITABLE NON-INVASIVE ALTERNATIVE TO BLOOD FOR HIV PREVALENCE TESTING, and may have an important role in epidemiologic surveillance.[59]

The Metpath Company in Teterboro, New Jersey, reports that testing urine for AIDS antibodies provides extremely accurate results among people from high and low risk groups.[60]

Urine is easily and painlessly collected. Accurate, rapid urine tests for AIDS have been developed. Using urine instead of blood for AIDS testing is safer for health care workers. Urine testing could readily and inexpensively be used on a mass scale to determine the prevalence of HIV disease in the population. *Testing urine for AIDS could be easily combined with drug testing in various occupations and other situations.*

HIV FOUND IN FLUID FROM SKIN BLISTERS

HIV has been isolated for the first time from the blister fluid of an AIDS patient. Speaking at the annual meeting of the American Academy of Dermatology, Dr. Nantaput Supapannachart of the University of Cincinnati School of Medicine, said the investigation was undertaken after a 37-year-old HIV-positive man with multiple skin lesions on the back of his hands expressed concern about whether his hand lesions might be contagious.

Samples of blister fluid were cultured and tested positive for HIV. Two months later, the fluid was retested and the results were again positive.

"HIV has been isolated in saliva, tears, alveolar [lung] fluid, and breast milk, but this is the first case in which HIV has been isolated from cutaneous blister fluid," said Dr. Supapannachart. She has reported her findings to the CDC and plans to evaluate additional HIV-positive patients with skin blisters. Dr. Peter Drotman, Assistant Director for the Public Health Division of HIV/AIDS at the CDC, said the findings were new to him, but not really surprising. "If HIV reproduces in lymphocytes, then one will find HIV when there is fluid that contains lymphocytes."[61]

MASS OUTBREAK OF HERPES CAUSED BY SKIN CONTACT

When two athletes are engaged in all-out combat on a mat where many others have also dropped their sweat and virus particles, the virus can get into the skin surface. A mat burn, a scratch, or a minor laceration can become a major herpes problem.
– William Wickett, Jr., M.D., *Herpes: Cause & Control*[62]

Two teenage athletes with herpes spread the viral infection to 58 others at a wrestling camp in Minnesota, the *New England Journal of Medicine* has reported. Epidemiologists from the Minnesota Department of Health reported that the virus was spread through skin contact. A walloping 67% of heavyweight wrestlers and 25% of lightweights attending the four-week training camp developed herpetic blisters of the face, arms, and upper bodies. Other symptoms included fever, chills, sore throat and headaches.

Five of the young athletes developed eye infections. Researchers said subsequent corneal damage remained a concern because the virus, which affects nerve cells, could cause recurrent herpes in the eye.

Transmission of herpes among wrestlers is referred to as *herpes gladiatorum*.[63] Recent surveys of athletic trainers "suggest that *herpes gladiatorum* is endemic among high school and college wrestlers, but the incidence of disease and optimal control methods remain unknown," the health officials reported. They said that prevention efforts should involve routine examinations of wrestlers for herpes-type skin blisters and *exclusion of anyone with a potential infection from competition*. "It is necessary to educate wrestlers, parents and coaches to increase their awareness of *herpes gladiatorum* as a serious health risk," the report said.[64]

DISCRIMINATION AGAINST PEOPLE WITH HERPES

It is clear that these health officials would actually disallow people with herpes from participating in sports involving extensive skin-to-skin contact. There has not yet been a public outcry protesting their advocacy of discrimination toward people with herpes. Civil liberties groups have not objected that such a discriminatory policy is unconstitutional, unfair, unkind or lacking in compassion because people with herpes would be made to feel socially ostracized and stigmatized.

AIDS TRANSMITTED DURING SPORTING EVENTS

During a soccer match in 1989, a 25-year-old man collided with another player, a drug abuser who was a carrier of HIV-1 disease.[65] *The AIDS virus was transmitted through direct contact at the brief moment of impact in which the players bumped heads.*

This disturbing case is not merely an isolated event. Dr. Donato Torre, one of the infectious disease specialists reporting the situation, stated:

OTHER CASES OF TRANSMISSION OF THE AIDS VIRUS FROM SPORTING EVENTS HAVE BEEN DOCUMENTED IN THE UNITED STATES AND BRITAIN.[66]

It is not feasible for athletes involved in vigorous contact sports to practice "universal precautions." Wearing a latex mask, gloves and rubber body suit is impractical. They interfere with sports performance, cause overheating and are likely to tear or break.

ATHLETES WITH AIDS ENDANGER OTHERS

Athletes who carry HIV disease can expose others to infective blood and blister fluid through the abrasive skin-to-skin contact involved in wrestling and other sports. An individual with HIV disease need not have pre-existing blisters or lesions to pose a risk; skin blisters can form and break during the course of competition, leaking HIV-infective blister fluid on the other participants. Abrasions, mat burns and scratches on the bodies of non-infected participants are vulnerable to infection by HIV-contaminated blood and blister fluid. The AIDS virus can also pass through intact skin via Langerhans cells located close to the surface of epithelial tissue.[67]

AIDS VIRUS MULTIPLIES IN THE SKIN

Researchers from the Laboratory of Tumor Cell Biology, National Cancer Institute, National Institute of Health, Bethesda, Maryland, and the Department of Dermatology, Department of

Otolaryngology, University of Vienna Medical School in Austria, indicate:

> ... ACTIVE VIRUS CAN BE RESCUED FROM THE SKIN OF HIV-INFECTED INDIVIDUALS.
>
> OUR FINDINGS CONCLUSIVELY CONFIRM that (I) Langerhans cells are an actual target for HIV infection and production, supporting the view that besides T cells, cells of the monocyte/macrophage lineage are a major target population of this virus (II) THE SKIN MAY SERVE AS A VIRAL RESERVOIR DURING THE COURSE OF HIV INFECTION.[68]

HIV INFECTS SKIN DURING "ASYMPTOMATIC" PERIOD

Virologists from the Department of Virology, Robert Koch Institute, Berlin, along with dermatologists from Oslo, Norway, state:

> Epidermal Langerhans cells from symptom-free ["asymptomatic"] HIV-positive individuals may be latently infected. In ARC/AIDS patients HIV has been demonstrated in the epidermis of the skin, and we have previously demonstrated that epidermal Langerhans cells [LC] can be infected in vitro with HIV, and that *THEY PRODUCE AND RELEASE VIRUS* into the culture medium.[69]

SKIN SATURATED WITH HIV

Specialists from the Institute for Tropical Medicine in Hamburg studied 150 biopsies from patients at different stages of HIV disease and determined:

> *Almost every cell in the basal layer of the skin* showed an unspecific positivity with p18 [p18 and p24 are core proteins of HIV]. ... The positivity of some Langerhans cells [LC] with p24 suggests *LC are target cells for HIV infection.*[70]

HIV DISEASE CAUSES SKIN LESIONS

Physicians from the University of Texas Southwestern Medical Center in Dallas, Texas, report that inflammatory disorders of the skin are common in the course of HIV disease.[71]

HIV disease can induce or exacerbate psoriasis, resulting in dry, cracked, scaling patches of skin which bleed when rubbed. Physicians A.P. Lozar, M.D., M.P.H. and H.H. Roenigk, M.D., of the Department of Dermatology, Northwestern University Medical School, Chicago, have reported severe psoriasis in patients with ARC/AIDS. The psoriatic lesions included skin pustules which were extremely difficult to eradicate. In one case:

> ... *more than 90% of the patient's body was covered with psoriasis.* Open sores in the gluteal area [buttocks], oral candidiasis [thrush] and recurrent herpes zoster infection of the left eye with severe pain was present. ...

One of our AIDS patients had giardial diarrhea [a parasitic disease, part of the "gay bowel syndrome"] and we decided not to let him use our PUVA phototherapy unit after he had an uncontrollable bout of explosive diarrhea and was considered contagious.

AIDS is becoming more prevalent in the population. We can expect to see patients with this syndrome who have associated dermatologic problems.

The researchers conclude:

Isolation of patients with psoriasis and AIDS from psoriatic patients without AIDS should be considered.[72]

HIV CAUSES SEVERE ACNE AND DERMATITIS

Seborrheic dermatitis of the face and scalp, eczema, and acneiform eruption [severe acne] are typical manifestations of HIV disease, and often prove resistant to treatment.[73] In one study, 58.6% of female patients with HIV disease had acneiform eruption.[74] The sebaceous [oil producing] glands appear to be involved in HIV disease. Yellowing of the toe nails is also frequently seen in patients with HIV disease.[75]

HIV INFECTS INTACT SKIN

Langerhans cells occur in skin and mucous membranes. . . . We therefore conclude that the accessory cells (target cells) for HIV are within these barriers themselves. THE ASSUMPTION THAT HIV INFECTION OCCURS EXCLUSIVELY THROUGH WOUNDS IN SKIN AND MUCOUS MEMBRANES INTO THE BLOOD CAN NO LONGER BE CONSIDERED VALID. Our results suggest that the Langerhans cells in the skin and mucous membranes are primary target cells for sexually transmitted HIV infection.[76]

There is a risk of transmission through intact skin as well as the mucous membranes of the eyes, nasal passages, mouth and the respiratory tract.[77]

HIV TRANSMITTED THROUGH DIFFERENT RECEPTORS

It had been previously thought that human cells had to have a certain type of receptor (CD4) or "docking" site in order to become infected with the AIDS virus. It is now known that HIV can utilize several cell surface receptors.[78] This has implications for the potential of different means of AIDS transmission.

AIDS TRANSMITTED THROUGH BREAST MILK

French researchers have documented HIV transmission through breast feeding.[79] HIV is present in the breast milk of "asymptomatic" HIV-infected mothers.[80] Healthy babies have contracted AIDS through imbibing contaminated breast milk. HIV transmission can occur without any blood contact (in the absence of cracked or bleeding nipples). Researchers from Madras Medical College and the Post Graduate Institute of Basic Medical Sciences in Madras, India, have documented a high rate of HIV-1 transmission from seropositive mothers to their nursing infants.[81] Other instances of HIV transmission through breast milk have been reported.[82]

SUMMARY

1.   The mouth of an individual carrying HIV acts as a viral incubator, fomenting the manufacture and multiplication of infective AIDS viruses.

2.   HIV-contaminated saliva is an infective body fluid. The AIDS virus has been found in "higher incidence and percentage" in salivary lymphocytes than those in blood. HIV-contaminated blood can transmit AIDS.

3.   HIV contained in saliva is not neutralized within the mouth of the infected individual because the normal "immunologic barrier" is eliminated.

4.   Intimate physical relations (deep kissing, etc.,) involving the saliva of an AIDS carrier should be avoided.

5.   Direct skin or mucous membrane (of the eye, mouth, nose, genitals) contact with the saliva of an AIDS carrier should be avoided.

6.   HIV-contaminated saliva which is sneezed or coughed into the air is infective. If the contaminated droplets come in contact with the surface of the eye or the membranes of the nose or mouth there is a danger of HIV transmission.

7.   The urine of AIDS carriers has been found to contain infective virus. Contact with HIV-infectious urine should be avoided.

8.   The AIDS virus survives outside the body for days to weeks in both dry and liquid form. HIV has been found to remain infectious outside the body after being dried out in a petri dish for ten days. This indicates that the HIV virus is a tough virus capable of surviving on inanimate objects for a prolonged period of time. Objects which have been contaminated with HIV-infective saliva should undergo appropriate disinfection procedures.

9.   Persons in occupations which require the performance of car-
dio-pulmonary resuscitation (CPR) involving mouth-to-mouth contact (e.g., policemen, firemen, paramedics, nurses) should be routinely screened for HIV infection. An AIDS-infectious individual
performing CPR has the potential of passing saliva contaminated
with HIV and other pathogens into the mouth of the recipient.

10.   Accurate, low-cost saliva and urine tests for AIDS have been
developed. These tests are safer for health care workers. The tests
are easy to perform and could be used for large-scale AIDS testing. A saliva assay for AIDS has been developed which is more accurate than conventional blood tests [ELISA].

11.   Saliva tests for AIDS are well-suited for screening dental patients. Testing urine for AIDS could be easily combined with drug
testing in various occupations and other situations.

CHAPTER FIVE

CONTAGIOUS SECONDARY DISEASES

Some virologists fear that a simple mutation in the AIDS virus itself could leave it armed with an ability to infect as the flu virus does now – via respiratory droplets spread by coughing or sneezing. HIV commonly infects macrophages, a kind of white blood cell often present in the lungs, notes Nobel Laureate Joshua Lederberg, president of Rockefeller University in New York City. Even a minor mutation might enable HIV to infect those cells via the respiratory tract.
– "Viruses: the Next Plague?" *The Washington Post*[1]

The potential for HIV to be transmitted through non-sexual interpersonal contact is one of the more unsettling aspects of the AIDS epidemic. AIDS advocacy groups, leading health officials and politicians have dogmatically denied the possibility of non-primary modes of HIV transmission. Most popular AIDS instruction materials include admonitions which read like a refrain from a script: "You can't catch AIDS through casual contact* . . . There is no risk of catching AIDS through coughing, sneezing or being in the same room as someone with AIDS . . . An AIDS patient is in greater danger of catching something from you than vice versa . . . The greatest danger is not AIDS, but ignorance, bigotry and fear."

These types of dogmatic assertions completely ignore the reality of the secondary diseases related to AIDS which are transmitted person-to-person. Pulmonary tuberculosis, for example, is a major secondary complication of HIV disease.

AIDS SPURRING GROWTH OF OTHER DEADLY EPIDEMICS
In the process of breaking down the immune system, HIV disease promotes the development of various contagious bacterial and

---

*"Casual contact" is a novel term developed specifically to belittle the possibility of HIV transmission through any means other than drug abuse or intimate contact. The term was not previously used to describe the transmissibility of any other communicable illness. It was not used to describe airborne or household transmission of the common cold, flu, hepatitis or TB.

The term "casual contact" inappropriately lumps together every non-primary form of HIV transmission. It erroneously implies that non-sexual contact with the body fluids of an AIDS patient, shaking hands or walking across the street from someone with AIDS pose the same level of risk.[2]

viral illnesses. These contagious diseases are difficult to eradicate in HIV-infected patients. Individuals whose contagious illnesses do not respond to medications remain infectious.

The weakened immunity caused by HIV disease allows the microbes causing these disorders to multiply at a ferocious rate. Individuals infected with HIV are likely to have high concentrations of the infectious organisms in their bodily fluids and secretions, increasing the risk of transmission to others.[3]

In addition to tuberculosis, there are a number of other communicable AIDS-related conditions which can be transmitted to healthy persons who are not infected with HIV. These infectious diseases can be spread through a variety of means apart from intimate relations and drug abuse.

Researchers from the Faculty of Medicine, University of São Paulo in Brazil, indicate that the AIDS epidemic will accelerate the growth of a host of virulent diseases in developing nations including:

Leishmaniasis, Chagas' disease, Malaria, Tuberculosis, Leprosy, Dengue, Yellow fever and parasitic disorders.[4]

In endemic areas, leprosy may represent another opportunistic infection of HIV disease.[5]

AIDS-RELATED INFECTIONS AND DISEASES

Pneumocystis carinii pneumonia is a common secondary lung disease among AIDS patients. Outbreaks of *p. carinii* pneumonia have occurred from AIDS patients to other immunocompromised patients. In Houston, AIDS patients who mingled freely with immunosuppressed cancer patients in the waiting room of a hospital transmitted the disease to other non-AIDS patients.[6]

Since the diseased patient may be able to transmit the infection to immunosuppressed patients, IT SEEMS PRUDENT TO AVOID RESPIRATORY CONTACT BETWEEN PATIENTS WITH PNEUMOCYSTOSIS AND OTHER SUSCEPTIBLE INDIVIDUALS, although such precautions are not recommended by the Centers for Disease Control. Such precautions might help prevent hospital clusters of pneumocystosis.[7]

P. carinii pneumonia can also be transmitted to premature and healthy newborn infants, because they have not developed resistance to disease.[8] The elderly are also at increased risk.

AIDS-RELATED DISEASES AND FOOD HANDLERS

It would seem prudent to ask that AIDS patients not engage in food preparation or handling for others, particularly if they have an intestinal infection.
– Dr. Sidney Finegold, President of the Infectious Disease Society of America[9]

When considering the issue of HIV transmission through food-handlers, most of the focus of attention is on whether or not an HIV-infected food handler would be able to transmit the virus through a cut and bleeding onto the food. HIV carriers are susceptible to skin lesions, cracks and sores which could ooze HIV, hepatitis B virus (HBV), hepatitis C and other blood-borne ailments. They are also at high risk of carrying serious bowel infections which are transmitted through food-handling and person-to-person contact.

HEPATITIS B TRANSMITTED AMONG BUTCHERS

Outbreaks of hepatitis B (HBV), which has very similar modes of transmission to AIDS, have been reported among employees in butcher shops.[10] Over a 13-month period, eight employees from two butcher shops developed acute hepatitis B. The source of the outbreak was an intravenous drug abuser with hepatitis B. The infectious carrier also spread delta hepatitis to two of the employees. Delta hepatitis can act in synergy with chronic HBV to cause fatal liver failure.[11] The wife of one of the infected butchers contracted hepatitis B.

The infectious disease specialists who analyzed the outbreaks reported:

> *All butchers reported that small full thickness lacerations occurred almost every day.* These were usually due to sharp bone edges, bled little and were not covered. Knife wounds were less common but tended to be more serious. Unless these appeared to need sutures, they were bandaged or covered with sterile plastic strips and work was resumed. *The cashiers, whose duties included wrapping the meat, reported occasional grazes from bone edges.* They also often assisted the butchers in the dressing of cuts.
> ... THE HIGH ATTACK RATE AMONG THE BUTCHERS ... CLEARLY INDICATES THE POTENTIAL FOR HBV TRANSMISSION WITHIN THIS OCCUPATION.[12]

AIDS VIRUS SURVIVES INTENSE HEAT TREATING

Canadian and American scientists have discovered that HIV-contaminated blood remains infective outside the body for many hours to days. Particularly significant is their finding that the *AIDS virus survives after undergoing dry heat treatment at 60 degrees centigrade (140 degrees Fahrenheit) for 30 hours.* Researchers from the Federal Centers for AIDS, McGill University, University of British Columbia, and the Centers for Disease Control in Ottawa, Canada and Atlanta, Georgia, state:

We conclude that, contrary to previous thinking, HIV can be transmitted by screened factor concentrates prepared with the shorter [30 hour] dry heat process.[13]

HIV-contaminated slicing equipment, knives, wrapping paper and surfaces would remain infective unless adequately disinfected. The continuous high volume of cutting and slicing makes it impractical to routinely autoclave knives and slicing blades and sterilize the cutting tables, meat hooks, etc., in between cutting various meats, fish and poultry. Given the inevitable risk of blood-to-blood exposure in these circumstances, it could be considered judicious to allow employers to require HIV testing for butchers.

DANGERS OF "THE GAY BOWEL SYNDROME"

Hepatitis viruses, enteric pathogens, and anorectal infections may commonly be transmitted by various sexual practices. Because of their larger numbers of sexual partners and sexual practices such as anilingus [oral-anal acts] and anal intercourse [sodomy], HOMOSEXUAL MEN ARE AT PARTICULARLY HIGH RISK OF ACQUIRING HEPATITIS B, GIARDIASIS, AMEBIASIS, SHIGELLOSIS, CAMPYLOBACTERIOSIS, and anorectal infections with Neisseria gonorrhoeae, Chlamydia trachomatis, Treponema pallidum, herpes simplex virus, and human papilloma viruses.[14]

AIDS patients and HIV high risk group members are very prone to contagious bowel infections. Male homosexuals in the United States and elsewhere are particularly susceptible to acquiring a variety of viral and bacterial bowel diseases which previously had been considered "tropical." A study in the *Scandinavia Journal of Infectious Diseases* found the majority of asymptomatic homosexual men in Sweden harbored intestinal parasites; many carried *Emtamoeba histolytica* and *Giardia lamblia*. The high prevalence of intestinal protozoas found among homosexuals in Sweden was ". . . quite comparable to those observed in homosexual men in North America."[15]

Enteric diseases are so rife in the male homosexual population they are referred to collectively in the medical literature as the "gay bowel syndrome."[16]

Infections associated with "gay bowel syndrome" are readily transmitted by infectious food handlers and through non-sexual, person-to-person contact. Conditions associated with this syndrome include:

Salmonellosis: A bacterial disease which causes food poisoning and gastroenteritis resulting in vomiting, abdominal cramps and voluminous diarrhea containing mucus and traces of blood. In infants and the elderly, lethal dehydration can result.[17] Salmonellosis is spread easily through infectious food handlers.

Giardiasis: A parasitic disease caused by the protozoan *Giardia lamblia*. It is transmitted among homosexuals primarily by oral-anal practices involving fecal contamination. *G. lamblia* can be transmitted through contaminated water, by direct person-to-person contact and infectious food handlers.[18] Giardiasis is a common cause of irritable bowel syndrome.[19] The *G. lamblia* protozoan has a large sucking disk which attaches to the lining of the small intestine in the human host. The organism is resistant to the concentrations of chlorine normally found in sanitized municipal water supplies.[20]

Symptoms include inflammation of the intestinal tract, frequent diarrhea, urgent loose stools, malabsorption and weight loss. Although some persons have a self-limited illness of several weeks duration, many have a more prolonged course, with waxing and waning symptoms and progressive weight loss. Resolution of symptoms is often slow in spite of drug therapies. Epidemics of giardiasis have also occurred in daycare centers.

Amebiasis: A disease of the colon caused by the parasite *Entamoeba histolytica*. In active amebiasis, the parasites directly invade the intestinal mucosa causing amebic colitis. The parasites can also travel via the bloodstream to produce metastic infections in the liver and other sites. Amebic colitis is characterized by ulcers that contain pus and parasites. Symptoms of amebiasis can mimic those of ulcerative colitis. Rupture of amebic liver abscess can cause peritonitis.

The manifestations of amebic colitis may be subtle or severe, ranging from mild watery diarrhea to explosive bloody dysentery. It is not uncommon for those with the disease to experience temporary remissions followed by reappearance of symptoms.

The treatment of amebiasis remains difficult. Different forms of the infection require different treatment regimens. Several of the drugs used to treat amebiasis have toxic side-effects.[21]

Campylobacter enteritis: *Campylobacter* infection usually results in an inflammatory, occasionally bloody diarrhea or dysentery syndrome. As many as two million Campylobacter enteritis (bowel inflammation) cases occur annually in the United States.

The transmission of *Campylobacter* infections is likely via the fecal-oral route. Fecal oral spread may occur by contact among animals, homosexual males and those in day care centers.[22]

Shigellosis: An acute bacterial infection of the intestinal tract causing diarrhea, cramping, fever, and painful defecation. The resultant rapid dehydration can be fatal in young children and the elderly. According to *Cecil's Textbook of Medicine*:

TRANSMISSION MOST OFTEN OCCURS BY CLOSE PERSON-TO-PERSON CONTACT *THROUGH CONTAMINATED HANDS* [e.g., shaking hands]. . . . During clinical illness and for up to six weeks after recovery, organisms are excreted in the feces.
THE MALE HOMOSEXUAL POPULATION IN THE UNITED STATES IS AT INCREASED RISK FOR SHIGELLOSIS, WHICH IS ONE OF THE CAUSES OF "GAY BOWEL SYNDROME."[23]

The onset of shigellosis is often very severe in children, producing a high fever and rapid fluid loss. Neurologic symptoms and signs, including delirium, headache and stiffening of the neck and back are common in young children who contract shigellosis. Individuals excreting shigellae should be excluded from all phases of food handling until negative cultures have been obtained from three successive stool specimens.

Cryptosporidiosis: A gastrointestinal tract infection characterized by watery diarrhea, abdominal cramps, malabsorption and weight loss. It is a severe, unremitting disease in immunocompromised patients such as those with AIDS.

Cryptosporidiosis has been reported in male homosexuals without AIDS. Nosocomial [in-hospital] spread of cryptosporidiosis as well as common occurrence of the infection in day-care centers and in household or other close contacts of index cases indicate that [NON-SEXUAL] PERSON-TO-PERSON SPREAD IS IMPORTANT. . . .
CRYPTOSPORIDIUM MAY ALSO BE TRANSMITTED BY INDIRECT EXPOSURE TO CONTAMINATED SURFACES, FOOD OR WATER. The cryptosporidial cyst is quite hardy. It is resistant to a number of laboratory disinfectants. . . .[24]

In the United States, most cases of *Cryptosporidium* infection are derived from a continuous human reservoir sustained by fecal-oral transmission.[25]

Rotaviruses: Rotaviruses have been detected in the diarrhea of HIV-infected homosexual males in Germany, caused by "sexual behavior with possible oral-anal transmission."[26] Rotaviruses cause acute gastroenteritis and are spread by contaminated food and person-to-person contact. Children and infants who develop rotavirus gastroenteritis are subject to severe dehydration.

TROPICAL DISEASES FOMENTED BY HOMOSEXUAL ACTS

In developing nations intestinal parasitism and other bowel ailments are prevalent because of poor sanitary conditions, such as sewage-contaminated food and water supplies.

Among male homosexuals, bowel diseases and infections are rampant because of oral-anal practices involving the ingestion of fecal matter.[27] In a type of oral-anal copulation, the tongue is inserted directly into the rectum. In medical terms, this unsanitary practice is referred to as anilingus (Latin, *anus* + *lingere*, to lick); in homosexual argot it is referred to as "rimming" or "brown-nosing." Infective virus and/or parasite laden secretions and fecal matter are ingested and swallowed in this manner. Anilingus is done as a deviant act per se, and as a prelude to anal-genital sodomy and "fisting." The practice of outright defecation/ingestion is also involved, a practice referred to by homosexuals as "eating scat" (Greek, *skatos*, dung, manure). Oral copulation (fellatio) performed after rectal sodomy and fecal contamination of the fingers and hands during homosexual acts are also means of spreading these diseases.

MASSIVE INCIDENCE OF PARASITISM

It is estimated that 30%-50% of practicing male homosexuals have contracted parasitic amebiasis as a direct result of practices involving fecal contamination.[28] In one homosexual bathhouse situation, there was an outbreak of parasites among patrons through the shared usage of an enema nozzle used for rectal douching.[29]
Dr. Hunter Handsfield, director of the STD Control Program Seattle-King County Department of Health, reports:

> Sexual transmission of amebiasis was initially suggested in reports of cutaneous amebiasis of the penis and perianal area. Subsequently both AMEBIASIS AND GIARDIASIS HAVE BEEN FOUND TO BE EPIDEMIC IN HOMOSEXUAL MEN, and in New York City E. histolytica, G. lamblia or both are found in 40% of homosexual men attending STD clinics. Similar prevalence figures have been reported in San Francisco, Seattle, and Cleveland.... ANILINGUS [ORAL/ANAL CONTACT] IS BELIEVED TO BE THE MAJOR MODE OF TRANSMISSION.[30]

Infectious disease specialists from the Tufts-New England Medical Center in Boston state:

> With the emergence of highly visible urban homosexual communities during the past decade, bathhouses and clubs where multiple, often anonymous sexual contacts are sanctioned have gained increasing popularity. This commercial mode of sexual access clearly enhances the uncontrolled circulation of intestinal pathogens in male homosexuals. . . .
>
> Although the increment in transmission may be largely ascribed to the homosexual community, THE POTENTIAL FOR WIDER DISSEMINATION [TO THE GENERAL PUBLIC] REMAINS. As Dritz has written of the San Francisco experience, "In 1979 . . . an average of 10% of all patients and asymptomatic contacts reported to the San Francisco Department of Public Health because of positive fecal samples or culture for amebiasis,

Giardia or Shigella infections WERE EMPLOYED AS FOOD HAND-LERS IN PUBLIC RESTAURANTS.

They conclude:

From the time of Moses there has been concomitant consciousness of the benefits to the public health of careful fecal disposal. Although man's technical ingenuity has achieved remarkable strides in the purification of our immediate domestic environment, the recent increase in transmission of intestinal infections among homosexual males offers new challenges in preventive medicine for physicians caring for these patients.[31]

As evidence of millennia-old basic sanitation guidelines, the physicians cite Deuteronomy 23:12,13: "Designate a place outside the camp where you can go to relieve yourself. As part of your equipment have something to dig with, and when you relieve yourself, dig a hole and cover your excrement" (NIV).

AIDS LINKED TO FECAL CONTAMINATION

In addition to the spread of intestinal parasites, the ingestion of blood-stained fecal matter may be a source of AIDS transmission among homosexuals. The pandemic incidence of hepatitis B among homosexual males has been fueled by anal-oral contact.

Unlike hepatitis A infection, fecal-oral spread was not considered an important route of transmission. Instead, HBV was thought to be transferred from acute or chronic carriers to other susceptible persons through shared toothbrushes, razors or fomites. *Quite the opposite appears to be true in homosexual men.* Oral-oral transmission [through kissing] may also occur if HBV gains entry through minute lesions in mucosal surfaces.[32]

The prevalence of AIDS among homosexuals has been associated with activities involving exposure to feces and past treatment for intestinal parasites.[33]

EDUCATIONAL EFFORTS YIELD DISAPPOINTING RESULTS

Articles in prominent medical journals have warned of the hazards of homosexual acts* involving fecal contamination for years prior to and after the onset of the AIDS epidemic.[34] The homosexual subculture has been inundated with reams of pamphlets and "safe

---

*Two major medical textbooks have been published detailing the relationship between homosexual behavior and bodily trauma and diseases: *Sexually Transmitted Diseases in Homosexual Men*, edited by David G. Ostrow et al., (New York: Plenum Books, 1983) and *The Acquired Immune Deficiency Syndrome and Infections of Homosexual Men*, by Pearl Ma and Donald Armstrong (New York: Yorke Medical Books, 1984). Jeanne Kassler, M.D., has written a concise paperback for laymen: *Gay Men's Health: A Guide to the AID Syndrome and Other Sexually Transmitted Diseases* (New York: Harper and Row, 1983).

sex" materials warning of the dangers of various "unsafe" acts.

In spite of these monumental and costly efforts to alter unsanitary behavior, the incidence of diseases transmitted by fecal-oral contamination among male homosexuals has remained abysmally high.

In 1988, researchers from the Johns Hopkins University School of Medicine and the National Institute of Allergy and Infectious Diseases reported:

> During the past 10 years, there has been an increasing appreciation of the medical problems of homosexual and bisexual men. In particular, THE HIGH RATES OF ENTERIC INFECTIONS IN THIS GROUP HAVE BEEN REFERRED TO COLLECTIVELY AS THE "GAY BOWEL SYNDROME." A VARIETY OF BACTERIA, VIRUSES AND PROTOZOA HAVE BEEN IMPLICATED, including . . . enteric pathogens traditionally ASSOCIATED WITH THE FECAL-ORAL ROUTE OF TRANSMISSION. . . . These observations presumably reflect epidemiologic patterns particular to gay men: multiplicity of contacts, *distinctive [sic] sexual practices*, and high rates of asymptomatic infection.
>
> We studied 388 homosexual or bisexual men from the Baltimore-Washington area to define the spectrum of enteric [bowel] pathogens carriage in a population at high risk for "gay bowel syndrome" in association with HIV infection. . . .
>
> Approximately 12% of the asymptomatic men harbored at least one enteric pathogen; the most frequently recovered were *C. trachomatis*, herpes simplex virus, and *Giardia lamblia. MEN CARRYING A PATHOGEN WERE MORE LIKELY TO BE HIV SEROPOSITIVE (48%) . . . AND MORE LIKELY TO HAVE A MUCOPURULENT EXUDATE [PUS-LIKE DISCHARGE]. We recovered an agent of enteric disease from 68% of gay men with diarrhea or proctitis. Campylobacter species, . . . herpes simplex virus, C. trachomatis, G. lamblia and Shigella* species were identified most frequently.[35]

AIDS FACILITATES BOWEL DISEASE

The weakened immune resistance induced by HIV disease can allow noxious intestinal microbes to "colonize" the body:

> Since 1981, the recognition of AIDS has added a new dimension to infectious disease complications in this population . . . diarrheal disease is found in a substantial proportion of patients with AIDS of the "AIDS-related complex [ARC]." *Immune function may play an important role in susceptibility to enteric pathogens in terms of either colonization or disease expression.*[36]

UNSANITARY ACTS DONE IN PRIVATE
CAN HAVE PUBLIC CONSEQUENCES

Hepatitis A is an inflammation of the liver which has spread like wildfire among homosexual males though behaviors involving fecal contamination. Hepatitis A is easily transmitted through infectious food handlers and direct person-to-person contact.[37] The infection can have grave, even fatal consequences when contracted by a woman during pregnancy. Massive outbreaks of hepatitis A caused by infected food handlers have occurred in different areas of the United States.[38] In describing a mass outbreak of hepatitis A in Multnomah County in Oregon, researchers stated:

> Increased surveillance in food service establishments and schools might have prevented outbreaks from a common source in the general population; however, an increase of sporadic cases in the non-drug-using population clearly occurred.[39]

In the study, "Linked Outbreaks of Hepatitis A in Homosexual Men in Food Service Patrons and Employees," investigators from the Centers for Disease Control compellingly documented the means by which "the sexual practices [oral-fecal contact] of homosexual men . . . enhance transmission of hepatitis A." The report describes how homosexual food handlers with hepatitis A spread the disease to other workers and customers.[40]

HEPATITIS A SKYROCKETS AMONG HOMOSEXUALS

In 1986, the journal *Medical Clinics of North America* reported:

> HOMOSEXUAL MALES HAVE AN EXTRAORDINARILY HIGH INCIDENCE OF HEPATITIS A. On an annual basis, at least 5 to 7 percent of homosexual males will acquire hepatitis A. Risk factors for hepatitis A include length of homosexual activity, number of sexual contacts, and oral-anal sexual contact. . . .[41]

In recent years, the incidence of hepatitis A has skyrocketed among homosexual males in New York City, Denver, San Francisco, Canada, and as far away as Australia. The CDC reported that oral-anal acts ("rimming" etc.,) were the main means of spread. Data from the NYC Health Department revealed that the annual number of reported hepatitis A cases among homosexuals between 1989 and 1991 jumped a staggering 400%; a four-fold increase in hepatitis A was also reported in Montreal.[42]

Hepatitis A is highly contagious and readily transmitted by person-to-person contact.[43] Food handlers with infectious hepatitis A can expose vast numbers of people.

10,000 PEOPLE EXPOSED
THROUGH THREE FOOD HANDLERS

The Centers for Disease Control (CDC) statistics show that *the incidence of hepatitis A has been rising in several western states as well as Pennsylvania and Maryland.*

In February 1990, *the discovery of hepatitis A in three food handlers* prompted city and state health officials to offer mass immunization to residents of several counties in Eastern Pennsylvania. . . .

Over a four-week period, combined efforts resulted in *approximately 10,000 people* receiving immune serum globulin (IgG). . . .

This was *one of several infectious disease emergencies* the community has faced in the recent past. Recognizing that *future incidents of this type are likely to occur,* one 435-bed community hospital devised an infectious disease emergency policy that allows for rapid deployment of personnel and services in event of an infectious disease outbreak.[44]

In addition to the danger to public health, the cost of coping with hepatitis A can be expensive for businesses with infectious carriers. The Worthington Hotel in Ft. Worth, Texas received close to 700 bills for injections to help prevent or lessen the severity of hepatitis A after a food handler in the banquet kitchens was confirmed to have the disease. Anyone who ate one of the 11,000 meals served through the hotel's banquet service over a two-week period could have been exposed to the virus.[45]

British researchers report that, "saliva is a convenient and satisfactory alternative to serum for the diagnosis of hepatitis A infection." If and when it becomes widely available, a saliva test for hepatitis A might be used to periodically screen food handlers to help prevent transmission of the disease to patrons.[46]

HEPATITIS C: "A SLEEPING GIANT"

Hepatitis C virus (HCV): This newly discovered virus is thought to be the main cause of bloodborne non-A, non-B hepatitis.[47] Infection with hepatitis C can have grave long-term consequences. People who contract hepatitis C through a blood transfusion have a 50% likelihood of developing chronic hepatitis, which can lead to fatal cirrhosis.[48] Women who contract hepatitis C during pregnancy are particularly vulnerable to developing fatal liver failure.[49] There is no vaccine to prevent the development of non-A, non-B hepatitis.

Infection with non-A, non-B hepatitis is a major problem for blood transfusion recipients and hemodialysis patients; a screening test for hepatitis C is likely to help reduce, but not entirely prevent, the incidence. Presently one antibody, anti-HCV, is detectable and appears only weeks to months after infection or onset of the disease.[50]

Dr. Joseph Feldschuh states:

Receiving foreign [other than one's own] blood from several anonymous sources—the average transfusion consists of 5.4 components—poses manifold risks to the human body. . . .

*Approximately one out of every ten individuals who receives a blood trans-
fusion will contract hepatitis. . . .*

The overwhelming majority of transfusion-associated hepatitis cases – 90
percent, or about a quarter of a million people in the United States each
year – become infected with non-A, non-B hepatitis from a blood transfusion.

Cirrhosis is a chronic liver disease that is irreversible. It occurs in 15 percent of non-A, non-B cases. . . .

Death from cirrhosis of the liver is a painful, wasting condition. The individual loses weight because he becomes unable to eat and digest his food.
The body becomes progressively yellow and the abdomen swollen with fluid
as the victim shrinks down and consumes his own muscles. Such a person in
effect, dies from starvation, despite the presence of food.

. . . The new Chiron test only detects one of the viruses that causes
hepatitis non-A, non-B, a virus tentatively called virus "C." There are many
viruses that attack the liver – remember that hepatitis non-A, non-B refers to
an unknown number of multiple organisms – and it remains to be seen
whether this new, previously unidentified virus "C" is the cause of a significant amount of non-A, non-B hepatitis . . . *as of today the nation's blood
supply remains dangerously threatened by hepatitis.*[51]

There is a significant incidence of hepatitis C among HIV-infected drug abusers and homosexuals. A high percentage (>70%)
of HIV-infected drug abusers in New York are co-infected with
hepatitis C.[52] Forty-one percent of male homosexuals presenting to
an inner city emergency department in Baltimore had markers for
hepatitis C.[53] German physicians report that 33% of HIV positive
homosexuals have evidence of infection with hepatitis C.[54]

Hepatitis non-A, non-B has been increasingly problematic
among homosexuals, drug abusers and AIDS patients.[55]

Researchers from Australia have reported that 62% of intravenous drug abusers and 34% of male homosexuals attending
bathhouses are carriers of hepatitis C.[56]

AIDS INCREASES THE INFECTIVITY OF HEPATITIS C

Hepatitis C can be transmitted through heterosexual relations.[57]
The frequency of HCV transmission to sexual partners is 500%
higher when HIV is also transmitted, suggesting that *the immune
deficiency caused by HIV can enhance the infectivity of hepatitis C.*[58]

Types of non-A, non-B hepatitis can be transmitted by contaminated food and water.[59]

Non-A, non-B hepatitis can also be transmitted by person-to-
person contact apart from sexual relations or drug abuse.[60]

An article in the *American Journal of Medicine* refers to hepatitis
C as a "sleeping giant:"

In the United States, non-A, non-B hepatitis accounts for 20-40% of acute
viral hepatitis. Although it has traditionally been considered a transfusion-
associated disease, non-A, non-B hepatitis is more likely to occur outside the

transfusion setting. Surveillance data from the Centers for Disease Control show that in 1988 . . . 40% OF PATIENTS WITH NON-A, NON-B HEPATITIS HAD NO KNOWN SOURCE OF EXPOSURE.[61]

Hepatitis C cases involving "no known source of exposure" involved people who did not use injectable drugs, did not have household exposure to someone with the disease, did not have sexual exposure to multiple partners, were not involved in medical or dental employment involving frequent blood contact. They contracted the disease through some means other than defined risk behaviors, most likely through person-to-person contact with infectious carriers or through contaminated food.[62]

HIV-related immune deficiency can facilitate active replication and transmission of hepatitis C, indicating that HIV carriers with hepatitis C can more readily transmit the disease to others.[63]

HEPATITIS C FOUND IN DENTISTS

Hepatitis C has appeared among dentists treating AIDS patients and HIV high risk group members. In addition to occupational exposure to blood, studies suggest that exposure to saliva and possibly other body fluids could contribute to the risk of transmission.[64]

KAPOSI'S SARCOMA: HAZARDOUS TO PUBLIC HEALTH

Kaposi's sarcoma (KS) is an invasive vascular cancer frequently seen among homosexual AIDS patients. The cancer causes unsightly purplish-brown spots on the face, neck, armpits, eyes, mouth, torso, arms, legs and around the genital area.[65] KS tumors can develop in the lungs, lymph nodes, liver, stomach, spleen and intestines.

KS has also been seen in homosexual patients not infected with the AIDS virus, indicating that *another infectious agent apart from HIV has a critical role in the development of Kaposi's sarcoma.*[66]

British researchers have uncovered substantial evidence that the agent for Kaposi's sarcoma is spread by homosexual practices involving the consumption of excrement:

> Our findings show that sexual practices in which there is substantial contact with faeces are the main determinants of Kaposi's sarcoma risk in homosexual or bisexual men with AIDS. The association between Kaposi's sarcoma and insertive rimming [analingus] was especially strong; THIS PRACTICE, more than any other activity, WOULD FACILITATE THE DIRECT ORAL TRANSMISSION OF AN INFECTIOUS AGENT.[67]

Insertive "fisting," a common homosexual practice in which the fist and forearm are shoved through the rectum into the colon, has also been cited as a risk factor for Kaposi's sarcoma.[68]

Researchers from the United States Centers for Disease Control have confirmed the link between acts involving fecal contamination and Kaposi's sarcoma. They requestioned homosexual or bisexual men with AIDS:

> The physicians asked, "Considering all the episodes of sexual contact with male partners during the past year [before onset of symptoms associated with AIDS], about what percentage of these episodes involved putting your tongue in your partner's rectum? Similarly phrased questions addressed how often the patient had put his fist or penis in a partner's rectum in the previous year.

They reported their data, "are consistent with the hypothesis that KS is caused by an agent that may be transmitted via fecal-oral contact."[69]

KS TRANSMISSION THROUGH "INADEQUATE HYGIENE"

These findings have several important implications. The agent for KS is distinct from HIV and is sexually transmitted. Human excrement should be properly disposed of rather than ingested. Transmission of the agent for KS may not be limited to deviant sexual practices:

> That sexual practices in which there is contact with faeces is the main determinant of Kaposi's sarcoma risk in homosexual men with AIDS does not imply that the same is true for others with AIDS-related Kaposi's sarcoma. NON-SEXUAL FAECAL CONTACT–FOR EXAMPLE, THAT ASSOCIATED WITH INADEQUATE SANITATION–MIGHT BE AN IMPORTANT MEANS OF TRANSMISSION OF THE AGENT....
> THE POSSIBILITY THAT THE AGENT OF KAPOSI'S SARCOMA MIGHT BE TRANSMITTED BY BLOOD PRODUCTS ALSO NEEDS TO BE CONSIDERED....
> Our results suggest that the agent of Kaposi's sarcoma is a microorganism that is transmitted primarily by contact with faeces.[70]

The reality that "inadequate hygiene" can be an "important means" of KS transmission is disconcerting. Hepatitis A is readily transmitted by infectious food handlers via minute amounts of contaminated fecal particles on their fingers and hands. Individuals who carry the agent for KS are likely to be excreting it in their stool and possibly other body fluids, thereby creating the potential for non-sexual transmission through "inadequate sanitation."

Furthermore, HIV itself directly infects the lining of the intestines. Since the fecal material of AIDS patients can be laced with bloody discharge, human excrement must be considered an "other body fluid" infectious for HIV disease as well as Kaposi's sarcoma.

BLOOD SUPPLY ENDANGERED
Homosexual males who test negative for HIV antibodies may be carriers of the KS agent and could transmit the deadly disease through donating blood. It is medically imperative that all homosexual males—including those who are not infected with HIV—be prohibited from donating blood because of their risk of transmitting Kaposi's sarcoma and other infections.

HEPATITIS B (HBV)
Hepatitis B virus infection (HBV) is a major cause of acute and chronic hepatitis, cirrhosis and liver cancer. Hepatitis B infection reached pandemic proportions among male homosexuals for years prior to the AIDS epidemic. The high rate of HBV provided a clarion early warning sign of the dangers associated with homosexual conduct.[71]

Studies show that between 50 and 75 percent of homosexual males have or have had hepatitis B and at least 5 to 10 percent are chronic carriers. This rate is 50 to 100 times higher than the national average of 0.1 percent.[72] A prodigious 90% of male homosexuals demonstrate chronic or recurrent viral infections with herpesvirus, cytomegalovirus (CMV) and hepatitis B.[73] "In the United States, homosexual men have a higher prevalence of hepatitis B infection than any other group."[74]

Intravenous drug abusers also have a high rate of hepatitis B.

HOUSEHOLD CONTACTS AT HIGH RISK
Hepatitis B infection is not limited to homosexuals and IV drug abusers. Transmission of hepatitis B occurs through heterosexual relations and person-to-person contact. The CDC reports:

> HBV infection can occur in settings of continuous close personal contact such as in households. . . . HOUSEHOLD CONTACTS ARE AT HIGH RISK of acquiring HBV infection.[75]

QUESTIONS ABOUT THE HEPATITIS B VACCINE
A vaccine against hepatitis B has been developed. The earlier version of the vaccine was derived from plasma and acceptance of the vaccine had been hindered by the fear of possible AIDS transmission. The new form of the vaccine is derived from recombinant yeast cells, "No human or animal plasma or other blood derivative is used in the preparation of recombinant HB vaccine."[76]

The CDC recommends that health care and dental workers at risk receive hepatitis B vaccine.[77] While not diminishing the critical importance of the HB vaccine in disease prevention, uncertainties about the long-term protective efficacy of the vaccine remain.

Although most people receiving HB vaccine develop protective antibodies, as many 5%-7.5% do not.[78] The incidence of non-response is increased in persons age 40 and above.[79] Obesity, regardless of age also increases the risk of being a non-responder.[80] In addition, the level of protective antibodies drops rapidly in the years following vaccination. Physicians from Duke University Medical Center in North Carolina report:

> Twenty-five percent of our [hepatitis B] vaccine recipients had subprotective levels [within] two years after their last vaccine dose, and *this proportion increased to over 60% after three and a half years.*[81]

Further research is needed to determine whether the marked drop in protective antibody levels results in an increased risk of acquiring HBV disease.[82] The efficacy and long range health implications of repeated HBV vaccine booster shots have not yet been established.

HEPATITIS B REACTIVATED DURING AIDS

Researchers from the National Cancer Institute have found evidence of hepatitis B in 84% of intravenous drug abusers and 82% of homosexual/bisexual males with HIV disease.[83] Chronic hepatitis is more severe in homosexual males with HIV disease.[84]

The markers of HBV active replication are present at a significantly higher degree in patients with HIV disease.[85] HIV affects the immune response to hepatitis B virus infection and may prolong HBV replication.[86]

Hepatitis B virus has reappeared in individuals with HIV who previously had hepatitis B antibodies.[87]

Response to hepatitis B vaccine is seriously impaired in individuals infected with HIV disease leaving them vulnerable to acquiring the disease.[88]

HEPATITIS B MORE CONTAGIOUS DURING AIDS

Australian public health officials have reported that in individuals with HIV disease,

> . . . *GREATER VIRAL REPLICATION MAY MAKE IT [HBV] MORE CONTAGIOUS* and resistant to antiviral therapy.[89]

The fact that hepatitis B can become "more contagious" during the course of HIV disease indicates that *the household members and other close personal contacts of AIDS carriers with active HBV infection are at very high risk of contracting hepatitis B infection.*

Hepatitis B virus is shed in all body fluids by individuals with acute or chronic infection and by asymptomatic carriers. Infection with hepatitis B is a prime occupational hazard for health care and dental workers. The sexual contacts of hepatitis B carriers are also at risk of acquiring the disease.

HEPATITIS B VIRUS IS VERY HARDY

Similar to HIV, hepatitis B is an extremely tough virus which remains infective outside the body after drying and storage at 77 degrees Fahrenheit for one week.[90] Environmental surfaces in clinical laboratories are frequently (34%) positive for HBsAg.[91] HBV has proven very resistant to most commonly used disinfectant agents.[92] A study in the *Journal of the American Medical Association* reported that contaminated file cards have been implicated in the transmission of hepatitis B.[93]

Hepatitis B has been transmitted through human bites, indicating that saliva can be infectious.[94]

HEPATITIS B SPREAD BY PERSON-TO-PERSON CONTACT

At least 30% of patients with hepatitis B cannot be associated with an identifiable risk factor.[95] This high rate of hepatitis B – almost one out of three cases – among persons with no known risk factors indicates that person-to-person spread is a major means of transmission. The incidence of hepatitis B rose significantly during the 1980s and currently 300,000 cases of the disease are reported annually in the United States. Approximately 100,000 of these cases occur in people who were unknowingly exposed to hepatitis B carriers.[96]

MYCOBACTERIUM AVIUM INTRACELLULARE

Organisms of *Mycobacterium avium intracellulare* (MAI) cause pulmonary disease in humans and are frequently encountered among AIDS patients. Virulent forms of MAI have been cited in the course of AIDS, according to researchers from the National Jewish Center for Immunology and Respiratory Medicine, Denver, Colorado.[97] This illness can also be transmitted to healthy individuals without HIV disease. Inhalation of infectious aerosols (through breathing) is the major route of transmission. [98]

MANY AIDS CARRIERS CARRY HTLV-1 AND HTLV-2

Many individuals with HIV disease have now been found to be carrying other types of viruses which cause paralysis and leukemia.[99] Studies involving the families of HTLV-1 carriers indicate:

... sexual, maternal-child, and/or *close family contact* as routes of transmission.[100]

DEADLY NEW MICROBES ISOLATED IN AIDS PATIENTS

Researchers from the Armed Forces Institute of Pathology and the National Institutes of Health have isolated a newly identified pathogen which was labeled a "Virus-Like Infectious Agent" (VLIA-sb51) from an AIDS patient. Four monkeys were inoculated with VLIA-sb51. None of the monkeys developed opportunistic disease but all four developed wasting syndromes and died within 7-9 months.[101] A high prevalence of infection (52%) with the previously unrecognized microbe has been detected in the blood of patients with AIDS.[102]

It has been suggested that an AIDS associated infection is related to the concurrent epidemic of chronic fatigue syndrome. Victims of chronic fatigue syndrome suffer profound exhaustion and swollen lymph glands. The syndrome seems to be transmitted like the common cold – by coughing, sneezing, household contact – and patients have transmitted the disease to household members.

> More than a hundred physicians and 3,000 nurses have come down with the illness; almost all of them have treated AIDS patients. Many of them are concerned that AIDS patients are spreading the mysterious illness.[103]

New forms of retroviruses have been isolated which have been derived from the lymphoma tissue of AIDS patients in the United States.[104]

CMV RISK TO PREGNANT WOMEN

> It clearly would be wise to keep certain personnel ... such as immunosuppressed or pregnant individuals from working with AIDS patients. ... Pregnant women should also avoid contact with AIDS patients because of the risk of infection with cytomegalovirus as well as the risk of AIDS itself.
> – Dr. Sidney Finegold, President of the Infectious Disease Society of America[105]

Cytomegalovirus (CMV) is a viral infection which can infect the unborn baby via the placenta. CMV has been implicated in several thousand cases of congenital birth defects annually in the United States.[106]

> An average of 30,000 CMV-infected infants are born annually in the United States. ... Of the infected infants, 10 percent have severe multiple organ system disease which damages the brain, perceptual organs, lungs, liver and blood; in a few instances it results in death soon after delivery. In the survivors, severe debilitating brain damage, blindness, and deafness are common.[107]

Cytomegalovirus is a member of the herpes virus group. It is transmitted through semen, urine, blood and saliva. A high percentage of homosexual males and AIDS patients shed CMV. Ninety percent (90%) of practicing homosexual males demonstrate chronic or recurrent infection with herpesvirus, cytomegalovirus (CMV) and hepatitis B.[108]

The severe birth defects which can result when CMV is contracted during pregnancy make it imperative for women who are or suspect they are pregnant to avoid close contact with AIDS carriers.

PNEUMOCOCCAL PNEUMONIA

Pneumococcal pneumonia is a bacterial infection of the lungs caused by *Streptococcus pneumoniae* which occurs with increased frequency among HIV carriers. The illness is usually characterized by sudden onset, high fever, shaking chills, pleuritic chest pains and *a racking cough that raises thick blood-stained sputum.*

Among AIDS patients treated at the Memorial Sloan-Kettering Cancer Center in New York City, physicians have found a 600% higher incidence of pneumococcal pneumonia than in the general population.[109]

Other researchers have found that homosexual males at high risk of HIV disease have weakened resistance to pneumonias due to *S. Pneumoniae* or *H. influenzae*.[110]

There is a marked increased in the incidence of bacterial pneumonia associated with HIV disease in drug abusers, including those who have not reached end-stage AIDS.[111]

SPUTUM TINGED WITH HIV-CONTAMINATED BLOOD

Cough occurs in more than 90% of patients with pneumococcal pneumonia. It may be dry at first, but soon the patient begins to raise sputum *which is blood-tinged or bloody* in about 75% of the cases. *The blood is usually well mixed throughout the sputum* rather than streaked on the surface, because bleeding occurs directly into the exudate from the alveoli (the tiny "air sacs" in the lungs). This gives the sputum a characteristic "rusty" or "prune juice" appearance. Chest pain is common and frequently severe.

The overall case fatality rate for untreated pneumococcal pneumonia is about 25% (1 out of 4). Treatment with penicillin has reduced the overall mortality to about 5% (1 out of 20). In elderly patients with chronic heart or lung disease the fatality rate approaches 50%. Persons contracting *the disease in old age or infancy, who are in advanced stages of pregnancy, or who have a delay in treatment are also at increased risk of severe, life threatening complications, even with penicillin treatment and intensive care.* If the bacteria enters the blood stream, the mortality is between 30%-76% even with the most intensive modern medical care.[112]

In addition, there are virulent strains of pneumococcal pneumonia which are resistant to treatment with antibiotics.[113] A pneumococcal vaccine against various types of *S. pneumoniae* has been developed but not all vaccinated persons will produce protective levels of antibody, and infections caused by types contained in the vaccine have occurred after vaccination.[114]

Pneumococcal pneumonia *is spread by the inhalation of infectious respiratory secretions coughed into the air.* Carriers of HIV disease with this type of pneumonia will cough sputum imbued with HIV-contaminated blood into the air. Sputum contaminated with HIV-contaminated blood should be considered infectious.

Inhalation of sputum or spray containing HIV-infective blood particles cannot be considered a particularly healthful event.

According to the U.S. Centers for Disease Control (CDC):

> . . . the skin (especially when scratches, cuts, abrasions, dermatitis or other lesions are present) and *mucous membranes of the eye, nose, mouth,* and possibly *the respiratory tract should be considered as potential pathways for entry of [HIV] virus.*[115]

SUMMARY
AIDS-RELATED SECONDARY ILLNESSES POSE SERIOUS HEALTH HAZARDS

AIDS high risk group members and individuals with HIV disease are frequently beset with other infectious conditions which are readily spread by person-to-person contact.

Employers should be allowed to take these contagious illnesses into account with regards to AIDS-infected employees who have direct or indirect contact with the public. For example, AIDS-infected medical workers are at heightened risk of acquiring infections from patients. They are also at risk of transmitting HIV-related illnesses to the patients they are treating. AIDS-infected cooks and food handlers are susceptible to a variety of harmful secondary infections which can be transmitted through food.

Private businesses, now redefined as "public accommodations" under the American with Disabilities Act, should be permitted to consider the serious secondary health hazards associated with AIDS with respect to infectious customers, patients and visitors.

CHAPTER SIX

AIDS AND INSECTS

However secure and well-regulated civilized life may become, bacteria, protozoa, viruses, infected fleas, lice, ticks, mosquitoes and bedbugs will always lurk in the shadows ready to pounce when neglect, poverty, famine or war lets down the defenses.
– Dr. Hans Zinsser, *Rats, Lice and History*[1]

Several years ago, leading scientific experts from the Los Alamos Research Laboratory in New Mexico warned:

> HIV may become capable of infecting an even wider variety of cell types . . . and may become pathogenic [able to cause disease] more rapidly . . . *different modes of transmission may arise: insect vectors*, colostrum [early breast milk], *or respiratory aerosols* [through breathing], for example. HIV may develop resistance to AZT and future antiviral drugs. Tests for the presence of HIV may not detect newly evolved variants.[2]

Studies have since confirmed most of the researchers' concerns. It is now known that HIV has the ability to infect a broad spectrum of cells. AIDS is transmissible through breast milk. HIV has developed resistance to AZT and other anti-viral drugs.[3] Numbers of people have developed AIDS but repeatedly test negative for the AIDS virus on the most sensitive DNA tests.[4]

Given their accuracy in predicting other disturbing facets of AIDS, the scientists' concern regarding HIV transmission through insects merits serious consideration.

INSECT TRANSMISSION OF HEPATITIS B

Hepatitis B and AIDS have very similar modes of spread. There is compelling evidence that mosquitoes play an important role in the transmission of hepatitis B in the tropical regions of South America, Africa and Asia.[5] Mosquitoes have also been implicated in the transmission of hepatitis B in a non-tropical urban area of the United States.

Researchers from the New Jersey Medical School have presented a study in the *Journal of the American Medical Association* supporting the role of mosquitoes in an epidemic of hepatitis:

> Persons who resided in a high population density area developed a long-incubation type of hepatitis following a period of unusually heavy mosquito

infestation, in which *each patient received multiple mosquito bites three months earlier*. There was no history of drug addiction, contact with jaundiced individuals, receipt of injections, or ingestion of shellfish. . . .

A high frequency of sporadic cases of viral hepatitis in New Jersey, where there is a continuing problem with mosquito infestation, led us to resume our studies of mosquitoes and viral hepatitis.

Infected Pools of Mosquitoes

Two hundred fifty-one pools of mosquitoes were caught in 15 separate trap sites in parks of Essex County, New Jersey, and examined for the presence of hepatitis B (HB Ag). *Ten of the pools were HB Ag-positive.* These were found at trap sites in parks adjacent to areas of high population density and low economic level, after periods of crowding over a weekend. . . .

Squashing Mosquitoes Could Spread Infection

Mosquitoes caught in areas with a high frequency of hepatitis B antigenemia are expected to be antigen-positive from both tropical and non-tropical experiences. . . . *This could contribute to the dissemination of hepatitis if feeding is interrupted and the mosquito is squashed by a second non-infected victim.* . . . If amplification of the infective agent occurs in mosquitoes, the risk of transmission of viral hepatitis by this means could be increased.

The researchers conclude:

Our observations indicate THAT MOSQUITOES, IF ABUNDANT, MAY PLAY A ROLE IN THE SPREAD OF VIRAL HEPATITIS AND IN THE HIGH INCIDENCE OF THIS DISEASE.

. . . *[L]ocal outbreaks of hepatitis of the type that initiated our interest in this matter make it desirable to consider this as a potential route for dissemination of this disease.* Moreover, the finding of HB Ab-positive mosquitoes in traps in or adjacent to parks following weekends of crowds EMPHASIZES THE NEED TO FOCUS FURTHER ATTENTION ON CONTROL OF MOSQUITOES TO PREVENT THE SPREAD OF DISEASE IN AN URBAN SETTING.[6]

BEDBUGS: MORE DANGEROUS THAN MOSQUITOES?

Bedbugs have been implicated as a blood-sucking vector of hepatitis B. The medical journal *Gastroenterology* presented a study which found:

. . . in the bedbug, HBsAg remained detectable throughout a 5-week testing period. Moreover, titers rose during the last week, when blood meal digestion was complete, *suggesting possible replication of the antigen.*

. . . juvenile bedbugs fed HBsAg when in the fourth or fifth week instar stage still contained antigen after molting. These studies suggest that BEDBUGS MAY POTENTIALLY BE A MORE DANGEROUS SOURCE OF HEPATITIS B TRANSMISSION THAN MOSQUITOES.[7]

The British medical journal *Lancet* has reported a study by leading South African virologists in which bedbugs were allowed to feed on HIV-contaminated blood:

> The known routes of transmission of AIDS are also common to those of hepatitis B virus, with which HIV shares several epidemiological features. *There is strong evidence for mechanical transmission of hepatitis B virus by the common bedbug. Similar transmission of HIV by bedbugs may be a cause of infection in African children.* . . .
> The survival of HIV for one hour in the common bedbug following the feed on a blood-virus mixture suggests that *mechanical transmission of the [AIDS] virus between human beings could be carried out by bedbugs.*[8]

HIV FOUND IN MANY SPECIES OF INSECTS

Researchers from the Pasteur Institute's Viral Oncology Unit in Paris have reported:

> We have studied THE PRESENCE OF HIV-RELATED SEQUENCES IN MORE THAN 200 INSECTS from endemic areas for AIDS in Central Africa. . . . Viral sequences have been found among insects from urban or suburban areas, directly or indirectly in contact with humans. POSITIVE INSECTS INCLUDED MOSQUITOES, ANTLIONS, TSETSE FLIES, COCKROACHES, TICKS AND BEDBUGS. Squash blot analysis indicated that UP TO 30% OF MOSQUITOES FROM ENDEMIC AREAS CONTAINED SUCH VIRAL SEQUENCES. Studies on mosquitoes also suggested a transovarian transmission of the viral genes since positive results were observed in both males and females.[9]

Although denying that the insects were a vector, researchers from the Pasteur Institute and the Laboratory of Molecular Virology, University of Paris, presented another study two years later:

> Screening of *MORE THAN 5,000 INSECTS* captured in Central Africa has revealed . . . the presence of HIV-1 related sequences in the DNA of insects belonging to NUMEROUS SPECIES.[10]

It may beg the question, but if there really is no concern over insect-borne transmission of HIV, why did researchers from the one of the world's premier virology institutes expend the time, finances and meticulous effort needed to screen and analyze 5,000 insects? This type of intense effort implies more than a passing interest in HIV and entomology.

These studies indicate that certain areas with a high incidence of AIDS are swarming with "numerous species" of insects carrying HIV-1 sequences in their DNA.

According to scientists from the Virology Section, Department of Microbiology, Middlesex Hospital Medical School in London and elsewhere, in Africa the AIDS virus "appears to be transmitted through heterosexual contact or exposure to blood through *insect bites.* . . ."[11]

TICKS, SAND FLIES AND KISSING BUGS
Dr. Ricardo Veronesi, Professor of Infectious Disease at the University of São Paulo, Brazil, and President of the Brazilian Society of Infectious Disease, is certain that insects are a vector of HIV:

> Mosquitoes may not be involved in AIDS transmission now in Brazil, but *I am absolutely convinced that they will be within a few years.* I worry about ticks, sand flies and kissing bugs. *I AM ONE HUNDRED PERCENT CONVINCED THAT MOSQUITOES OR SOME OTHER INSECTS ARE INVOLVED IN AFRICA,* although certainly they are not the primary mode of transmission.[12]

NATURE'S FLYING HYPODERMIC NEEDLES
Dr. Max Klinghoffer, M.D., President of the American Civil Defense Association, writes:

> Mosquitoes do transmit malaria; dengue fever; filariasis (sometimes called elephantiasis); yellow fever; and many types of encephalitis. Why is there such certainty that the mosquito (or other biting or stinging insect) cannot carry the AIDS virus? When the mosquito inserts her mouth parts into her victim (the "mosquito bite," or "sting") she injects some of her saliva in order to keep the blood fluid. She then drinks her meal. But if her victim brushes her away before she finishes her meal, and if she then completes her feast on another victim, why would it not be possible to transmit the virus from the first to the second victim?
>
> There are recorded cases of medical personnel becoming HIV positive following an accidental needlestick. *The mosquito might be described as nature's hypodermic needle.* It is premature to arbitrarily state that stinging and biting insects cannot spread AIDS.[13]

Tropical disease specialists Mark Whiteside, M.D., and Caroline MacLeod, M.D., direct the Institute of Tropical Medicine in Miami, Florida. The physicians have carefully evaluated the high rate of AIDS in Belle Glade, Florida, and other areas and maintain that insects can be a significant vector of AIDS.[14]

AIDS AND LICE
The AIDS virus may also be transmitted by insect vectors such as mosquitoes, bedbugs, or lice.
– African and British AIDS researchers[15]

Lice are tiny blood-sucking insects that thrive on the body of the human host. Infestation with lice is called pediculosis. Lice are vectors of typhus, a virulent infectious disease. Lice acquire the typhus organisms through feeding on the blood of an infected human (murine typhus is spread from rats to humans by fleas). The organisms multiply in the gut of the louse. The lice pass feces saturated with typhus bacilli (*R. prowazekii*). Infection occurs when the human host scratches the affected area of the bite and the feces enter the skin. Fecal particles excreted from the lice can dry out and become airborne. When clothes contaminated with lice and feces are shaken out an infectious aerosol is created. When inhaled, the infectious organisms penetrate cells in the mucous membranes. Nurses and other medical personnel are at risk of inhaling airborne particles when they handle or remove clothing from a patient.[16]

Deborah Altschuler of the National Pediculosis Association has expressed concern that lice may also be able to transmit the AIDS virus.[17] Dr. David Taplin, a microbiologist and professor of dermatology at the University of Miami, is director of the University's field epidemiology research team. He performs clinical trials for pharmaceutical companies and spends several months a year in the tropics conducting research and testing delousing products. Dr. Taplin will not conduct any experiments with insects in a clinic setting with patients.

"I wouldn't want to be working with an obligate blood-sucking parasite and an AIDS patient and wake up one morning to find the louse sucking on my neck. You want about a Class 100 security–sterile lab, complete isolation–to even consider such tests," he says. But he thinks the tests should be done. . . . Lice feed six or seven times a day–steadily sipping [on blood]. *A louse can move from one head to another within minutes and resume feeding.*

"A lot of energy is going into AIDS research with flying insects, which is fine," Taplin says. "But *just as much work should be going into research on an arthropod that lives in human skin–and on human skin alone–and that will move from one person to another* when that first person throws a fever." Moreover, as the louse feeds, it immediately excretes the meal in blood form on the host, and Taplin thinks it is a fair question whether virus might persist in that blood as it dries.[18]

AIDS AND FLEAS

Dr. William T. O'Connor has expressed concern that fleas might be a vector of HIV transmission:

In the same realm of concern is the possibility that *fleas could carry and transmit the virus via their mouth parts.* Bedbugs have been shown to carry active AIDS virus on their mouth parts for at least one hour. In light of that, a valid preventative recommendation would be not caring for the flea-bearing animals of AIDS virus carriers. *One recalls that the greatest plague known to man [bubonic plague] was spread by fleas.*

Certain species of fleas prefer to live on humans and jump on other people to take blood meals. . . .

Be especially careful about letting your children contact other children who may have lice or fleas. These are blood-sucking creatures and their mouth parts must be assumed to be contaminated with blood-borne pathogens and capable of transmitting disease.

Cockroaches are known to carry up to 29 species of bacteria, 4 unspecified strains of poliomyelitis virus, 2 fungi, 2 protozoans and the eggs of 7 helminths (worms) all known to be disease producing in humans.[19]

MEDICAL WORKERS CONTRACT SCABIES

The scabies (Latin, *scabere*, scratch) mite has four pairs of legs and infests humans by burrowing into the skin. Since the mite reproduces on humans it can maintain a continuous infestation. Fertile female mites make tiny tunnels into the skin and lay eggs as they dig in. Scabies offspring move out to the surface and enter hair follicles. Scabies infest the skin. Common sites include the sides of the fingers, the skin in between the bottom of the fingers, the wrists, elbows, skin around the nipples, genitals, abdomen, thighs and buttocks.[20]

Scabies is highly contagious and is transmitted through skin contact with an infested individual (including shaking hands) or by touching clothing recently worn by a carrier.

Patients with AIDS are susceptible to a severe infestation with scabies, a condition called crusted scabies (it is also called Norwegian scabies but affects patients in any country).

An outbreak of Norwegian scabies occurred among 40 medical workers on a designated AIDS ward in London. The infested medical workers then inadvertently spread the mites to their partners and other close contacts. It was not disclosed if the affected medical workers were tested for AIDS.[21]

Italian researchers suggest Norwegian scabies be considered an "opportunistic infestation" of AIDS patients and urge that stringent precautions be taken to prevent spread of the mites to health care workers.[22]

INSECT TRANSMISSION: NOT TO BE TAKEN LIGHTLY

Arboviruses are viruses which are transmitted by various arthropods (insects) such as mosquitoes, flies, lice, bedbugs and ticks. There are nearly 500 insect-borne viruses and at least 90 of these infect humans.[23] Dr. Robert Shope is the Director of the Yale Arbovirus Research Unit and the pre-eminent arbovirologist in the world. Dr. Shope asserts that the potential for insect transmission of AIDS warrants further investigation:

Insects were known to transmit retroviruses long before AIDS came along. There are retroviruses in horses transmitted by biting flies. *To hypothesize that AIDS might be transmitted by flies or other insects is perfectly logical and within the realm of possibility.* I don't think people should believe it until it is proven, and if it is not proven we should not believe it. But *I think studies should be done. I don't think we can explain all cases of AIDS.*[24]

CHAPTER SEVEN

AIDS AND TB:
A LETHAL COMBINATION

This is an impending public health nightmare; we are heading back to the middle ages. We no longer have the upper hand in the fight against TB. We had a disease that was preventable and curable, which is now being taken over by organisms resistant to prevention and cure.
– Dr. Lee Reichman, President of the American Lung Association[1]

Because TB is transmitted by the airborne route, persons at highest risk for acquiring tuberculosis are "close contacts," e.g., persons who sleep, live, work or otherwise share air with an infectious person through a common ventilation system.
– U.S. Centers for Disease Control(CDC)[2]

The recent emergence of multiple drug-resistant strains of M. tuberculosis among patients with HIV infection and their close contacts is alarming and has serious public health implications.
– Margaret A. Fischl, M.D., University of Miami School of Medicine, commenting on reports indicating that multidrug-resistant tuberculosis is spreading through hospitals in the United States. The resistant strains progress quickly, killing up to 89% of infected patients.[3]

CDC: "TB OUT OF CONTROL IN THE UNITED STATES"
People are obsessed by the possibility of casual transmission of the AIDS virus. I think there should be a real concern about a far more likely possibility: the casual transmission of TB.
– Dr. John Mills, of the University of California, San Francisco, warning that once TB is reactivated, it is highly contagious and can be readily spread through the air.[4]

In an article entitled "HIV and Tuberculosis – An Old Plague Returns with Added Fury," Dixie E. Snider, M.D., Director of the Tuberculosis Control Program at the CDC, states:

The re-emergence of TB is . . . secondary to the HIV pandemic. . . . A statistical overlap is developing between HIV-infected and TB-infected [individuals] and there are big troubles ahead.[5]

Individuals with HIV disease are highly susceptible to developing forms of tuberculosis which do not respond to anti-TB drugs. Outbreaks of these deadly strains of tuberculosis are increasing with alarming frequency across the United States.

Particularly dangerous forms of tuberculosis have struck in 13 states, including Texas, and *the spread of the disease is out of control,* federal health officials say.

Strains of the bacterium that are resistant to the standard anti-tuberculosis drugs have caused deadly outbreaks in five states and at least one case in eight other states. The more common form of the infection is also spreading rapidly in many states.

The data were presented at a two-day meeting of health officials and tuberculosis experts from the federal government and 46 states.

"At no time in recent history has tuberculosis been of such great concern as it is now, and legitimately so, because tuberculosis is out of control in this country," said Dr. Dixie Snider, the CDC's top expert on tuberculosis.

Dr. William Roper, head of the CDC, called reports of the disease's spread "very sobering."

. . . Federal health officials say the outbreaks chiefly involve people infected with HIV. . . .

The latest outbreak was at Elmhurst Hospital in the Queens section of New York City, where the drug-resistant form was diagnosed in 13 cases; 11 were fatal. Elmhurst is the fourth hospital in New York state where multiple drug-resistant tuberculosis [MDR-TB] cases have been detected in recent months.

In this outbreak, federal health authorities said *85% of the tuberculosis patients were also infected with HIV.*

But experts said *the disease could be a threat to everyone,* particularly health care workers or others in close contact with people with tuberculosis.[6]

During the Industrial Revolution of the 18th and 19th centuries, tuberculosis was a leading cause of death among young people throughout the world. The disease was known as the White Plague because its victims were left ashen-faced and emaciated. In the United States, cases of TB had steadily declined and the airborne scourge appeared on the verge of being eradicated. Concurrent with the emergence of the AIDS epidemic, the number of new reported cases of TB began escalating.

TB PLAGUE RETURNING WITH A VENGEANCE

In some African cities 80% of the hospital beds are allocated to AIDS patients and at least half of these patients have tuberculosis. Dr. Michael Merson, director of the World Health Organization's (WHO) Global AIDS Programme, told participants at the 6th International Conference on AIDS in Africa, *"TB is a veritable epidemic within the AIDS pandemic."* In addition to Africa, AIDS is spawning a resurgence of tuberculosis in South America and the United States.[7] AIDS-associated TB is burgeoning in Rio de Janeiro, Brazil.[8] Tuberculosis among AIDS patients has shown increasing trends in Mexico.[9]

WHY AIDS INCREASES THE RISK OF TB

Many HIV carriers are also infected with the bacterial parasite (*Mycobacterium tuberculosis*) which causes tuberculosis. HIV disease impairs the immune system and permits dormant TB organisms to break loose and multiply. As the lungs deteriorate, abundant amounts of TB bacilli are brought up in the sputum. Individuals with TB who delay seeking treatment can become highly infectious. "*The organisms multiply and when they cough . . . they're coughing out millions of organisms,*" according to Dr. William Rom, Chief of Pulmonary Medicine at New York's Bellevue Hospital.

Dr. Rom said he recently treated a short-order cook with TB who had lost 70 pounds. "His boss thought he was looking a little thin so he brought him here. The man probably had the active disease for six months or longer and just didn't seek medical attention until it got very advanced. He was certainly exposing others."[10]

Although just beginning to come to light in most of the popular press,[11] AIDS-associated tuberculosis has been on the rise for over a decade.[12]

> Recent reports have described an increase in cases of tuberculosis in several urban centers. To investigate the possible relationship between tuberculosis and the acquired immunodeficiency syndrome (AIDS), we reviewed case records at a New York City hospital between 1978 and 1985. *The yearly rate of tuberculosis more than doubled* during the study period; *this increase was entirely attributable to cases among patients with AIDS or AIDS-related complex* and parenteral drug users, a group at high risk for the development of AIDS. Patients with AIDS and tuberculosis were younger and more frequently men than other patients with tuberculosis, and were more likely to have extrapulmonic disease. *In the majority of patients, tuberculosis occurred prior to confirmation of CDC-defined AIDS.*[13]

HIV carriers with pre-existing TB infection are at high risk of manifesting active tuberculosis. HIV carriers exposed to TB are vulnerable to developing aggressive forms of the disease. According to Donald E. Kopanoff of the CDC's TB Division, "Not only are they going to be highly susceptible to infection, *they are also more likely to progress directly to active disease.* They can't fight it off."[14]

AIDS CARRIERS TEST NEGATIVE ON TB SKIN TEST

Because HIV disease alters the body's immune response, HIV carriers are likely to test negative on the standard TB skin test even when they have active, contagious tuberculosis. This impaired response is known as anergy.[15] The *Journal of the American Medical Association* notes:

> Studies have shown that the standard tests for detection of tuberculosis are unreliable when used in persons infected with HIV.[16]

Among people not infected with HIV, the standard skin test is very useful for diagnosis, although between 5 to 20 percent of those with newly diagnosed cases of TB may have a negative response to the initial test.[17]

HIV carriers are prone to other lung ailments which can mask the presence of TB on a chest x-ray. Physicians from NY Medical College state:

> The frequently atypical chest x-ray and the occurrence of skin test anergy *may mask the diagnosis of pulmonary tuberculosis* in the HIV-infected patient. The lack of early institution of respiratory isolation in these patients may pose an increased risk of transmission of TB to health care workers. A high index of suspicion for TB in HIV-infected patients will be essential in preventing nosocomial [in hospital] outbreaks of TB.[18]

LACK OF MANDATORY TESTING SPURS DRUG RESISTANCE

In many states, doctors cannot test for HIV without the patient's special written permission. Many individuals who carry HIV refuse to be tested.[19] The medical workers treating them are not aware they have HIV disease. Consequently, in HIV carriers with tuberculosis who test negative for TB, treatment is delayed. This delay gives TB organisms more time to multiply and amplifies the spread of the disease to others.

Due to their impaired immunity, patients with HIV disease and tuberculosis require prolonged treatment with a battery of anti-TB drugs. When a physician is not allowed to determine if a TB patient has HIV, the patient may only be put on the standard anti-TB drug regimen. Consequently, the TB organisms are not eradicated and build resistance to drugs.

The super-powerful forms of TB which do not respond to treatment are referred to as multidrug-resistant tuberculosis (MDR-TB). TB which cannot be cured is fatal.

MANY TB PATIENTS ARE NONCOMPLIANT

Another major factor in the acceleration of drug-resistant TB is the refusal of people with TB to undergo appropriate treatment. Many active TB carriers are HIV-infected intravenous drug abusers and mentally troubled vagrants who are unable or unwilling to comply with the disciplined drug regimen required to treat the disease.[20]

Tuberculosis is also a growing problem among AIDS-infected homosexuals. Out of 1452 TB/AIDS patients identified by the New York City Department of Health, 49% were homosexual.[21]

Out of 181 TB patients who were discharged from one hospital in New York City, an overwhelming 96% of the HIV positive patients did not return for follow-up treatment.[22] Without continuous treatment, patients with active tuberculosis are prone to develop drug-resistant strains of the disease. Tuberculosis – including the potent, incurable forms of the disease – can be transmitted to anyone.

Physicians from Harlem Hospital and Columbia University College of Physicians and Surgeons, state:

> . . . poor compliance is a key factor leading to frequent readmission and probably *many secondary cases* [of TB]. . . . *New strategies are needed* to treat patients most likely to have HIV and TB.[23]

The rise of drug-resistant TB among AIDS carriers is a growing international problem.[24]

STANDARD TB CONTROL MEASURES ABANDONED

The "new strategies" necessary for containing the spread of tuberculosis are not exactly novel. In the not-too-distant past, people with contagious tuberculosis who refused to comply with treatment were compulsorily detained. They were quarantined and treated until they no longer posed a health threat to others.

In today's political climate, efforts at quarantining noncompliant patients with tuberculosis have been met with stiff resistance. Civil liberties and AIDS advocacy groups argue that such measures constitute a violation of the civil rights of persons with AIDS/TB.

BLEAK PROSPECT OF TREATMENT

Unlike standard TB, the prognosis for drug-resistant tuberculosis is grim. The cost of treatment is staggering.

An old and curable disease is starting to become incurable again.

The United States is courting disaster unless it expresses renewed concern for tuberculosis, according to one of the nation's leading TB specialists.

*The number of TB cases is on the rise, and many are drug-resistant and
difficult to treat,* said Dr. Michael Iseman of the National Jewish Center for
Immunology and Respiratory Medicine in Denver, Colorado. The cost of
treating patients with multiple-drug resistant TB can run as high as *$250,000
per patient,* and *47% of those treated for MDR-TB at the Center have not re-
sponded to treatment.* "We're seeing young patients *die* of TB when it should
be easily treatable, Iseman said.[25]

HOW TB AFFECTS THE BODY

Tuberculosis is characterized by the formation of small round lesions (tubercles) in the affected organs. Tuberculosis of the lungs
is known as pulmonary tuberculosis. In addition to the lungs, almost every organ and tissue in the body can be involved in tuberculosis: the heart, kidneys, intestines, genital tract, eyes, larynx,
bones, joints, brain and central nervous system.

The usual site of TB's initial onset is the lungs. During active
disease, the lungs are eaten away or "consumed" by the TB parasites. In times past TB was called "consumption."

The deterioration of lung tissue produces caseum (Latin,
"cheese"), a substance with the consistency of soft cheese. Breakdown of the lesion occurs when the caseum is softened and lique-
fied and then expelled through the bronchial system by coughing
and breathing. This process results in the formation of pus-filled
cavities in pulmonary tissue ("holes" in the lungs).

TB CAN BECOME REACTIVATED

TB infection usually begins in the lungs and spreads to the lymph
nodes, then to the blood stream. Thus, disease can occur in any organ of the body. TB organisms which have been seeded in the
lungs may remain dormant for years only to reactivate during a period of lowered immune resistance. Between 5%-40% of people
without HIV disease who are infected with the TB microbe will
develop active disease over time, according to the CDC.[26] Older
persons and infants are especially vulnerable to progressing to life-
threatening disease.[27]

Many conditions are known to increase the risk for the activation of dormant TB. Periods of lowered immune resistance such as
caused by emotional stress, influenza (the "flu"), advancing age,
pneumonia, lung cancer, various types of surgery, dialysis, alcoholism, drug abuse, and other ailments can reactivate dormant lesions and unleash full-blown TB. The weakened immunity caused
by HIV disease is a major cause of reactivated TB.

Reactivated tuberculosis in adults tends to be chronic and is
characterized by the formation of cavities in the lung tissue.

The onset of the disease can be insidious, involving the gradual development of fatigue, weight loss and other symptoms. *Individuals can have active, infectious TB for a substantial period of time in the absence of obvious symptoms.* It is not possible to discern if a person is infectious for TB merely by overt signs of disease.

BLOOD-TINGED SPUTUM

In others, the onset may be acute and involve increasingly productive cough and blood-tinged sputum. Fever and night sweats can also occur. Sputum tinged with HIV-contaminated blood should be considered infectious.

TREATMENT FOR CLASSIC TB

Prior to the development of potent anti-tuberculosis drugs, TB sufferers were frequently confined to sanitariums [Latin, *sanitas,* health, sanity] for therapeutic reasons as well as to help curtail the spread of the disease.

Beginning with the discovery of the antibiotic streptomycin by Selman Abraham Waksman in 1945, major strides were made in conquering the disease. Along with streptomycin, the subsequent introduction of drugs such as isoniazid (1952), ethambutol (1961), rifampin (1966) and pyrazinamide had a dramatic impact on curtailing the incidence of the disease.

As anti-TB drugs became widely used, the growth of TB dropped drastically. TB patients treated with these drugs were rendered non-infectious within a matter of weeks to months and treatment shifted from hospitals to home settings. By the 1960s most TB sanitariums in the United States had been closed.[28]

CONVENTIONAL TB REQUIRES LENGTHY TREATMENT

Because of advances in medical "wonder drugs," tuberculosis came to be viewed as a relatively innocuous relic of years past. Tuberculosis, including the conventional variety, should not be regarded lightly. In individuals who are *not* infected with HIV, treatment for tuberculosis requires *at least six to nine months* of regular drug therapy with some very potent medications. Anti-TB medications can have serious side effects including kidney damage, nerve damage, hepatitis, and vision loss. Streptomycin should not be used to treat pregnant women because it can cause serious nerve damage in their children. Rifampin crosses the placental barrier during pregnancy and may be harmful to the developing infant.

Some experts believe that it only takes about two weeks of effective chemotherapy to render patients noninfectious. Others assert that "the evidence for this is inconclusive, and it is more reasonable to consider a patient with smear-positive sputum to represent a gradually diminishing risk until the smears are negative."[29]

Although in most cases conventional tuberculosis responds to drugs, it remains a very serious, potentially fatal, communicable disease. In persons with HIV disease, tuberculosis is particularly virulent and refractory to treatment.[30]

CONTROVERSIAL TB VACCINE

There is a TB vaccine, consisting of vaccination with bacille Calmette-Guérin (BCG), but its efficacy is controversial.[31] Vaccination with BCG does not prevent transmission of TB infection. A report in the *Reviews of Infectious Diseases* states: "Presently available vaccines have not proven to be reliable in producing resistance [against TB]."[32]

The U.S. Centers for Disease Control states:

BCG vaccination is no longer recommended for health-care workers or other adults at high risk for acquiring TB infection. In addition, BCG should not be given to persons who are immunocompromised, including those with HIV infection. [33]

MULTIDRUG-RESISTANT TB

The AIDS epidemic has fostered the growth of super-powerful strains of tuberculosis which cannot be cured by any known drugs. Studies from across the United States indicate that an alarmingly high percentage of TB cases involve drug-resistant forms of the disease.[34]

Close to fifty percent or more of healthy persons who contract multidrug-resistant TB will succumb to the disease. Among HIV carriers, the mortality rate from drug-resistant TB is even higher.

Medication used to treat MDR-TB can have greater toxic side-effects. The administration of ethionamide, for example, "is accompanied by rather severe gastrointestinal upset and occasionally by hepatitis, and allergic reactions are common." Cycloserine commonly causes aberrations of mental function and seizures.[35]

HOW TUBERCULOSIS IS SPREAD

TB is an infectious disease that is spread from person to person through the air. TB germs are put into the air when a person with TB of the lungs coughs, sneezes, laughs or sings.
– CDC, *The Connection Between TB and HIV*[36]

Pulmonary tuberculosis is a classic example of a contagious disease spread by the airborne route. TB infection is acquired by breathing in air that has been contaminated with microscopic TB organisms by a person with active disease.

In the medical textbook, *The Pathogenesis of Infectious Diseases,*
Dr. Cedric Mims states:

Respiratory Tract Infections
   In infections transmitted by the respiratory route, shedding [giving off of
infectious organisms] depends on the production of airborne particles
[aerosols] containing microorganisms. *These are produced to some extent in
the larynx, mouth, and throat during speech [talking] and normal breathing . . .*
more pathogenic [disease-causing] streptococci, meningococci and other
microorganisms are also spread in this way, especially when people are
crowded together inside buildings or vehicles. There is particularly good
aerosol formation during singing and it is always dangerous to sing in a choir
with patients suffering from pulmonary tuberculosis.
   Tubercle bacilli in the lungs that are carried up to the back of the throat
are mostly swallowed and can be detected in stomach washings, but a cough
will project bacteria in the air.
   Efficient shedding from the nasal cavity [nose] depends on an increase in
nasal secretions and on the induction of sneezing. IN A SNEEZE, UP TO
20,000 DROPLETS ARE PRODUCED and during the common cold, for
instance, many of them will contain virus particles. The largest (1mm diameter) fall to the ground after traveling 15 feet or so and the smaller ones
evaporate rapidly, depending on their velocity, water content and on the relative humidity. Many have disappeared within a few feet and the rest, including those containing microorganisms, then settle according to size. *The
smallest, although they fall theoretically at 1-3 feet per hour, in fact stay sus-
pended indefinitely because air is never quite still. Particles of this size are
likely to pass the turbinate baffles and reach the lower respiratory tract.*
   IF THE MICROORGANISMS ARE HARDY, AS IN THE CASE OF
THE TUBERCLE BACILLUS AND SMALLPOX VIRUS, PEOPLE
COMING INTO THE ROOM LATER ON CAN BE INFECTED.[37]

In a report citing the relationship between HIV disease and the
rising incidence of tuberculosis, the U.S. Centers for Disease Control (CDC) warns:

Because TB is transmitted by the airborne route [coughing, sneezing,
breathing], persons at highest risk for acquiring tuberculosis are "close contacts," e.g., persons who sleep, LIVE, WORK, OR OTHERWISE *SHARE
AIR* WITH AN INFECTIOUS PERSON THROUGH A COMMON
VENTILATION SYSTEM.[38]

Drug-resistant forms of tuberculosis are spread in the same
manner as conventional TB.

TB SPREAD THROUGH SKIN SORES

Persons with extrapulmonary TB can develop draining abscesses
(oozing sores) of the skin through which other people are liable to
become infected.[39]

EXAMPLES OF TB OUTBREAKS
The following examples illustrate the relative ease with which TB infection is transmitted under a variety of circumstances.

MALE TEACHER INFECTS 161 CHILDREN
It's like tuberculosis gets in your lung and rots it. This adult coughed on all the children and exposed them to the TB germ.
– Dr. Linda Fischer, chief medical officer of St. Louis County

In 1990, a male teacher with active pulmonary tuberculosis infected 161 out of 342 children (47%) at the Robinwood Elementary School in the St. Louis suburb of Florissant. Twenty-seven of the infected children developed active TB. Health officials said it was the worst TB outbreak in the area in twenty years.

The outbreak first became apparent when a member of the school's staff coughed up blood, a symptom of cavitating tuberculosis. Some of the children infected by the teacher developed fluid in their lungs and swollen lymph glands.

Vic Tomlinson, a staff member of the Missouri Department of Health, said the outbreak was consistent with an increase in tuberculosis nationally since 1986. "A lot of the people are under the impression that TB is dead. It's not."

Due to restrictive HIV confidentiality laws, health officials could not disclose whether the teacher also had AIDS.[40]

TB TRANSMITTED BY STUDENTS
A 13-year-old female seventh grade student with pulmonary tuberculosis in a South Carolina junior high school was inadvertently responsible for transmitting TB infection to 387 people. Forty-three percent of 900 people directly or indirectly exposed to the child were infected.

School teachers showed a seven-fold [700%] increase in the prevalence of positive skin-test reactions following the outbreak.

Tuberculin-reactor rates for seventh graders were substantially higher than for eighth graders. The more classes shared with the index patient, the higher the probability of being a reactor.

Among students who shared no classes with the index patient, the highest rates of tuberculin reactions were found for those who had entered a classroom immediately after the index patient had left it. Evidence of transmission on the school bus and in the church choir was also suggested.

The index case was found to be a missed contact of a previously identified case of tuberculosis. Since household contacts are at high risk for developing active disease, there is a need for meticulous and complete investigation and preventive therapy for all such persons, especially children.[41]

This case provides a striking example of how even one infectious child can casually transmit TB infection to a vast number of people. People became infected with the TB organisms by simply walking into a room and breathing the air after the girl had already left. Children sitting on the same school bus and members of her church choir also became infected.

Researchers from Germany report:

Tuberculosis was spread from a 15-year-old girl with open disease, treated for pneumonia with antibiotics for months and not separated from school, *to a further 77 children.* A two-and-one-half-year-old niece developed open perforating bronchial lymph node tuberculosis, 34 companions from school and sports developed closed active lymph node tuberculosis and 42 pupils showed suspect chest radiographs with positive tuberculin tests. All of them had to be treated.[42]

TB TRANSMITTED BY "MINIMAL EXPOSURE"

In a report entitled "Outbreak of Tuberculosis after Minimal Exposure to Infection," physicians determined by intensive contact tracing that an attendant at a swimming pool center was responsible for transmitting TB infection to 108 children ages 8-11 years old who had visited there. Sixteen of the children developed active tuberculosis.

The contact of these children with the index case was apparently minimal. Early detection, isolation, and treatment of infectious cases of respiratory tuberculosis and vigorous contact tracing should be given more priority in tuberculosis control.[43]

POTENT FORMS OF TB MAY BE MORE CONTAGIOUS

Some researchers have suggested that there are virulent strains of TB which can be more easily transmitted:

A case of miliary [disseminated] tuberculosis in a 4-year-old girl led to contact tracing, revealing *32 children with evidence of tuberculous infection. Three adult cases were also identified.* The source case was a mother who passed on the infection at two Christmas parties. *Limited exposure to the organism caused infection, suggesting a virulent strain.* . . . A range of complications of primary tuberculosis in the children was seen.

Side-effects of the chemotherapeutic agents used to treat TB was seen in most of the cases and 3 suffered substantial toxic effects. The limited range of agents suitable for use in young children was a serious problem.[44]

The CDC has reported an interstate outbreak of drug-resistant tuberculosis involving children in California, Montana, Nevada and Utah.[45]

TB OUTBREAKS IN NURSING HOMES
Patients, staff and visitors to nursing homes are susceptible to acquiring TB infection.

An outbreak of tuberculosis among elderly residents of a nursing home was caused by the presence of a highly infectious patient. . . . *Forty-nine of 161 previously tuberculin-negative residents became infected, and eight developed progressive primary tuberculosis including one who died. Also, 21 of 138 tuberculin negative employees were infected,* of whom one developed clinical tuberculosis. The fraction of elderly persons harboring a dormant tuberculosis infection today is smaller than generally thought. *If one of this group develops active tuberculosis, however, it may endanger 80% to 90% of fellow residents and employees.*[46]

The presence of active tuberculosis can be masked by symptoms which resemble those of other lung ailments. The patient who is not treated for TB will remain infectious.

. . . a patient with what was thought to be an episode of bronchitis or bronchopneumonia may die after having exposed a number of young health workers [and other patients] to tuberculosis in a country where it should have been eliminated several years ago.[47]

In one study, physicians found a 67% increase in TB infection among persons admitted to nursing homes.[48]

Nursing homes and mental hospitals across the country are being compelled to admit infectious AIDS patients, many of whom have dementia and are at high risk of developing drug-resistant strains of TB and other contagious diseases. Since patients with HIV disease and TB will likely show negative results on a TB skin test, the possibility of an AIDS patient with undiagnosed TB causing major spread of tuberculosis in a nursing home or psychiatric institution environment is substantial. Should AIDS patients be newly exposed to TB organisms from other residents, their weakened immune systems make them vulnerable to rapidly developing full-blown TB.

Older persons are liable to have their immune systems weakened by advancing age and are more susceptible to severe, life-threatening illness when exposed to various infectious diseases.

Dr. Dixie Snider, Director of the CDC's TB Control Department, warned in 1988 that a survey of 29 states showed that TB was on the rise in nursing homes.

Not that I want to alarm people, but there have been outbreaks of TB in nursing homes. Some family members are very devoted and stay many hours. Those folks are at risk. I think for these reasons the public has a vested interest [in preventing the spread of TB in long-term care facilities].[49]

TB SWEEPING PRISONS

The crisis of TB in prisons was underscored when twelve inmates and a guard died from deadly strains of the disease.[50] Four of the inmates were from the Auburn state prison in central New York and eight were from a prison in Queens. The prisoners reportedly were HIV carriers. The guard who died of TB had been overseeing the prisoners while they were hospitalized at the Health Science Center in Syracuse.

While it was not widely reported in the press, *the Syracuse hospital announced that 52 health care workers at the Health Science Center also became positive for TB.* New York state Corrections Commissioner Thomas Coughlin said TB has the potential for explosive spread among inmates:

> I am concerned for the health of the 60,000 inmates, their visitors, their families and communities. I am also concerned about the 28,000 employees of this department, their families and the public.

The incidence of tuberculosis among inmates in New York State correctional facilities skyrocketed over 700% from 1978 to 1988.[51] In a survey of TB cases reported during 1984 and 1985 by 29 state health departments, the incidence of TB among inmates of correctional institutions was more than 300% higher than the general population.[52]

Transmission of TB in correctional facilities presents a health problem for the institutions as well as for the communities into which they are released.

> Each year more than 8 million inmates are discharged from local jails, and more than 200,000 from state and federal prisons. Because the median age of inmates is relatively young – 27 years – the total lifetime risk for TB in persons infected during incarceration is considerable.[53]

> The increasing incidence of tuberculosis among prison inmates in association with AIDS and HIV infection will require enhanced TB control efforts within prisons and in communities from which inmates originate.[54]

COMPULSORY HIV TESTING OF PRISONERS IS CRITICAL

Under the highly restrictive AIDS secrecy laws of various states, physicians and prison officials are not allowed to test convicts for HIV without their specific written permission. The drastic rise in TB among prison inmates closely parallels the growth of HIV disease.

Prisoners who are HIV positive and carry TB will show little or no reaction on the standard TB skin test (due to anergy). *Without mandatory HIV testing, prisoners at high risk of manifesting deadly forms of TB will go undetected.* Prisoners with unsuspected tuberculosis endanger other inmates, staff, visitors and people in the communities to which they are released. It is critical that all prisoners be compulsorily screened for HIV upon intake.

A simple, low-cost urine test which provides immediate results could be readily used for mass screening of prisoners, including those in jails.[55]

TB OUTBREAKS IN MEDICAL FACILITIES

Patients with contagious TB can transmit the infection to hospital employees, patients and visitors.

Physicians from the Division of Tuberculosis Control, Centers for Disease Control, report the case of a patient with oozing TB sores who infected scores of others:

> Nine secondary cases of tuberculosis and 59 tuberculin skin test conversions [68 total infected] occurred after exposure to a hospitalized patient *with a large tuberculous abscess of the hip and thigh.* . . .
>
> Four of 5 surgical suite employees who assisted with incision and debridement of the abscess had skin test conversions, as did *85% of 33 employees on a general medical floor who recalled exposure to the patient* and 30% of 20 intensive care unit employees who recalled exposure. *The prevalence of tuberculin reactivity in visitors and other patients on two floors also showed a strong association with exposure to the patient.*
>
> A high concentration of *Mycobacterium tuberculosis* in the abscessed tissue, disturbance of the surface of liquid drainage from the abscess by irrigations and *by the agitated behavior of the patient,* and positive air pressure in the patient's room are factors that appear to have contributed to the high risk of tuberculosis transmission. . . .
>
> During the first three days after the operation copious drainage from the abscess area soaked the dressing continuously. The patient was agitated, confused, and complained of intense thigh pains. On more than one occasion, he completely removed the pus-soaked gauze dressing.[56]

Hospital visitors with active TB also pose a serious health risk to patients and staff.

> A 3-year-old girl was admitted to a children's hospital; subsequently her mother was found to have pulmonary tuberculosis with smear-positive sputum. . . . *30 inpatients, three outpatients, two sibling visitors and one staff member became infected.* . . . Altogether, three generations of infected children and adults were diagnosed amongst community and hospital contacts in this extended outbreak.
>
> These findings support current recommendations for the follow-up of highly susceptible CASUAL CONTACTS of cases of pulmonary tuberculosis with smear-positive sputa.[57]

PATIENT SPREADS TB TO 47 MEDICAL WORKERS

One patient with active tuberculosis who was treated at the emergency room at Parkland Hospital in Dallas, Texas, transmitted TB infection to 47 employees at the hospital. A resident physician developed cavitary tuberculosis after exposure to the patient. *An additional six workers in the emergency department developed active tuberculosis* as did an immunocompromised patient. Another employee case may have resulted from transmission by another worker who initially caught TB from the patient. Fifteen of the infected emergency room workers were found to have newly acquired TB infection after working on the same day the TB patient was admitted to the emergency room.[58]

DEADLY FORMS OF TB BREAKING OUT IN HOSPITALS

Patients with HIV disease have transmitted multidrug-resistant tuberculosis to other patients and health care workers.[59] In at least one instance, a health care worker with HIV disease died after contracting drug-resistant TB from an AIDS patient.[60] HIV-infected medical workers are at heightened risk of contracting and disseminating TB.

A substantial number of medical workers, including physicians, nurses and housekeeping staff, have contracted TB from AIDS patients.[61] Health care workers in AIDS units are at increased risk of acquiring TB infection.[62] Certain procedures used to treat lung conditions in AIDS patients cause violent spasmodic coughing which projects large numbers of infectious TB bacilli into the air. Airborne transmission of infectious diseases from AIDS patients to health care workers is a growing concern.[63]

DRUG-RESISTANT TB ENDANGERS THE PUBLIC

Deadly multidrug-resistant types of TB can be spread to other people without HIV disease and pose a dangerous threat to health care workers and the general public. Since 1990, hundreds of patients have contracted intractable TB at various hospitals in the United States. The death rate among the patients exceeds 72 percent.[64]

AIDS DEMENTIA COMPOUNDS TB CRISIS

Many AIDS patients who develop active TB experience psychiatric disorders as a result of HIV-related brain deterioration. Dementia compounds the difficulty of caring for these individuals in medical centers, mental hospitals, nursing homes, prisons and other institutional settings.

HIV/TB patients with memory loss, mental confusion, homicidal and suicidal tendencies, hallucinations, etc., are not able to comply with the therapy regimen required to render them non-infectious. When AIDS dementia is present in tandem with contagious TB, compulsory monitoring of such patients is necessary to prevent disease transmission to the general public.

TB INCREASINGLY COMMON AMONG AIDS PATIENTS

By 1989, physicians from Cabrini Medical Center in New York City stated, "Tuberculosis is now *frequently reported* in AIDS."[65] The Centers for Disease Control reported "TB is an important cause of morbidity in AIDS patients. *The HIV epidemic is probably a leading reason for recent increases in TB in young adults.*"[66]

AIDS-RELATED TB ENDANGERS EVERYONE

In New York City, the epicenter of the AIDS epidemic, cases of TB are being seen in record numbers. Hospitals in the area have been experiencing an explosive growth in patients with tuberculosis since the mid-1980s. At St. Clare's hospital in Manhattan the annual TB caseload soared 700% in a three-year period.

> The PPD conversion [positive TB skin test] among hospital staff demonstrates a spread of this [TB] agent in both the community and the hospital. . . . This hospital's increase in clinical cases suggests that THE RISE IN M. TUBERCULOSIS AMONG HIV POSITIVE INDIVIDUALS IS IMPACTING THE GENERAL COMMUNITY.
>
> Early, aggressive community screening and treatment procedures must be instituted to control this [TB] epidemic.[67]

TB EXPLODES IN NEW YORK

The *New York Post* carried a series of front-page stories depicting the monumental TB crisis in New York City. The series received little or no coverage from the national media.

> Tuberculosis is now so prevalent in New York City that everyone – regardless of status or wealth – is at risk of being infected. . . .
>
> The sheer magnitude of these people [contagious TB carriers] and the degree of infectiousness threatens to turn some parts of New York into virtual contagion zones.
>
> *"No matter where you are in New York City today, you can be at risk of becoming infected,"* said Dr. Lester Blair, pulmonologist at Beekman Downtown Hospital. *"Certainly in any close environment where someone is coughing with active TB you're at risk – in elevators, subways, buses and so forth,"* he said.[68]
>
> TB carriers are living, working and roaming everywhere in the city – even working as cooks in restaurant.[69]

Pete Hamill, a well-known columnist for the *New York Post*, only found out that he had contracted TB after undergoing lung surgery. He has no idea how or where he contracted the disease. Hamill did not have any of the usual severe symptoms – hacking, coughing, night sweats, fever, weight loss, or blood-tinged sputum. Doctors did surgery after finding a spot on his lung during a physical and discovered he had TB. Doctors told Hamill that he could have picked up the TB parasite overseas or anywhere in New York City. The 55-year-old columnist remarked that:

> We did, at one point, have a well-developed system of tracing people who have contagious diseases in this city. But today the AIDS phenomenon confuses that immensely.
>
> Trying to trace a person's movements to see where they might have picked up a contagious disease is now confused with the right to privacy.[70]

TB IS READILY TRANSMITTED

Dr. Dixie Snider, Director of TB Control at the Centers for Disease Control in Atlanta, has expressed deep concern about the rise of tuberculosis.

> I don't want to create sensationalism, but on the other hand, it is not fair to the public to pretend there is no risk. . . . *TB can be quite easy to get* if you are exposed to an infectious case. . . . Unless we take control aggressively it could get out of hand and cost us even more – not just in dollars, but in lives.[71]

A recent study of 1,853 homeless men in New York City found that 42.8% tested positive for TB infection. Dr. Stuart Garay, assistant clinical professor of medicine at New York University Medical Center, states:

> If a homeless person with tuberculosis coughs on you as you're giving him a quarter, those droplet particles are in the air for you to breathe. In fact, he may have coughed five minutes before he greeted you . . . tubercle bacilli remain suspended in the air for a period of time . . . if you're walking down the street and someone coughs on you, or if you're in the New York City subway system and someone is coughing, it is possible that you may develop TB.[72]

In certain areas of Brooklyn, *"tuberculosis is more rampant than in many Third World countries,"* according to Dr. Kildare Clarke, associate director of emergency medical services at Kings County Hospital in Brooklyn. Dr. Clarke and other physicians are concerned about the public's risk of becoming infected in emergency rooms. "Many times a patient sits for hours in an emergency room and you don't know he has TB," said Clarke.[73]

Dr. Lester Blair of Beekman Hospital has expressed even greater concern about the potential for mass dissemination of tuberculosis on the subways. "You have a large population who live in the subways and it's a very close environment during rush hour," he said. "There's no question about it. Because of the very nature of TB – it's a respiratory illness – commuters are going to be exposed."[74]

TB SPREADING AMONG CHILDREN

Other physicians are dismayed about the alarming spread of TB among school children. The TB infection rate among children at 26 city schools tested by the health department was 500% higher than the national average, prompting the city to institute mandatory TB skin testing for new students. "If TB were well-controlled, you would not have new cases in children," said Dr. Karen Brudney, medical coordinator of Manhattan and the Bronx for the Bureau of TB. "*Children shouldn't be getting it at all. It's a sign TB is increasing quite markedly.*" TB can result in scarring of the lung and loss of breathing capacity. It can cause infections of other parts of the body, such as meningitis – especially in children – that can go on to cause brain damage.

ONE MILLION NEW YORKERS CARRY TB

Dr. Jack Adler, Director of the NY City Health Department's Bureau of Tuberculosis, estimates that as many as one million New Yorkers – roughly one in seven – are infected with the TB microbe.[75]

VAST NUMBER OF HIV/TB CARRIERS AT RISK

Researchers from the Boston Department of Health and Hospitals, Boston University of Medicine and Public Health and Massachusetts Department of Public Health, state:

> . . . there is a *large reservoir of persons* with asymptomatic TB/HIV coinfection who are likely to progress to active TB.[76]

The U.S. Centers for Disease Control has warned that AIDS patients with active tuberculosis have been reported from across the United States:

> *The number of AIDS-TB patients in the United States will probably continue to increase* in direct proportion to the number of reported AIDS cases. While the great percentage of AIDS-TB patients are concentrated in a few states and large cities, *they have been identified in nearly all states.*[77]

Drug-resistant strains of tuberculosis are becoming increasingly prevalent and pose a dire health threat. Susceptible persons who contract these intractable forms of the disease are in extreme danger. According to the CDC:

> *No* drug regimens have proven effective in preventing progression to disease in persons infected with multidrug-resistant TB.[78]

TB FACILITATES TRANSMISSION OF HEPATITIS B

Hepatitis B and HIV have very similar modes of transmission. Prior to the onset of the AIDS epidemic, a mass outbreak of hepatitis B occurred in a hospital unit for the care of male patients with pulmonary tuberculosis:

> Sixty-four patients were studied of whom 37 were HB Ag positive. Hepatitis developed in at least 20 and was icteric [jaundiced] in 11. . . . A carrier state developed in 15 of 24 HB Ag-positive patients followed up for more than six months and was unrelated to the presence or absence of initial hepatitis. SPREAD OF HB AG TO DOMESTIC AND MEDICAL STAFF OCCURRED AND FOLLOWING THE DISCHARGE OF THE PATIENTS, HOUSEHOLD CONTACTS BECAME POSITIVE. Five, all wives of patients, developed jaundice. . . .
>
> Closure of the unit, isolation of HB Ag-positive cases with separate toilet and kitchen facilities, and discharge of patients when their respiratory condition allowed, resulted in prevention of further spread and eventually all patients were discharged from the unit.[79]

As discussed previously, hepatitis B can become reactivated and more contagious during the course of AIDS. AIDS patients with tuberculosis appear to be at heightened risk of transmitting hepatitis B. In addition, active tuberculosis could magnify the spread of HIV. AIDS patients with extrapulmonary TB can develop oozing skin abscesses contaminated with HIV. AIDS patients with pulmonary TB will cough TB/HIV-contaminated lung secretions into the air creating a risk of transmitting HIV as well as TB.

COULD TB FACILITATE THE SPREAD OF AIDS?

Individuals with HIV disease and pulmonary tuberculosis will cough up sputum containing infectious TB organisms and blood. Blood particles and other cells brought up from the lungs are likely to be contaminated with HIV. This raises the possibility that the AIDS virus could become airborne by "hitchhiking" in the sputum expelled by HIV patients with acute lung disease.[80]

HIV DIRECTLY CAUSES LUNG DISEASE

The ability of the AIDS virus to infect cells in the brain and cause dementia is well established. Less well known is the fact that *the AIDS virus directly infects and multiplies within the lungs causing inflammation and deadly forms of pneumonia.*[81]

Analogous to AIDS dementia, HIV disease of the lungs or "pulmonary AIDS" causes progressive deterioration of lung tissue resulting in death, even in the absence of secondary disease related to immunosuppression.[82] Pulmonary AIDS also induces the coughing up of phlegm and blood-tinged sputum.[83]

HIGH CONCENTRATION OF HIV IN LUNG SECRETIONS

In order to determine what is causing the symptoms of various respiratory ailments, physicians use a lung washing technique called bronchoalveolar lavage (BAL). A bronchoscope is inserted down the windpipe into one of the large air passages in the lungs and the lower respiratory tract is flushed with a sterile saline solution. The fluid is then suctioned out and analyzed for the presence of bacteria and viruses and for different types of cells.

Researchers from the University of Cincinnati, College of Medicine in Ohio who utilized this lung irrigation procedure with AIDS patients, have reported:

> Previous work in our laboratory has shown that HIV CAN BE RECOVERED FROM THE BAL FLUID [LUNG WASHINGS] OF ALL PATIENTS WITH AIDS.[84]

> ... HIV can be recovered in culture of the BAL fluid in most AIDS patients, unrelated to the type of pulmonary tissue. .... *All BAL fluid [lung washings] should be considered infectious.*[85]

In patients with pulmonary AIDS, the tissues of the lungs are infiltrated with an abnormally large number of white blood cells.[86] A significant proportion of these cells have been found to be infected with HIV.[87] French researchers have determined that the lung fluid recovered from patients with pulmonary AIDS has an 800% higher concentration of HIV-infected white blood cells than blood.[88]

Pulmonary AIDS causes hardening of lung tissue and hemorrhaging of the walls of the alveoli, the tiny grape-like units of "air sacs" in the lungs. "*Alveolar hemorrhage is a common event* during opportunistic infections or bronchial Kaposi's sarcoma in HIV-infected individuals. It can also occur without any detectable cause."[89] Hemorrhaging in lung tissue produces secretions containing HIV-infectious blood which will be brought up in the sputum.

HIV INFECTS LUNG CELLS

HIV-infected cells washed up out of the lungs of patients with pulmonary AIDS include alveolar macrophages. Alveolar macrophages are defensive scavenger cells which normally seek out, engulf, ingest and destroy pathogens which penetrate to the airways or alveoli. When alveolar macrophages ingest HIV, they are taken over by the virus and become a lethal reservoir of infection.[90]

INFECTIOUS LUNG SECRETIONS

HIV-infected cells are washed up out of the lungs during the lavage process. HIV-infected cells in lung and bronchial secretions are also dredged up and expelled through coughing and breathing. Pulmonary tuberculosis causes sputum contaminated with TB bacilli and HIV-infected cells to be coughed up into the air. In laboratory studies, normal alveolar macrophages from healthy persons become infected when brought in contact with HIV.[91]

INHALATION OF HIV-INFECTED SECRETIONS

When HIV-infected secretions are expelled into the air, larger droplets can be inhaled by another person and deposited inside their nose and mouth. The mucous membranes of the mouth and nose are lined with octopus-like Langerhans cells which reach out and capture invading viruses. Langerhans cells become infected when they capture HIV.[92]

When very tiny particles (1 to 3 microns in diameter, called "droplet nuclei") containing TB organisms are inhaled, they can reach the air sacs (alveoli) in the lungs.

According to the report, "Problems Associated with Aids," printed by the British House of Commons:

... IF AN AIDS VIRION IS INHALED INTO THE LUNG it is engulfed by an amoeba-like macrophage on the lung of the alveoli [air sacs]. It has been shown repeatedly in the laboratory that the Aids virus readily infects macrophages, and the virus replicates within them, THEREBY ENABLING INFECTION OF PEOPLE TO BE INITIATED BY THIS ROUTE.

... Chronic lymphoid interstitial pneumonitis is a well recognized variety of pneumonia caused directly by infection of the lungs with the Aids virus. It is similar to the pneumonia of maedi-visna in sheep and is particularly common in children with Aids. WHEN ASSOCIATED WITH PULMONARY TUBERCULOSIS, A VERY COMMON COMPLICATION OF AIDS, IT IS INEVITABLE THAT COUGHING WILL PRODUCE SOME AEROSOLS CONTAINING TUBERCLE BACILLI AND THE AIDS VIRUS. After the fluid in the aerosols evaporates, the minute dry flakes containing tubercle bacilli and the Aids virus float in the air indefinitely and both remain infectious for days.[93]

LENTIVIRUS IN SHEEP SPREAD THROUGH AEROSOLS

A number of studies of pulmonary AIDS in humans have pointed out its similarities to progressive pneumonia lentivirus disease in sheep.[94] Researchers from the National Institutes of Health and elsewhere report that their studies of adult patients with pulmonary HIV disease ". . . together with the knowledge that lymphocytic *pulmonary lesions may be caused by lentiviruses in humans and animals* suggest that HIV plays a significant role" in the development of pulmonary AIDS.[95]

While drawing the close parallels of lentivirus disease of the lungs in sheep and humans, virtually all these studies inevitably avoid mentioning how pulmonary lentivirus disease in sheep is transmitted.

The report on AIDS to the British House of Commons notes:

> The normal route of transmission of the maedi-visna lentivirus between adult sheep is by *respiratory aerosols* when they are crowded closely together in winter shelters. Maedi-visna is not a sexually transmitted disease of sheep.[96]

In the treatise, *Slow Virus Diseases of Animals and Man*, P.A. Palsson described the transmissibility of maedi lentivirus disease among sheep:

> Maedi was successfully transmitted to healthy sheep by direct contact between healthy and diseased animals by contaminating their drinking water with faeces from diseased animals and by injecting material from typically infected lungs and lymph nodes *intranasally* [into nasal passages] and intravenously. . . .
>
> In advanced stages of maedi the presence of the viral agent can be demonstrated regularly in various organs. Occasionally maedi virus has also been demonstrated in nasal swabs from such sheep. During the clinical course of [maedi disease], *fits of dry coughing are occasionally seen and thick mucous is often seen in the larger bronchi.*
>
> *Transmission of maedi by the respiratory route as a droplet spread of the infectious agent while animals are in close contact* is considered from field experience to be the most likely way the disease is spread naturally.[97]

Numerous studies have determined that maedi-visna is readily transmitted through nasal passages and the respiratory tract.[98] Uninfected lambs deprived of milk from infected ewes still have been found to contract the infection. A number of sheep with maedi demonstrate a copious nasal exudate (runny nose) which apparently contributes to sheep-to-sheep transmission.

HOUSEHOLD CONTACTS OF HIV/TB PATIENTS AT RISK

A study of the household contacts of AIDS carriers with tuberculosis indicates that they have a greatly increased incidence of acquiring HIV.

Along with members of the Sida (AIDS) Project in Zaire, researchers from the Cornell University School of Medicine, NY and the Mt. Sinai School of Medicine in New York, reported the results their HIV transmission from AIDS patients with active TB to their household contacts.

The study excluded:

- household contacts who were ever transfused (excluding transmission through blood transfusions)
- spouses of the TB patients (excluding sexual transmission)
- children ages four or younger (excluding children who contracted AIDS from their mothers at birth or through breast feeding)

Household contacts of HIV positive patients with TB and HIV negative patients with TB had similar rates of pulmonary M.Tb. However, *The HIV-1 prevalence was significantly greater [300% higher] in household contacts of HIV positive TB patients when compared to household contacts of HIV negative TB patients.*[99]

In excluding the possibility of transmission of HIV through blood transfusion, sexual contact and birth, it is evident that another means of HIV transmission occurred from the AIDS patients with TB to their household contacts. It is entirely plausible that AIDS was transmitted through HIV-contaminated aerosols produced by the labored breathing and deep coughing accompanying TB.

NOBEL LAUREATE URGES CAUTION

Dr. Joshua Lederberg is a renowned, highly respected American biochemist who was awarded the Nobel prize for discoveries concerning genetic recombination and the organization of the genetic material of bacteria. He is also President of Rockefeller University in New York City. In an enlightening treatise presented in the journal *Social Research*, Dr. Lederberg asserts:

. . . the progress of medical science during the last century has obscured the human species' continued vulnerability to large-scale infection.

. . . Unlike other virus infections which leave some survivors immune to further attack, *there is nothing in the natural history of AIDS to point either to a cure or to a vaccine*. . . .

The long latent period multiplies the opportunity for spread; the victim may be unaware of carrying the virus, even less his contacts. . . . The targeting of the immune system also encourages the seeding of other infections – we are already starting to see a recrudescence of tuberculosis in the United States and aggravations of syphilis and a host of opportunistic organisms rarely ever seen before. . . .

What are the odds of the virus learning the tricks of airborne transmission? The short answer is, "No one can be sure."

However, given its other ugly attributes, IT IS HARD TO IMAGINE A WORSE THREAT TO HUMANITY THAN AN AIRBORNE VARIANT

OF AIDS. NO RULE OF NATURE CONTRADICTS SUCH A POSSI-
BILITY; THE PROLIFERATION OF AIDS CASES WITH SEC-
ONDARY PNEUMONIA MULTIPLIES THE ODDS OF SUCH A
MUTANT, AS AN ANALOGUE TO THE EMERGENCE OF
PNEUMONIC PLAGUE....

*... and with so much at stake we must multiply our vigilance for evidence
of extraordinary channels of spread.*[100]

TB MORE DEADLY THAN BUBONIC PLAGUE

Individuals with HIV/AIDS are at high risk of manifesting contagious deadly forms of TB.[101] As early as 1987, a TB epidemic
broke out among nurses treating AIDS patients at a hospital in
Urbana, Illinois. Physicians found "abundant" TB bacilli after obtaining a sample of lung fluid from a 48-year-old male AIDS patient. Dr. Thomas Schrepfer, a family physician and chairman of
the Carle Foundation Hospital's quality assurance committee, explained that AIDS heightens the transmissibility of TB:

*... THE SHEER NUMBER OF ORGANISMS THAT THRIVE UNDER
AN AIDS PATIENT'S WEAKENED IMMUNITY CAN INCREASE THE
CONTAGION RISK TO OTHERS* – including healthy people. "The more
organisms you're exposed to, the more difficult it is to fight them off."[102]

The survival rate for people who contract these tough strains of
TB is far worse than that of bubonic plague.*

In an editorial entitled "Tuberculosis – The Plague of the '90s?"
Dr. Theodore C. Eickhoff, M.D., writes: "It is most likely these
problems [outbreaks of multidrug-resistant TB] are already
widespread and will spread to all parts of the country in the relatively near future."[103]

When people contract incurable TB from breathing the contaminated air exhaled by an infectious AIDS carrier they will die a
ghastly and painful death – even without catching HIV.

---

*With prompt drug treatment, the mortality rate for bubonic plague is less than
5%.[104] In contrast, *the fatality rate for multidrug-resistant TB among healthy people
is over 50%*; among HIV carriers it is much higher.[105]

CHAPTER EIGHT

WHY PATIENTS ARE AT RISK

I'd like to say that AIDS is a terrible disease that we must take seriously. I did nothing wrong, yet I'm being made to suffer like this. My life has been taken away. Please enact legislation so that no other patient of a health care provider will have to go through the horror that I have.
  – AIDS victim Kimberly Bergalis' final statement to members of Congress,
    urging the enactment of laws requiring AIDS-infected health care workers
    to notify their patients. The 23-year-old young woman and four other pa-
    tients contracted AIDS from their dentist.

The sad story of Kimberly Bergalis is just the tip of the iceberg.
  – Dr. Sanford Kuvin, Vice-Chairman of the National Foundation for Infec-
    tious Diseases[1]

FIVE PATIENTS INFECTED BY THEIR DENTIST

*If this man had the courage and the medical dignity to admit he had AIDS, we
would have been spared. There is morally no reason for Kim to be dying and
for me to be feeling terrible.*
  – Barbara Webb, a 65-year old grandmother and retired school teacher who
    was among the five victims of dentist David Acer. Mrs. Webb is fighting an
    AIDS-related pleurisy that fills her lungs with fluid.

Pretty young Kimberly Bergalis had no idea the dentist treating
her had AIDS. Two years after having some routine dental work,
she developed a lung ailment and underwent a complete physical.
The doctor started asking her if she had engaged in pre-marital
relations or had ever used illegal drugs. The answer was no on
both counts. "What's going on here? Why all these types of questions?" the young woman asked. That is when the physician
dropped the bombshell. She had a pneumonia common among
AIDS patients. Blood tests confirmed the presence of HIV. Kimberly had AIDS.
    The young woman and her parents were devastated. A devout
Roman Catholic, Kimberly had refrained from pre-marital relations. She came from a happy, middle-class family and had never
used heroin or crack. How could this have happened?
    Health department workers who questioned Kimberly could not

find any exposure factors and called in the Centers for Disease Control. For three long weeks, CDC investigators grilled the young woman about her past.

"We kept going over certain things, and I asked, 'What about the dentist?'" said Kimberly. "Because at the time it was only a rumor that he had AIDS. But I was told they were not investigating that."

The investigators' repeated questioning implied she was being less than candid in regard to her personal life. To confirm her statements, Kimberly underwent a pelvic exam.

FINDING OUT ON THE EVENING NEWS

Unbeknownst to the Bergalis family, the CDC investigators *were* aware that her dentist had AIDS and had been looking into his situation. The restrictive AIDS secrecy laws of Florida prohibit health officials from informing patients their health care provider has AIDS.[2]

"*I first heard about my case on the evening news,*" said Kimberly, referring to a news broadcast discussing a report issued by the CDC which said an unnamed Florida woman apparently contracted the disease from her dentist.

Her dentist, Dr. David Acer, a homosexual, had letters sent out informing his patients that he had AIDS–*three days after he died.* Suddenly, the pieces of the terrible nightmare came together. "There was this anger toward God," said Kimberly. I really didn't have anyone I could put the blame on. I even had crazy thoughts. I go to the beach a lot and I thought maybe I stepped on a hypodermic needle. You just go crazy trying to figure out how this happened."

Dr. Sanford Kuvin, vice chairman of the Board of Trustees of the National Foundation for Infectious Diseases, carefully analyzed the case and agreed that she contracted AIDS from her dentist. "This is a young, beautiful articulate woman. I interviewed Kimberly and I saw no risk factors."[3]

Although media attention focussed primarily on Miss Bergalis, it was soon learned that the dentist had infected *four other patients* before his death.

Five unsuspecting patients had contracted the fatal disease despite the dogmatic assurances by the Surgeon General's Office:

> *There is no danger of AIDS virus infection from visiting a doctor, dentist,* hospital, hairdresser or beautician. AIDS cannot be transmitted non-sexually from an infected person through a health or service care provider to another person. . . . *You may have wondered why your dentist wears gloves and perhaps a mask when treating you. This does not mean he has AIDS or that he thinks you do.* He is protecting himself from hepatitis, common colds or flu.[4]

INFECTIOUS MEDICAL WORKERS ARE A CONCERN

Eileen Moran, editor of *RT Image*, the nation's largest news-magazine for radiological technologists, writes:

While it is of grave concern to health care workers that of those who have HIV infection, 5 percent were infected in the health care setting, it is also of concern that of those contaminated workers, 100% are contagious within the health care setting. *They are exposing not only fellow workers, but also the patients whose health they are dedicating their lives to protect.*[5]

DOCTORS WITH HIV DEMENTIA ENDANGER PATIENTS

Dr. James S. Fulghum, III, M.D., of the North Carolina Neurosurgical Society, asserts:

Of particular interest to me as a neurosurgeon in active clinical practice is the question of the responsibility of a physician to disclose a physical or mental impairment to the patient should that impairment place the patient at some degree of risk. The risk may involve direct surgeon-to-patient transfer of the AIDS virus *or it may involve professional incompetence....*

Assuming that the risk is low of direct transmission of the HIV virus from surgeon to patient, shouldn't a more appropriate issue be that of impairment of the physician to do the job? IS IT APPROPRIATE FOR HIV-POSITIVE INDIVIDUALS WITH AIDS DEMENTIA COMPLEX TO BE OPERATING A JET AIRCRAFT, MAKING SURGICAL DECISIONS, PERFORMING PROCEDURES USUALLY ASSOCIATED WITH FINE MOTOR SKILLS, AND FUNCTIONING IN OCCUPATIONAL CATEGORIES IN OUR SOCIETY USUALLY ASSOCIATED WITH GREAT RESPONSIBILITY?...

One wonders what the definition of an impaired physician is if it doesn't include AIDS dementia complex.[6]

WOUNDS ENDANGER WORKERS AND PATIENTS

CDC researchers who studied the risk of skin wounds involving blood during 1382 surgical procedures observed 99 injuries. The percentage of surgical procedures with one or more bloodletting injuries varied according to area of service:

gynecology	10.1%
cardiac	9.3%
general surgery	7.7%
trauma	4.6%
orthopedics	3.6%

The wounds observed were caused by suture needles or another sharp object held by a co-worker and associated with the fingers used to hold tissue being sutured (sewn together). The researchers concluded:

In 29% of the injuries THE SHARP OBJECT RECONTACTED THE
PATIENT'S OPEN WOUND AFTER INJURING THE HEALTH CARE
WORKER, RESULTING IN POSSIBLE EXPOSURE TO THE
WORKER'S BLOOD.

PERCUTANEOUS INJURIES [skin wounds] ARE COMMON DUR-
ING SURGERY; additional measures to protect HCWS [health care work-
ers] and patients from blood-borne pathogens are needed.[7]

A study of 200 caesarian sections found that the obstetricians'
surgical gloves were punctured during 54% of the procedures.[8]

INFECTIOUS DENTIST TREATED OVER 1000 PATIENTS

Cases involving AIDS-infected medical and dental workers are
coming to light with alarming frequency.

In Delaware, dentist Raymond Owens, 61, received his diagnosis
of AIDS in 1989 but continued to work on patients until weeks before his death in March of 1991. Unlike Dr. David Acer, the homosexual dentist in Florida who posthumously notified his patients, Dr. Owens *never* told patients he was carrying the fatal disease. His obituary in local newspapers cited the cause of death as
"pneumonia." State health officials found out Owens had the disease only when a personal acquaintance contacted them after his
death, according to Lester Wright, Director of the Delaware Division of Public Health.

The state sent certified notification letters to 1200 patients of
the deceased dentist offering free AIDS tests.[9]

PATIENTS OF INFECTED ORAL SURGEON NOTIFIED

Hundreds of unsuspecting patients were treated by an AIDS-infected oral surgeon in Detroit before he died of the disease. A
neighbor, Mike Zollick said the death was "a scary deal, especially
when you know that the AIDS virus can incubate for 10 years.
How would you know?" Michelle Kott, 28, who had four wisdom
teeth pulled by Dr. George Fredrickson, told the *Detroit News* she
was "shocked." "I was a little scared," she said. "I guess I still am. I
haven't decided what I should do. My parents are concerned, but
they haven't decided what I should do either." Fredrickson is at
least the fourth Michigan dentist known to have AIDS and the
second to have died, following Dr. Thomas Snedeker, age 40, of
Grand Rapids.[10]

RURAL RESIDENTS SHOCKED

Residents of the central Illinois community of Nokomis (pop.
2,500) were stunned by the revelation that the town's only dentist
had died of AIDS. The dentist's widow wrote a letter which

appeared on the front page of the local newspaper confirming that her husband Gary Darr, age 37, had died of the disease. She said the "only possible way" her husband contracted the disease was from an infected patient. Local residents expressed sympathy for Darr's widow and three children but there was also angry questioning of why *it took almost nine months* for the dentist's patients to learn the real cause of his death.[11]

Representative Penny Pullen, a former member of the President's Commission on AIDS and a stalwart advocate of sound public health measures, asserted that it would have been more appropriate for patients to have been informed of his condition prior to undergoing invasive procedures. Pullen said more than 194 Illinois health care workers have tested positive for AIDS and 126 of them have died from the disease, including another dentist who was not identified.

Pullen pointed out that a much larger number of other health care workers are carrying HIV disease. "Not all of these health care workers perform invasive procedures but the health department has no policy to deal with those who do." she said. "What about the patients of the other AIDS-stricken dentist who died last August?"

Pullen was subsequently instrumental in the passage of a state law establishing mandatory procedures to notify the patients of AIDS-infected health care workers. The law provides similar notification to physicians and others who have performed invasive procedures on an infected patient.

AIDS AND BRACES

Robert A. Engel, a Florida dentist who specialized in orthodontics and often worked with children, notified 750 of his patients that he was HIV positive and was closing his practice. "I am sorry for any anxiety this may cause to anyone," he remarked in a one-page letter. He reassured his patients that he had followed CDC guidelines. Similar to Dr. David Acer, the Florida dentist who infected five of his patients, Engel wrote, "I feel no patients could have been infected by me."[12]

CANADIAN SURGEON HAD AIDS FOR FIVE YEARS

A surgeon in Guelph, Ontario performed at least 700 operations over five years while carrying AIDS, an Ontario coroner's investigation revealed. When Dr. Patee was diagnosed, he was afflicted with AIDS-related dementia, said Deputy Chief Coroner James Young. Three other physicians in the Canadian province, including one surgeon, are known to have AIDS, according to Dr. Richard

Schnabas, Ontario's chief medical officer of health. Prior to his death, Dr. Patee performed an average of 140 operations a year at Guelph General Hospital and a smaller number at St. Joseph's Hospital in Guelph.[13]

SURGERY PATIENTS OFFERED FREE AIDS TESTS

Officials at Johns Hopkins Hospital in Baltimore, Maryland, offered free AIDS tests to about 1,800 patients operated on by a surgeon who died of AIDS.

Dr. Rudoph Almaraz, a cancer surgeon, died at the age of 41. His family refused to confirm that Dr. Almaraz died of AIDS, but the family's lawyer Marvin Ellin told the Sunday *Sun* of Baltimore, "He had AIDS and he died of AIDS."

Mr. Ellin said Dr. Almaraz told him *he was exposed to the disease when blood from an AIDS patient squirted into his eyes and mouth during an operation* in New York about seven years previously while Dr. Almaraz was on a fellowship at the Memorial Sloan-Kettering Cancer Center.

A Sloan-Kettering spokeswoman said that the hospital did not have records that would indicate Dr. Almaraz contracted AIDS when he practiced at the hospital from July 1 to December 1, 1983.

"We have no record at this time. We have not uncovered any blood incident report," said Suzanne Raussenbert, Sloan Kettering's vice president for public affairs.

Dr. Timothy Townsend, Johns Hopkins Hospital's senior director for medical affairs, said the hospital made repeated efforts, several months before he died to determine Dr. Almaraz's illness amid rumors that he had AIDS.

The letter offering free AIDS tests will not name Dr. Almaraz because neither the doctor nor his family would discuss the nature of his illness. . . . [14]

Cancer surgeons treat many patients who are immunosuppressed due to the debilitating effects of the disease and anti-cancer therapies. Immunosuppressed patients are highly susceptible to the various opportunistic diseases that frequently beset AIDS carriers such as CMV, toxoplasmosis, *P. carinii* pneumonia, bowel parasites, tuberculosis, etc. Even if the patients of an AIDS-infected health care provider do not contract HIV or hepatitis B (which can reactivate in highly contagious form during the course of AIDS), they are vulnerable to contracting other HIV-related secondary diseases. In patients with severely weakened immune systems, these other infections can be as deadly as AIDS itself.

GYNECOLOGIST DIES OF AIDS

Benny Waxman, M.D., was about to complete 14 years as associate chairman of George Washington University's obstetrics and gynecology department when he died of AIDS. The 59-year-old physician had been married and fathered four children. He was also a practicing homosexual.

He didn't tell his patients he had the disease, even though he knew it for years before his death and even though *he continued to perform what the medical profession calls "invasive procedures."* He also didn't tell officials of George Washington University Hospital; they found out only months before he died. . . .

Meanwhile, George Washington Hospital *has lost two more of its doctors to AIDS*, according to its clinical director.[15]

An AIDS-infectious gynecologist-obstetrician performs intrusive procedures in which patients are vulnerable to viral and bacterial exposure. Pelvic and rectal exams, normal deliveries, cesareans, episiotomies and hysterectomies involve contact with mucous membranes and blood. Glove punctures are not uncommon during involved surgical operations, especially during obstetric procedures.[16] *A single drop of a physician's or nurse's AIDS-infected blood oozing into the patient's open abdominal cavity or vaginal membranes could transmit the disease.*

FAMILY PHYSICIAN WITH OPEN SORES AND HIV

In Minneapolis, Minnesota, an AIDS-infected family physician who had open sores and lesions on his hands informed 328 patients that he may have exposed them to the fatal disease. Dr. Philip Benson, a family physician, said he double-gloved while delivering babies and during other procedures. However, since a significant percentage of gloves have tiny holes and can break, stretch or tear during surgical procedures, wearing gloves is not a sufficient precaution, said Minnesota state epidemiologist Dr. Michael Osterholm.

Health officials are trying to contact the patients *who underwent invasive procedures such as surgery, deliveries and oral, rectal or gynecological exams* during that time.

Patients could not have been notified without Dr. Benson's permission, said Stephen Kelley, chairman of the Minnesota Board of Medical Examiners public policy committee.[17]

PATIENTS AT CHILDREN'S HOSPITAL NOTIFIED

Officials at Children's Hospital Medical Center in Akron, Ohio notified 59 patients that they were treated by an HIV-infected physician during his residency at the hospital. The physician, who hospital officials refused to name because of the state's restrictive HIV confidentiality laws, had assisted in numerous surgical operations over a one-month period. He was later employed at Fairview General Hospital near Cleveland. He died of AIDS about a year and a half after leaving the hospital in Akron. Officials at another area hospital chose not to inform patients of the physician that he had AIDS.

PATIENTS OF ORTHOPEDIC SURGEON TEST POSITIVE

In Philadelphia, officials at Mercy Catholic Medical Center informed 1050 patients that they had been operated on by an orthopedic surgeon infected with HIV. The patients were offered free AIDS tests; three out of 330 of the patients who had themselves tested were positive for HIV. The hospital later released a statement alleging that the infected patients had a history of "high risk behavior." The sensitive DNA "fingerprinting" test which would reveal if the surgeon and his patients carried the same form of the virus was not conducted. A hospital spokeswoman declined to give out information on how the surgeon contracted the virus.

NEW TEST TRACKS THE SPREAD OF VIRUS

A team of researchers from the U.S. Centers for Disease Control have developed an extraordinarily precise means of determining if individuals are infected with the same unique form of the AIDS virus. Analogous to fingerprints, each strain of virus has its own distinctive genetic markings. When an individual transmits HIV to someone else, the unique genetic "fingerprints" of the virus he has transmitted can be detected and traced back to him. The DNA "fingerprinting" test enabled researchers to determine that Kimberly Bergalis and four other patients were actually infected by the same dentist and not another source.[18] Another patient of the dentist was also found to be HIV positive, but the genetic "fingerprints" of the virus he carried were so different from that of the dentist that it was determined he was infected by someone else.

The CDC researchers state:

> We have developed a novel approach to study the transmission and evolution of individual HIV strains. This technology will play an important role in our understanding of the spread of HIV through the population.[19]

The scientists were able to use this advanced type of genetic "fingerprinting" test to track down the type of virus found in a person who contracted AIDS from a blood transfusion to homosexual donors who carried the same unique strain of the virus.

In order to accurately assess the possibility of worker-patient transmission, investigators must utilize the sensitive DNA "fingerprinting" test and compare the types of viruses in the AIDS-infected health care worker and the infected patients. When this sensitive DNA test is not performed, health officials can claim that the patients became infected through "other risk factors." Even when patients have other risks of exposure, the test should be performed to accurately determine whether they may have contracted HIV from the health care worker treating them.

CRUEL AND UNUSUAL PUNISHMENT

Besides the five victims of Dr. David Acer, dozens of other patients of AIDS-infected health care providers have been found to be infected with HIV. In many cases, health officials have refused to conduct the sensitive DNA testing necessary to determine if they carry the same strain of HIV as the health care worker treating them. One particularly disturbing situation involves two AIDS-infected dentists, Dr. Victor J. Luckritz and Dr. Herman Dale Scott, who treated thousands of unsuspecting prison inmates in Maryland.

Dr. Victor J. Luckritz's friends and colleagues say he carried his fatal disease with humor and dignity. And, we would add, with reckless disregard for the health and safety of others, if assertions that the Baltimore dentist who died of AIDS May 7 often wore no surgical gloves while treating about 4,000 Maryland inmates are correct. . . .

Though Dr. Luckritz's friends and fellow parishioners at the church he attended knew he was stricken with the deadly disease, the dentist didn't see any duty to inform his patients or his employer. He blithely went about his duties as chief dentist at the Maryland Penitentiary between June 1988 and April 1990, risking his patients' lives while violating his companies "infection control procedures," which required the wearing of gloves, among other sanitary practices.

Dr. Luckritz's employer and patients learned that he had AIDS only through a death notice published in the Baltimore Sun three days after he died.[20]

At least 33 of the inmates treated by the dentists were found to be infected with HIV. Health officials have declined to conduct the sensitive tests necessary to determine if they were infected by the dentist. Greg Shipley, a spokesman for the Maryland Division, alleged that using the more sensitive test would "be too expensive." "There is nothing we can conclude as far as how or when they [the prisoners] contracted this infection," Shipley said.

Lack of certainty is precisely the reason why health officials should conduct the more sensitive tests. With a disease as devastating as AIDS, it is imperative that the risk of virus transmission from infectious health care providers to patients be thoroughly investigated, not glossed over. With the billions of dollars being funnelled into the interminable cause of "AIDS research," there is more than enough money available to conduct the sensitive testing needed to carefully examine cases involving AIDS-infectious health care providers and their infected patients.

Moreover, compelling vulnerable prisoners to undergo invasive dental procedures by AIDS-infected dentists can be viewed as a form of cruel and unusual punishment.

INVESTIGATIONS STALLED

Not surprisingly, there has been a great deal of foot-dragging when it comes to investigating cases involving possible HIV transmission from physicians and dentists to patients. In the Maryland prison situation as well as in a number of other cases, public health officials have balked, stalled and outrightly refused to do the sensitive testing needed.

WHY HEALTH OFFICIALS BALK

The tragic case of Kimberly Bergalis and four other less publicized fellow patients of Dr. David Acer caused an enormous public outcry. The public overwhelmingly wants the right to be informed if the health care worker treating them is carrying AIDS.

Despite the outcry, the U.S. Congress and most states have been unwilling to pass legislation requiring mandatory HIV testing of medical and dental workers. If a few more cases involving patients contracting HIV from medical workers were brought to light, public outrage would reach a fevered pitch. The furor would result in the enactment of laws requiring mandatory AIDS testing of medical and dental workers. Likewise, medical and dental workers could utilize the wave of public outrage to demand the right to test patients.

These forms of mandatory testing are anathema to political special interest groups whose members constitute the largest percentage of reported AIDS cases in the United States. Medical and dental facilities which have employed AIDS-infectious workers also face massive lawsuits if it is demonstrated that patients contracted HIV from one or more of their employees. Consequently, there has been a massive amount of political pressure poured on to quash investigations involving patients who may have contracted AIDS from dentists or physicians.

WHY HEALTH CARE WORKERS
SHOULD BE SCREENED FOR HIV
"DO NO HARM"

There is a common disturbing denominator in most cases involving AIDS-infected medical and dental personnel. Patients learn about the provider's condition only *after* undergoing procedures through which they could have become infected.

Dr. Sanford F. Kuvin asserts:

ALL HEALTH CARE PROFESSIONALS INVOLVED IN INVASIVE PROCEDURES SHOULD HAVE THEMSELVES TESTED FOR HIV AND MAKE THEIR STATUS KNOWN TO THEIR PATIENTS. Similarly, patients who will be undergoing invasive procedures should be tested and make their status known to those treating them. A central principle of medical ethics is "First, do no harm." How can a physician or dentist know that he or she will do a patient no harm if he or she might be a carrier of HIV."[21]

AIDS CARRIERS CAN TRANSMIT HEPATITIS

HIV is transmitted in similar modes to hepatitis B virus (HBV). Many AIDS carriers are at high risk of manifesting reactivated hepatitis B. During the course of HIV infection, "greater viral replication may make it [HBV] *more contagious* and resistant to antiviral therapy."[22] "HIV affects the immune response to hepatitis B virus and may prolong productive HBV replication."[23] In addition to the risk of transmitting HIV itself, AIDS-infected health care providers pose a risk of transmitting hepatitis B to patients. Hepatitis B causes severe liver inflammation and can lead to liver cancer, cirrhosis and death.

MEDICAL WORKERS SPREAD HEPATITIS B

According to infectious disease specialists from the University of North Carolina, health care workers who are hepatitis B carriers

. . . appear to be at low risk for transmitting hepatitis B to their patients. *However,* occasionally HBsAg-positive physicians, dentists, oral surgeons, obstetric-gynecologic surgeons, and nurses have been implicated in the transmission of HBV to *multiple patients.*[24]

The New England Journal of Medicine has reported:

Over a four-year period in a five-county area, *71 patients with clinical hepatitis B had dental work performed* in the two to six months before their illness. *Fifty-five cases were traced to a single oral surgeon.* Seventy-nine per cent of these patients were positive for hepatitis B surface antigen (HBsAg) and most had no other recognized source of hepatitis. *An investigation of the implicated dentist uncovered no gross inadequacies in instrument sterilization or general dental procedures*; however, the dentist was found to be an asymptomatic carrier of HBsAg of the same subtype (ay) as nine of 11 of his patients who had hepatitis and whose serums were available for testing.[25]

Other cases of HBV transmission from dentists to their patients has been officially reported.[26] In one instance, two out of the nine patients treated by their dentist died of fulminant hepatitis B.[27]

"UNIVERSAL PRECAUTIONS" FAIL

Researchers from the Hepatitis Branch, Division of Viral Diseases at the CDC have reported a case in which five patients developed acute hepatitis B within four months after major operations by the same obstetric-gynecologic surgeon. The obstetrician was allowed to resume his surgical practice but "was required to obtain written informed consent from patients, *to double glove, and to employ appropriate surgical techniques to avoid injury.*" Despite wearing a surgical mask and double surgical gloves, seven months later *another* patient contracted hepatitis B after undergoing a cesarean section. The surgeon was then excluded from major operations.[28]

LARGEST OUTBREAK OF HEPATITIS B IN MEDICAL HISTORY

Despite the advent of "universal precautions," the year 1991 saw the largest nosocomial (hospital acquired) outbreak of hepatitis B in medical history. *An astounding 213 of 2,331 patients became infected with hepatitis B virus* after being treated by Ft. Myers, Florida, dermatologist Dr. Robert Boudreau. State health officials claimed the outbreak was generated by unsterilized equipment used to treat a patient with hepatitis B. It is difficult to fathom, however, how there would have been enough virus left from one patient on a piece of equipment to infect over 200 other people. The dermatologist has since closed his office and refused to comment on the outbreak. It was not disclosed if the dermatologist had hepatitis B or AIDS or whether the patients were also tested for HIV.[29] Regardless of how the hundreds of transmissions took place, this case illustrates the high infectivity of a blood and body fluid borne virus in a medical setting.

HIV-INFECTED DOCTORS POSE MULTIPLE RISKS

Medical and dental workers with HIV disease are subject to developing a variety of secondary diseases which can be transmitted to patients. They are at high risk of manifesting contagious forms of hepatitis, pneumocystis pneumonia (which poses serious health risks to immature infants and patients with weakened immune systems), cytomegalovirus (CMV), bowel parasites, and other infectious illnesses related to AIDS and high risk groups (see Chapters 4 and 5).

. . . The transmission of the AIDS virus to patients is not the only serious risk associated with the practicing HIV-infected physician.

Because brain damage ultimately occurs in almost 100% of symptomatic AIDS cases, *clinically ill physicians may not be able to practice effectively.* In fact, one study detected subtle cognitive and behavioral defects in about 40% of carefully evaluated "asymptomatic" HIV carriers.

AIDS-INFECTED PHYSICIANS ALSO CAN INFECT IMMUNO-SUPPRESSED PATIENTS WITH POTENTIALLY FATAL OPPORTUNISTIC INFECTIONS. Moreover, AIDS carriers are assumed to be infected and contagious with cytomegalovirus (CMV), which can cause devastating congenital neurological defects.

Organized medicine has placed its trade union role ahead of patient safety on the issue of the HIV-infected physician.
– Mark I. Klein, M.D., Berkeley, California[30]

Medical and dental personnel with HIV-induced brain deterioration pose serious hazards to patients. Cognitive dysfunctions such as memory loss, mental confusion, etc., are likely to interfere with their ability to accurately assess patients' medical conditions and make them liable to prescribe inappropriate, potentially life-threatening medications. The inability to perform a job task adequately and safely is also a consequence of HIV brain deterioration. Physicians with HIV dementia are at increased risk of performing treatment in a manner which endangers the lives of patients (see Chapter 3).

French researchers using a variety of neuropsychological tests found:

Psychometric abnormalities do exist *early* in HIV disease in almost *all* HIV-infected patients.[31]

NEUROMUSCULAR DISEASE COMMON IN HIV CARRIERS

Researchers from the National Institute of Neurological Disorders and Stroke, National Institutes of Health, Bethesda, Maryland, state:

Recent estimates show symptoms of neuropathy [nerve disease] or myopathy [muscle disease] in up to 80% of infected adults. *A neuromuscular disease can occur in all stages of HIV infection*, can coincide with HIV seroconversion, or can be the only clinical indication of a chronic, silent HIV infection.[32]

HIV-related disease of the nervous system results in slowed reaction time, tremors and impairment of fine motor skills. These impairments can have a detrimental affect on the ability of medical and dental workers to perform procedures competently and safely. Moreover, *HIV disease of the brain and nervous system can cause health care workers to perform procedures in a manner which heightens the danger of transmission of HIV and other AIDS-related infections*. It has been suggested that AIDS dementia may have been a factor in Dr. David Acer's transmission of the disease to five of his dental patients.[33] It is noteworthy that Acer did wear a mask and gloves. None of the infected patients recall Acer injuring himself during the course of their treatment. It is possible that the dentist had a particularly infectious form of HIV which was transmitted despite adherence to "universal precautions."

SHODDY ROOT CANALS AND AIDS

Mary Lynne Desmond thought she had found the perfect dentist. Philip Feldman, a graduate of the School of Dental Medicine at the University of Pittsburgh, had an engaging manner and seemed meticulous. Soon Desmond, a fourth grade teacher who lives in Coram, N.Y., and her two children, husband, sister and brother-in-law, all became Feldman's patients. *"But in the last five or six years, he changed," Desmond recalls. "He did three shoddy root canals on me and even left a drill bit in one tooth."*[34]

Feldman, 45, died of AIDS-related pneumonia. His decreasing competence may have been related to HIV-related brain deterioration. Health officials are attempting to determine if he infected any of his patients with HIV.

HEALTH CARE WORKERS WITH HIV DEMENTIA MAY DENY THE PROBLEM

One of the symptoms of HIV brain deterioration is proneness to accidents. Another characteristic of HIV-dementia is denial: the individual affected is unable or unwilling to acknowledge that they are experiencing mental problems.

If an AIDS-infectious nurse, dentist, pharmacist, etc., accidentally pricks his finger on a hypodermic or intravenous needle, his brain impairment can make him less likely to notice the injury at all or until *after* he has inserted the contaminated needle into the arm or gums of the vulnerable patient.

A dentist or physician with HIV brain deterioration is prone to mental slowing and loss of fine motor skills, making them more liable to sustain bloodletting cuts, puncture wounds and other injuries during an invasive procedure. Conversely, since HIV disease of the CNS causes a slowing in reaction time they would be less likely to withdraw their injured hand or bloodied instrument rapidly and carefully enough to prevent leakage of infective blood into the bleeding mouth or open body of the patient.

Since HIV dementia causes denial, the affected worker may not be aware that their work skills are impaired and that they are endangering the lives of patients. *HIV-induced cognitive impairment coupled with denial poses a deadly two-edged threat in the medical workplace.*

A COMPASSIONATE SURGEON SPEAKS OUT

Dr. G. Edward Rozar, Jr., M.D., a cardiac surgeon who unknowingly contracted HIV disease from a patient, shares this sobering testimony:

> I voluntarily stopped seeing surgical patients within days of learning my HIV status. . . .
> OUR PRIMARY GOAL MUST BE TO PROTECT OUR PATIENTS.
> . . . Beyond the risk of transmission, there's also the fact that practitioners in advanced stages of infection will in all likelihood have impaired functioning, since 75 to 80 percent of patients who die of AIDS show central nervous system deterioration. DISCOVERING AND ACKNOWLEDGING INFECTION EARLY ON, AND RELINQUISHING THE SURGICAL TOOLS WELL BEFORE IMPAIRMENT BECOMES AN ISSUE IS OBVIOUSLY THE SAFEST COURSE.
> The usual objections to HIV testing for doctors strike me as illogical. Yes, there's the "window period" – during which a recently infected person may test negative – but that's hardly a valid excuse not to test. As for the alleged costliness of routine screening, the Army has been doing it since 1985, at only about $3 per sample, with a turnaround time of less than 72 hours.[35]

"BLIND" PROCEDURES INCREASE DANGER

Dr. F. S. Rhame, writing in the *Journal of the American Medical Association*, cautions:

> Procedures involving blind by-feel manipulation of sharp instruments in body cavities are hazardous and *make instances of HIV transmission likely* considering the occurrence of surgeon-to-patient and patient-to-surgeon hepatitis B infection. "Hospitals should keep isolates of a surgeon's viral strain to help prove *most* detected HIV infections are not related to the surgery, he warns."[36]

A more prudent approach would require pre-operative preventive medicine. Rather than keeping a sample of an AIDS-infectious surgeon's strain of HIV on hand while letting him continue to risk infecting patients, hospitals should suspend his operating room privileges.

PATIENTS OFFERED FREE TB TESTS

> Rockford, Illinois – Nearly 200 patients have been offered free health tests to determine whether they were infected with tuberculosis by an anesthesiologist, officials said.
> The mailings from five Rockford-area hospitals and a medical group, went out to the 191 patients treated by the anesthesiologist between June 13 and October 4.
> At this time, we suspect only a very small percentage of the tests will be positive, said Dr. Gary Rifkin, a Rockford doctor specializing in infectious diseases who was involved in the mailings. . . .

"We're not making a big thing of this medically," Rifkin said.
The name of the Rockford anesthesiologist who has the disease has not been released.[37]

Although it was not disclosed if the physician had AIDS, this case underscores the risk posed by health care workers with contagious tuberculosis.

HIV-INFECTED WORKERS CAN SPREAD TB

Pulmonary tuberculosis has become a significant problem among the asymptomatic HIV-positive population.[38] Health care workers with HIV disease are at substantial risk of developing tuberculosis. TB is highly contagious and can be readily transmitted to patients and other staff members. HIV-infected health care workers are also vulnerable to contracting tuberculosis from infectious patients.

Testing health care workers for TB alone is insufficient to uncover the presence of infection among those who carry HIV disease. The impaired immune response (anergy) caused by HIV produces false negative results on the TB skin test, even in the presence of active, contagious tuberculosis. *Health care workers with unsuspected HIV disease and active TB are likely to remain undiagnosed until after exposing vulnerable patients, staff members and hospital visitors.* In the interest of safeguarding the health of the patients entrusted to their care, hospitals should require mandatory HIV and TB screening of health care personnel.

AIDS-infected health care workers are also more susceptible to acquiring tuberculosis and other infections from patients. They in turn can then transmit these infections to other patients.

PATIENTS FORCED TO PLAY RUSSIAN ROULETTE

At present, medical and dental patients are compelled to play viral Russian roulette. Patients should have the right to know if the individual putting his hands inside their body, injecting them or cutting them open is carrying AIDS.

Routine, periodic mandatory AIDS testing of all medical and dental personnel who perform invasive surgical procedures would help prevent the spread of HIV and related diseases (hepatitis, TB, etc.,) to vulnerable patients. *Obligatory mass screening of medical and dental personnel would also uncover other unidentified cases of occupational transmission of HIV to health care workers.*

Hospitals should consider cancelling the operating room privileges of any surgeon or nurse who is HIV-positive or refuses to be tested. At the very least, AIDS-infectious surgeons and dental professionals should be required to obtain written informed consent from patients prior to performing invasive examinations and procedures.

MOST AIDS-INFECTIOUS HEALTH CARE WORKERS ARE "UNDERGROUND"

The CDC has officially reported that over 8,000 health care workers have been diagnosed with end-stage AIDS. This number includes over 637 physicians, 42 surgeons, 156 dental workers, 1,199 nurses and an assortment of paramedics, technicians, therapists and dieticians.[39] The federal agency estimates that *an additional 50,000 health care workers* are infectious carriers of HIV disease, a figure that has been challenged as *"just the tip of the iceberg."*[40]

Most of these infectious medical and dental workers are currently "underground." Many of them have engaged in behaviors at high risk of HIV but may not know or acknowledge that they are infectious carriers of the disease. *Mandatory HIV screening would help bring those carrying the disease to the surface where their condition could be assessed by medical and dental peer review panels.*

PHYSICIANS: A NEW HIGH RISK GROUP FOR AIDS?

Dr. E. Douglas Whitehead, assistant clinical professor of urology at the Mount Sinai School of Medicine in New York City, asserts:

> *Physicians dealing with blood and human secretions,* particularly surgeons and physicians doing invasive procedures, *may represent a heretofore unrecognized high risk group for HIV positive status,* due to the high frequency of needlestick injuries, and torn surgical gloves. *Clearly, if we are ignorant of our HIV status, but are HIV positive, we may inadvertently subject our patients to direct physician-to-patient transmission of the AIDS virus,* just as our HIV positive patients may subject us to direct patient-to-physician transmission of the AIDS virus.[41]

Out of rational humanitarian concern for the safety of patients as well as health care workers, it is critical that medical and dental personnel undergo periodic mandatory AIDS screening. Rapid, accurate, low-cost urine or saliva tests could be used for this type of regular mass screening. The modest cost ($5-$10) of the test could be borne by health care professionals as simply another occupational expense.

COURTS RULE PATIENTS HAVE A RIGHT TO KNOW

A Pennsylvania appeals court has ruled that a hospital can warn patients being treated by a doctor with HIV disease despite the physician's claim that it would violate his privacy. The physician was in the obstetric/gynecology residency program at a Harrisburg hospital.[42]

Previously, a New Jersey court affirmed that a surgeon infected with HIV disease must inform patients before operating on them. Superior Court Judge Philip S. Carchman, in a ruling believed to be the first in the nation, found a patient's right to know outweighs a surgeon's right to privacy. His decision came in a lawsuit brought by the estate of the late William Behringer, M.D., against the Medical Center in Princeton. Dr. Behringer, an ear, nose and throat specialist, said he contracted the disease while performing an emergency tracheotomy on a patient. Upon learning that Behringer was HIV positive, the hospital asked him to give up invasive surgery. When he declined, the hospital insisted that he require his patients to sign a consent form which said they knew he was infected with the AIDS virus and that there was "a potential risk of transmission." The hospital maintained that the requiring of written informed consent was "reasonable and proper" and that it had "an obligation to protect the interests of the patients it serves." The judge ruled:

> If there is to be an ultimate arbiter of whether the patient is to be treated invasively by an AIDS-positive surgeon, *the arbiter will be the fully informed patient. The ultimate risk to the patient is so absolute, so devastating,* that it is untenable to argue against informed consent, combined with a restriction on procedures which present any risk to the patient.[43]

PREVENTING MEDICAL TYPHOID MARYS

British orthopedic surgeon Dr. Justin Cobb asserts:

> *Both doctors and nurses generally have obligation to see . . . that patients are not being operated on by the surgical equivalent of Typhoid Mary.*
> *To find that one had been operating on people for years spreading the disease [AIDS], would be grim.*
> For the average patient, contact with us is as close as they will get to the fast lane. We know that clinical viral hepatitis is four times more common in American hospital employees than in the general population and 10 times higher among British surgeons than among the general population of London.
> So BEING IN A HIGH RISK PROFESSION I THINK WE SHOULD ALL HAVE MANDATORY ANNUAL BLOOD TESTS FOR HIV state and to confirm the active immunization against hepatitis B. . . .[44]

PHYSICIANS FOR MORAL RESPONSIBILITY

Dorsett D. Smith, M.D., Physicians for Moral Responsibility, University of Washington Medical School, Seattle, states:

> I find little difference between the HIV-infected homosexual or intravenous drug abuser who continues to have unrestrained sexual activity and the surgeon who is infected and continues to practice surgery.[45]

CHAPTER NINE

HEALTH CARE WORKERS UNDER SIEGE

I had always told my patients that living with HIV is an emotional roller coaster, and now I have experienced this first-hand.
   – Dr. Patricia Wetzel, chief of the AIDS unit at John Peter Smith Hospital in Ft. Worth, Texas. Dr. Wetzel accidentally contracted the fatal disease from a patient.

On April 11, 1989, AIDS became a subject of keenest concern to me. That was the day I found out, as the result of a routine insurance company physical, that I was HIV-positive. My only risk factor: I was a cardiac surgeon.
   – Dr. G. Edward Rozar, Jr., of Marshfield, Wisconsin. Dr. Rozar unknowingly contracted HIV from a patient in 1985 at a hospital in Pittsburgh, Pennsylvania.

In the early years of the AIDS epidemic, we made many efforts to reassure health care personnel that the risks of caring for AIDS patients were extremely low and limited only to HIV transmission. THAT IS CLEARLY NO LONGER THE CASE.
   – Theodore C. Eickhoff, M.D., Chief Medical Editor, *Infectious Disease News*[1]

PHYSICIAN PASSES VIRUS TO WIFE AND CHILD

A young British doctor learned to his dismay that he had transmitted the AIDS virus to his wife only after the couple's four-month-old son died of the disease. The couple had themselves tested for AIDS two days after the child succumbed to pneumonia. Only then did the physician realize he had contracted HIV disease through working with infected patients. The London *Daily Mirror* reported:

> Yesterday the curtains were closed at the couple's three bedroom home in a Liverpool suburb. Colleagues of the surgeon said he was an outstanding physician who was destined for a top medical position.
> His son, born two weeks before Christmas, died of severe pneumonia in the intensive care unit at Liverpool's Alder Hey Hospital.[2]

171

After returning to England two years previously, the physician continued his practice, operating on over 200 patients before he learned he was HIV positive. He believes he probably contracted the virus while operating on AIDS-infected patients in Zambia, although he might have become infected through operating on patients in Liverpool. The doctor informed hospital administrators upon learning of his diagnosis and voluntarily stopped doing surgery. Letters were immediately sent out to his patients offering free AIDS tests.

Besides the risk to patients, this tragic case highlights a crucial reason why health care workers should have themselves regularly tested for HIV: *they could unwittingly transmit the fatal disease to their spouses and children.*

AIDS STRIKES IOWA NURSE

Barbara Fassbinder, a 32-year-old nurse in the farming community of Monona, Iowa (pop. 1530), received the fateful news that she was HIV positive after attempting to donate blood. Her infection was traced back to an incident six months previously when she had applied pressure with a piece of gauze to a male patient's IV puncture site for about 10 minutes. Afterwards she learned that the patient had died of AIDS. Transmission of the virus apparently occurred through some tiny nicks in her skin she acquired while gardening.

Local resident Ted Balekos commented that after Mrs. Fassbinder decided to go public with the news, "everybody was stunned. There was sorrow. She's such a beautiful person for that to happen to."[3]

HIV PUTS END TO PROMISING SURGICAL CAREER

Dr. Edward Rozar, Jr., learned he was HIV positive after an insurance physical. He believes that transmission occurred during a surgical residency at Allegheny Hospital in Pittsburgh in May of 1985. In retrospect, he recalls experiencing mononucleosis-like symptoms and other classic signs of acute HIV infection. Since there was no routine HIV testing of patients, Dr. Rozar does not have a clue as to the patient from which he contracted the fatal disease. "It's impossible to say which needle stick or blood spatter was responsible for transmission," he said.

Just four months before finding out he had HIV disease, Dr. Rozar along with his wife, Donna and their five adopted children, then all under age 6, moved to Marshfield, Wisconsin, where he had joined the surgical staff.[4]

WOULD YOU BOARD A PLANE IF ...

Tragic cases like these have occurred across the United States. Health care workers are frequently told the concentration of HIV in blood is very low and exposure to HIV-contaminated blood poses only a "low risk" of infection. However, researchers from the San Diego Medical Center in California using sensitive DNA tests:

> ... detected a *very high percentage* (greater than 10%) of peripheral blood mononuclear cells (PBMCs) containing HIV sequence in seropositive individuals. This reflects a *substantially higher percentage* of PBMCs actually infected with HIV than previously reported.[5]

According to the official estimate, *only* one out of 250 needlestick exposures results in HIV transmission.[6] In occupations where exposure occurs more frequently, such as surgery, the risk is higher. One study estimated that 1 out of 50 to 100 surgeons in New York City will become infected with HIV over the course of their careers.[7] Another study suggested that for surgeons who are exposed repeatedly, the risk may be as high as six percent (1 out of 16 exposures could result in HIV infection). Dr. Robert Sharrar, M.D., M.Sc., Assistant Health Commissioner of Medical Affairs at the Philadelphia Department of Health and a nationally recognized expert in public health, explains:

> Let me put the risk of HIV infection for a single exposure in perspective. One out of 250 isn't very high, but if the risk for airplane crashes was that high, you wouldn't get on the plane. THE RISK IS A LOT HIGHER THAN WE LIKE TO ADMIT.[8]

According to the eminent British venereologist Dr. John Seale:

> It is probable that, as with so many viraemic diseases, *a single virion introduced directly into the blood will regularly transmit infection.*[9]

Although AZT has been recommended following an individual's exposure to HIV, *there has not been a single documented case of the drug preventing infection after the virus has been transmitted.* AZT first-aid treatment failed to prevent HIV infection in a 58-year-old monogamous heterosexual man in a hospital who was accidentally given an intravenous injection with a syringe containing blood from an AIDS patient. The hapless patient was started on AZT within 45 minutes after he was accidentally stuck and continued receiving the drug for several weeks, but it was of no avail.[10] The AIDS virus integrates in the genetic material of cells shortly after infection occurs.[11] As discussed in Chapter 2, HIV infection is a permanent, inexorably fatal condition.

NOTORIOUS UNDER-REPORTING
Scores of health care workers are officially acknowledged as having contracted AIDS through occupational exposure.[12] Larry Gostin, executive director of the Boston-based American Society of Law and Medicine, has said the true number of medical and dental workers who have contracted HIV disease in the workplace could be up to *five times greater* than the CDC's official count.

Dr. Hacib Aoun, a Baltimore physician who contracted AIDS through cutting his finger on a test tube containing blood in 1983 commented, "I practically had to beg for the CDC to come and evaluate the situation. It was months and months before they came. It's still not counted, even after it was acknowledged by the hospital."[13]

According to David Bell, Chief of the CDC's AIDS activity and hospital infection program:

> We know they're *notoriously under-reported*. Basically, nobody knows how many health care workers have been infected [with HIV] on the job.[14]

A study in the *Annals of Emergency Medicine* found a high incidence of under-reporting of contaminated needlestick injuries among emergency health care workers, indicating that "*current estimates of the incidence of occupationally acquired HIV-1 infection are low.*"[15] There is a great deal of sensitivity and even politics behind the under-reporting. Once health care workers perceive that they have a significant risk, they are going to be asking for things that certain special interest groups don't want to happen, such as mandatory AIDS testing of all hospitalized patients.

VIRUSES AND BACTERIA PENETRATE GLOVES
Researchers from the Johns Hopkins University School of Nursing studied the efficacy of latex and vinyl gloves as barriers to microorganisms. They designed laboratory experiments to test the permeability of vinyl and latex gloves to bacteria (*S. marcescens*).

> In most health care settings, vinyl gloves are provided to protect personnel from contaminated materials. However, NO EVIDENCE OF PROTECTIVE EFFICACY EXISTS.
>
> We conclude that high inocula of bacteria *can penetrate gloves*, particularly vinyl, during routine clinical manipulations *in the absence of obvious damage* to the gloves.[16]

Viruses are smaller than bacteria. If bacteria can permeate surgical gloves, infective viruses can as well.

> In the largest study to date of hospital gloves, researchers have found some brands leak more than *30 per cent of the time*, which could allow easy passage of viruses responsible for AIDS, hepatitis and other diseases.[17]

SENSITIVE TESTS REVEAL MOST GLOVES LEAK

About 60% of a random sample of 680 surgical gloves leaked before and during use in a study in San Antonio, Texas. *All of about 100 examining gloves studied had perforations or thinned areas that would permit the passage of molecules the size of viruses.* The University of Texas research was done in operating rooms and dental clinics using a new electronic detector test twice as sensitive as the usual test of filling gloves with water and seeing whether they dribble. The electronic test showed that double gloving still had a leak rate of 25%.[18]

Edward L. Gershey, Director of Laboratory Safety at Rockefeller University, states:

> The AIDS problem has created an environment where everyone from health care workers to school teachers is relying upon examination gloves for protection from infectious materials. Our study on the effectiveness of these gloves in excluding virus particles *highlights the need for caution* on the part of those who rely upon these gloves for protection. . . .[19]

"UNIVERSAL PRECAUTIONS" FAIL TO PROTECT

Standard "universal precautions" involve the avoidance of direct skin exposure to blood and body fluids. This entails always wearing gloves, not recapping needles, disposing of contaminated needles and bandages in receptacles designated for biohazardous material, and autoclaving or otherwise disinfecting equipment and reusable garments and bed sheets.

"Universal precautions" have proven woefully inadequate in preventing hepatitis B transmission to oral surgeons and other health care workers.

Researchers from the Hepatitis Branch, Division of Viral Diseases at the Centers for Disease Control, have reported:

> A survey of 434 oral surgeons was conducted to examine risk factors for hepatitis B virus (HBV) infection. Overall, 112 (26%) [1 out of 4] of the participants demonstrated serologic evidence of past or current infection with HBV. . . . The strong correlation between years in practice and seropositivity WAS UNAFFECTED BY REPORTED USE OF GLOVES, FACE MASKS, OR EYE SHIELDS. THE USE OF GLOVES AND OTHER PROTECTIVE DEVICES DOES NOT APPEAR TO OFFER SUBSTANTIAL PROTECTION AGAINST HEPATITIS B EXPOSURE IN ORAL SURGEONS. . . .[20]

These findings have chilling implications for the health and safety of oral surgeons, dentists and other medical professionals. HBV and HIV have similar modes of transmission. As documented previously, there is high concentration of infective white blood cells in the saliva of patients with HIV disease. Infectious

HIV has been detected in the plasma of AIDS patients in higher concentrations than is commonly suggested.[21]

A National Institutes of Health study reported that among anesthesiologists in practice for several years, the incidence of hepatitis B is an appalling 43%. The CDC estimates that 12,000 health care workers become infected with hepatitis B annually.[22]

If an unvaccinated health care worker is exposed to HBV, they can receive hepatitis B immune globulin (HBIG) to help prevent their progression to active hepatitis.[23] There is no such fail-safe medication available to prevent the development of AIDS in HIV-infected health care workers.

Although touted as an effective primary "universal precaution," gloves are hardly a foolproof preventive against transmission of hepatitis B or HIV. Vinyl and latex gloves are subject to undetectable holes, tearing and stretching.[24]

Repeated handwashings and usage of gloves causes chapped skin, and contact dermatitis which facilitate entrance of virus into susceptible epidermal cells.

Razor sharp scalpels, wires and needles readily pierce gloves and skin permitting entrance of HIV-contaminated blood and other body fluids.[25]

HIV infection can occur during blood-to-blood contact. The virus can be transmitted through intact or chapped skin via Langerhans cells.[26] Double and triple gloving is recommended to make it more difficult for a scalpel or other sharp instruments to slice through into the skin. The downside of triple gloving is that it reduces tactile sensitivity and interferes with the surgeon's ability to feel for the presence of internal abnormalities during various surgical procedures. In addition, triple gloving is not impervious to scalpel slices or piercing by wires, needles and sharp bone fragments.

SURGEONS AT HIGH RISK

There is a world of difference in the perspective of politicians, bureaucrats and armchair medical theorists who issue sanguine advice about "universal precautions" and glibly dismiss the danger of HIV transmission and that of medical workers in the trenches. Surgeons not infrequently are up to their elbows in blood while handling razor sharp glove-piercing instruments. In many procedures blood is everywhere, splattering surgical garments, eye glasses and surgical masks, and spraying into the air.

A study presented in the *British Medical Journal* describes the high frequency of blood exposure which surgeons face:

It is an everyday occurrence for surgeons to find at least one hand stained with
the patient's blood at the end of a major procedure. We were, however, surprised to find that *the incidence is almost 50%* and is not necessarily related
to experience. Furthermore, *in only 44 of a total of 78 contamination inci-*
dents was the surgeon aware that he had perforated his glove; this was a
needlestick injury in every case except one in which the assistant's scissors
were at fault.
      Clearly, the bigger the operation the greater the risk of blood contami-
nation for the surgeon. In general surgery, where the "no-touch technique" is
largely inappropriate, this problem is not only exceedingly common but
probably unavoidable as it often goes unnoticed.[27]

There are industrial grade masks and full body plastic smocks
and suits which help prevent blood and body fluid contamination
of the head, neck, torso and legs. These suits become brutally hot
and enervating under the glaring spotlights of the operating room
and in the intensive work of surgery itself. It is impractical to compel surgeons to wear such suits for every patient. Without routine
AIDS testing of patients, surgeons are compelled to treat every patient as HIV positive. The suits are cumbersome and can slow
down surgery creating an increased risk for the patient[28] and giving
them less time to devote to other patients – including non-AIDS
patients – who also require care. A glove composed of steel mesh
has been developed for surgeons but it greatly interferes with sensitivity and can still be pierced with the thin needles used during
surgery. Surgery requires tactile sensitivity, dexterity and alacrity in
handling sharp instruments interchangeably.

HIV MIST IS INFECTIOUS

A study presented by Stanford researchers in the *Journal of Virol-*
ogy has documented that infectious AIDS viruses are aerosolized
or "misted" into the air during various surgical procedures. Human
papilloma virus (HPV) which causes venereal warts, has been detected in the fumes generated during laser surgery for wart re-
moval. HPV warts are seen to develop in the noses of physicians
and operating room staff exposed to HPV misted into the air during laser surgery.[29]
      Similarly, HIV particles contained in the fine mist generated
during various surgical procedures pose a health hazard if
breathed into the nose or mouth[30] or absorbed into the skin or the
surface of the eyes. AIDS viruses pass easily through the fibers of a
surgical mask.[31]
      Dentists have voiced similar concerns about the expulsion and
misting of the virus when using high speed drills. High-speed dental handpieces permit the retention of potentially infective saliva
which can be sprayed into the mouth of the next patient.[32] Heat

treating high-speed handpieces should be an essential component of standard safety procedures.

AIDS PATIENTS CAN TRANSMIT SECONDARY INFECTIONS

AIDS patients with *P. carinii* pneumonia who were in the waiting room of a cancer clinic transmitted the pneumonia to other immunosuppressed non-AIDS patients.[33]

As described previously, AIDS patients are prone to developing highly contagious and virulent types of hepatitis B and non-A, non-B hepatitis.

Cytomegalovirus (CMV) is a widespread infection among AIDS patients which can have devastating consequences for an unborn infant if contracted by a woman during pregnancy.[34] *Prior infection with CMV does not confer immunity and reinfection may occur.*[35] A report published in the journal *Infection Control*, warns:

> Because of the seriousness of the disease [AIDS], PREGNANT WOMEN SHOULD AVOID CARING FOR DIAGNOSED [AIDS] CASES, especially since cytomegalovirus (CMV) is a common infection in AIDS patients.[36]

Toxoplasmosis is a protozoan parasite which is found in cat feces and is also a common secondary infection in AIDS. Pregnant women are cautioned not to change kitty litter because of the risk of contracting toxoplasmosis which can cause hydrocephalus, blindness, mental retardation and death if passed on to their babies. *Pregnant women are also at risk of contracting toxoplasmosis from AIDS patients and passing the infection to their unborn children.*

A report in the *American Journal of Medicine* "strongly urges" seronegative pregnant medical personnel to transfer from areas of the hospital where there is a significant incidence of hepatitis B.[37] AIDS patients are at high risk of manifesting highly contagious forms of hepatitis B.[38]

Hospital employees, patients and visitors who are pregnant should avoid contact with AIDS patients with parvovirus B19,[39] an infection which can cause severe complications and death in preborn infants. Pregnant women should not share a hospital room with an AIDS patient. *Pregnant health care workers should not be required to work with AIDS patients in a hospital or in a home health care setting because of the risk of devastating birth defects and death.*[40] It is inhumane to force pregnant medical and dental workers to be unnecessarily exposed to deadly infectious diseases. *There is more than one life at stake when a pregnant health care worker is exposed to HIV and its related infections.*

WHY PHYSICIANS MUST BE ABLE TO TEST PATIENTS

In many areas of the country, medical and dental professionals are being legally denied the right to know if the patients they are treating have a 100% fatal infectious disease.

Dr. Edward R. Annis, former president of the American Medical Association, states:

> Several states have established absurd statutes denying physicians the right to test for the presence of HIV antibodies without written permission from the patient. When confronted with a sick patient, a physician can call upon a vast array of tests to rule out heart disease, liver disease, cancer and most sexually transmitted diseases. But testing for AIDS has been declared off-limits without approval from the patient. Not only does this position violate the basic principles of public health, but it also ignores proper medical practice and common sense.[41]

NEED FOR PROPER DIAGNOSIS

In order to diagnose and provide appropriate treatment for any medical disorder, physicians need to be able to determine which condition(s) they are treating.

A basic principle of medicine is that it is the duty and responsibility of the trained health professional to determine which tests are medically necessary. In endeavoring to diagnosis the health status of patients, physicians will routinely run an array of tests. These can include an overall physical exam, analyses of blood and urine, EKGs, x-rays, CAT-scans and other diagnostic procedures.

Authorization to run these exams is granted as part of a routine general consent form. If a patient is experiencing chest discomfort, it can be symptomatic of a myriad of conditions ranging from simple muscle strain to bronchitis, pneumonia, heart problems, lung cancer, etc. A physician does not present the patient with a complex smorgasbord of blood tests and intricate diagnostic techniques for them to pick the ones they suppose may be a good idea. It is incumbent upon the trained medical professional to diagnose what is wrong and to treat the patient accordingly or make a referral to an appropriate specialist.

A physician may be held liable for damages if his failure to run the appropriate test(s) results in a delay or lack of treatment which causes harm to the patient.

PHYSICIANS FORCED TO PLAY DEADLY GUESSING GAME

When physicians are denied the right to routinely screen for HIV disease, they are forced to play a deadly guessing game of diagnostic hide-and-seek.

It is dangerous for patients with HIV disease because unless physicians know their condition, they will not be alerted to look for the numerous primary and secondary ailments to which AIDS patients are susceptible. Some of these conditions may be treated or ameliorated if caught in time.

Health conditions caused by HIV disease can mimic those of other illnesses – illnesses and disorders which require different types of treatment and medications for someone with HIV disease than for someone who is not infected.

Prohibiting a physician from knowing if a patient has HIV disease can result in ill-advised procedures being performed which do more harm than good. It is medically inappropriate for someone who is immunocompromised to undergo certain medical procedures. Their weakened immunity makes them less able to cope with the trauma of surgery itself and susceptible to developing bacterial infections. These infections can prove deadly in patients with HIV disease. Various vaccinations are contraindicated in individuals with HIV disease because they induce illness rather than prevent it.

ANTI-TESTING POLICIES CAN BE DEADLY

Among other hazards, denying physicians the right to screen for HIV disease can be deadly for others because unsuspected HIV patients with active tuberculosis will test negative (due to anergy) on the standard TB skin test. Outbreaks of multidrug-resistant tuberculosis are being seen with alarming frequency among physicians, nurses, other medical workers and patients.[42] Recent outbreaks have involved more and more patients in institutional settings and propagated rapidly, according to Sam Dooley, M.D., of the CDC.[43] In one hospital an alarming 46% of internal medicine physicians became infected with TB.[44] Media reports – including those in medical periodicals – depicting physicians treating AIDS patients with TB rarely show them wearing masks to prevent inhalation of infectious TB microbes.[45] Yet, federal health officials recommend wearing air-tight masks in order to filter out TB bacteria. Dr. Dixie Snider of the CDC says there is some controversy over the masks' effectiveness but that they still should be worn.

Mandatory HIV screening of patients would uncover individuals at high risk of TB and facilitate the implementation of rigorous isolation procedures to control the spread of the disease in medical facilities.

EXPOSING THE MYTHS REGARDING AIDS TESTING
Aggressive homosexual and AIDS advocacy groups have been successful in prompting legislators to pass laws banning physicians from routinely testing for AIDS. They use a number of appealing but erroneous arguments to support their claim that mandatory HIV screening of patients should be prohibited:

CLAIM 1: Since the standard AIDS screening test only detects the presence of antibodies it is not diagnostic ("doesn't mean anything"). The test frequently yields "false positive" results and can create unfounded anxiety in patients.

REALITY: Dr. James Slaff, former medical investigator at the National Institutes of Health, comments:

> Another semantic game played by advocates of "moderation" is the claim that "we do not really know the significance of seropositivity" [i.e., a positive blood test for antibodies to the AIDS virus]. *THAT IS ALSO RIDICULOUS.* If the blood test is performed rigorously, and if an initial positive outcome is confirmed by another test [such as the Western Blot – which is standard if the ELISA is positive], we *do* know the significance of seropositivity. In 999 out of 1000 cases, *it means that the individual is infected with the AIDS virus!*
>
> Infected individuals should consider themselves infectious [capable of infecting others] . . . they should refrain from sex, postpone marriage and not bear [conceive] children. . . . They may at any time, without warning, develop AIDS or ARC.[46]

Individuals who test positive on the AIDS antibody test have not merely been "exposed" to HIV. The reason they *have* AIDS antibodies is because AIDS viruses have been present a sufficient time for antibodies to develop. They are not merely "infected with the virus that can cause AIDS" nor are they "healthy carriers" who are likely to remain "asymptomatic." A positive AIDS antibody test indicates that the AIDS virus is permanently entrenched within the genetic material of cells. Individuals infected with the AIDS virus actually have HIV disease, an infectious, progressive, uniformly fatal disorder.

CLAIM 2: THE "NEGATIVE WINDOW." The possibility of a "negative window" is used to promote "universal precautions" rather than universal testing of patients. If a patient has a negative test for HIV antibodies but is in fact carrying the virus, it is suggested that health care workers would have a false sense of security and fail to take the appropriate precautions. They should therefore treat all patients as though they have AIDS because they can never really be sure which ones are infected even if the patients were routinely tested.

This argument is based on findings that a certain percentage of individuals who are infected with the AIDS virus test negative on the standard AIDS antibody test. The lag between the time of HIV infection and the development of antibodies is referred to as the "negative window." The lag time or "negative window" can be as brief as 4 weeks or as long as 3½ years – in at least one instance it was 7 years.[47]

The AIDS Antibody Test and the Blood Supply

REALITY: It needs to be underscored that the standard AIDS antibody test is used to screen and protect the nation's blood supply. Since universal AIDS antibody testing of blood was implemented, the incidence of reported newly acquired HIV infections through blood transfusions has dropped drastically.[48] This does not mean the test is perfect and that no HIV-infected antibody-negative blood ever slips through. It does mean that the test has been effective in greatly reducing the units of HIV-contaminated blood going into the general supply.

Public health spokespersons who oppose mandatory HIV testing of patients – ostensibly because of the "negative window" – do not similarly claim that universal mandatory HIV screening of blood donors should be banned and all blood treated as though it was "universally HIV-infectious." The same health experts who are reassuring the public that universal mandatory testing of blood donors has rendered the chance of getting AIDS from a blood transfusion as remote as getting hit by lightning *simultaneously* claim that the test is not sensitive enough to be used for routinely screening patients!*

The double talk of public health savants aside, it is entirely legitimate to acknowledge that though the possibility of a subset of HIV-infected individuals in the "negative window" exists, it does not forestall the need for routine mandatory AIDS antibody testing of patients. Informing physicians and other health care workers as to which patients are *known* to have HIV disease would not preclude their taking prudent infection control procedures with all patients. It means they could exercise the intense caution required in dealing with patients known to have a 100% fatal communicable disease – patients who are also prone to have infectious secondary ailments, such as drug-resistant tuberculosis.

---

*Although prudent physicians are judicious in recommending blood transfusions for their patients, it would be unconscionable to insist that no blood be tested for HIV antibodies.

Dr. Marcia Angell, senior editor of the prestigious *New England Journal of Medicine*, states:

> Screening all hospital patients would allow doctors and nurses to be especially alert against accidentally infecting themselves when treating virus carriers.[49]

Rapid, economical tests are in the diagnostic pipeline which will reveal the presence of virus within a few days to a few weeks after infection with HIV disease has occurred. When allowed to be used, they will rapidly and firmly close the "negative window."[50]

Medical Workers' Rights Under Siege

In some states, if a health care worker–including a surgeon or nurse–is exposed to the blood or body fluids of a patient such as through a scalpel wound, needlestick injury, etc., they are prohibited from knowing whether the patient is infected with HIV. Unless the patient *deigns* to be tested and grants special written permission, the medical worker is left in the dark as to their risk. Many high risk group members spurn being tested[51] or letting exposed medical worker(s) know their HIV status. The anxious medical workers at risk are told instead to have *themselves* periodically tested for HIV without being allowed to know whether they were actually exposed to the virus! This type of shroud of secrecy makes a mockery of sound medical practice and is a violation of the worker's right to know if they have been exposed to a toxic substance in the workplace.

Where is the cry for *compassion* for the endangered medical workers who are left in anguished uncertainty as to whether they have been exposed to an infectious, 100% fatal disease?

Test Could End Agony of Uncertainty

Even when the exposed worker is informed that the patient is AIDS infectious, they are left in an agonizing quandary. Should they immediately start taking AZT, DDI or other drugs which can have toxic side effects when they do not know if they have actually been infected? It may be weeks, months or even years after they have contracted HIV disease before they test positive on the standard AIDS antibody tests. Should they forego intimate relations with their spouse and having children for months to years in the interim? Should they immediately forego performing or assisting in invasive surgical operations so as to avoid accidentally transmitting HIV to patients?

Fortunately, *there are tests which have been developed which detect the presence of infinitesimal amounts of HIV within an extremely short period of time after HIV infection occurs.* This includes the polymerase chain reaction (PCR) test which uses methods similar to those of DNA fingerprinting which police have used to match a person's DNA against a sample obtained at a crime scene. The test allows scientists to multiply up to a million times the amount of genetic information in a blood sample, making it much easier to find genes from the AIDS virus within a person's DNA. "This test is among the most exciting advances in helping locate and measure the AIDS virus," states Dr. Samuel Broder, director of clinical oncology at the National Cancer Institute and a leading AIDS researcher."[52] Due to political pressure and other factors, these tests are only officially available for "research purposes." However, in the case of health care workers as well as other non-medical people who have reason to suspect they may have been exposed to the virus, they can speak with their physician in order to obtain these other tests.

The PCR test has proven exceptionally useful in determining whether infants born to seropositive mothers are infected with HIV.[53] A significant percentage of HIV-antibody negative heterosexual partners of known HIV carriers have been found to actually be infected with the virus by PCR analysis.[54]

The test can be a godsend for individuals who know or have reason to believe they have been exposed to HIV disease, but have tested negative on the standard AIDS antibody tests (ELISA confirmed by Western Blot). Persons with occupational exposure such as medical and dental personnel, paramedics and law enforcement officers may want to use the test. Rather than being compelled to live a state of grating uncertainty while undergoing periodic testing for up to three and one half years or longer, they can learn whether or not they have been infected with HIV very soon after their exposure.

The cost of the test is roughly $175, a cost which could be significantly reduced if it was utilized in large quantities and subsidized with some of the vast funds being exerted on "AIDS research" and "AIDS education."

As ironic as it may seem, there is an inordinate amount of political pressure being poured on by homosexual and AIDS advocacy groups to stymie the availability and usage of tests which permit the rapid, early detection of HIV infection. Although early diagnosis can help the treatment of HIV disease, the overriding concern of these groups is to prevent any type of compulsory or routine screening for HIV. The ready availability and mass usage of such tests would knock out the underpinnings of one of the main arguments against routine obligatory testing: the possibility of a prolonged "negative window."

AIDS and the "Right to Privacy"

CLAIM 3: *Allowing physicians to test patients for AIDS without their special written approval violates the patients' "right to privacy."* AIDS advocacy groups claim that no one – not even a physician – really needs to know if patients have HIV disease. It should be left up to the at-risk patients to decide whether it is in *their own* best interests to be tested.

REALITY: When an individual seeks medical treatment, he is implicitly giving the physician the right to perform the tests deemed medically necessary to determine his medical condition. *The very nature of medical diagnosis requires the patient to forego keeping his medical condition a secret from the physician attempting to assess his condition and administer appropriate treatment.*

Allowing a medical professional to analyze a patient's blood or other body fluids for physical abnormalities, viruses and other organisms is not a matter of violating the so-called "right to privacy"; it is absolutely essential to sound medical practice, treatment and diagnosis.

Moreover, a patient with a 100% fatal, infectious disease should not have a "right" to keep knowledge of that disease a secret from the physician or dentist treating him.

CLAIM 4: Patients should not be routinely screened for HIV disease because a positive test would result in the loss of their jobs.

REALITY: Under the federal Americans with Disabilities Act (ADA), terminating or refusing to hire an individual solely on the basis of their HIV status is considered illegal unless they are in an occupation where HIV disease/AIDS is determined (by EEOC investigators or the courts) to pose "a direct threat the health or safety of himself/herself or others."[55]

Individuals experiencing HIV disease and related disorders which pose a threat to the health or safety of others in a given occupation (such as a pilot with AIDS dementia or a food handler with AIDS-related bowel parasites and tuberculosis) *should* be removed from that position or if appropriate, reassigned to another position where they do not endanger other people.

A truly caring individual would *want* to know if they have physical or mental disorders which could endanger the health and safety of others in the workplace.

Provision of Insurance is Based on Risk Factors

CLAIM 5: Patients should not be routinely screened for HIV disease because a positive result would interfere with their ability to obtain life, health or disability insurance.

REALITY: The provision of insurance coverage must be based on sound actuarial risk principles for a company to remain solvent and retain the ability to pay claims to its policyholders. An individual with repeated offences for driving under the influence of alcohol or drugs is at a much higher risk for future accidents and can be denied automobile coverage. Cigarette smokers cost more to insure because they have a greater susceptibility to cancer, heart disease and other serious ailments.

Policyholders Must Be Protected

Individuals who discover they have *any* terminal or life-threatening illness do not have an intrinsic "right" to then go out and obtain million dollar life insurance policies. If insurers were compelled to accept any and every applicant *carte blanche*, it would wreak financial havoc on the companies and their policyholders whom they are supposed to protect. In order to provide secure financial protection and benefits to their policyholders, insurance companies must remain financially stable. In Washington, D.C. an edict was passed prohibiting insurance companies from requiring AIDS testing. Scores of companies were compelled to stop accepting new applications from that area.

AIDS Insurance Fraud Costs Consumers Millions

During the course of the AIDS epidemic it became apparent that many high risk group members were finding out they were infected with AIDS through anonymous testing and then fraudulently obtaining large life insurance policies. As insurance companies began screening applicants using the AIDS antibody test, individuals who knew they were at risk circumvented having to take the blood test by taking out life insurance policies with various companies at amounts below those which required a blood test, a practice known as "stacking policies." If the standard maximum amount of insurance companies would provide without a blood test for AIDS was $100,000, individuals who knew or suspected they were HIV positive stacked up coverage under that amount with several different companies.

Dr. Paul Emtacher, medical director of the Metropolitan Life Insurance Company, has stated his company paid out a colossal $368 million in personal insurance claims for deaths caused by AIDS between 1985 and the middle of 1987 and that the liability costs for the disease were rising each year. "In the past two years [1985-1987], we have seen the average size of policies increasing significantly and we are seeing more people who are at high risk for AIDS apply for them," he said.

New York Life has released evidence that AIDS carriers were taking out life insurance policies after they were aware that they were terminally ill. The trend was evinced by a marked increase in the dollar amounts for death claims for AIDS and an inordinate percentage of claims on policies in force less than two years. From September, 1985 to February, 1987 the company had 110 claims totalling $7.1 million for AIDS-related deaths, as determined by death certificates. Fifty percent (50%) of the policies were in force less than two years, compared with an average of 13% for all life policies. Moreover, the average size of each policy was twice the amount of policies in force two years or longer. The company said that many more claims could have been included but that AIDS was not officially listed as the cause of death.

According to a spokesman for Metropolitan, the average amount of Metropolitan policies paid out to the beneficiaries of people who died of AIDS during 1986 was $68,000–three times (300% higher) the amount of policies involving other deaths.[56]

That type of fraud has now been guarded against by a sophisticated intercompany tracking system which screens out applicants who attempt to fraudulently obtain and stack coverage. Many companies now require HIV blood tests when applying for even low amounts of coverage. In the meantime, insurance fraud perpetrated by AIDS carriers unfairly cost companies and consumers hundreds of millions–perhaps even billions–of dollars.

The argument that individuals should refuse to be tested for HIV disease because if found to be positive they would not be able to take out more life insurance, is medically unsound, ethically wrong and smacks of fraudulent intent. Insurance underwriters have an obligation to protect their policyholders by taking AIDS into account when individuals apply for coverage just as they do for every other terminal disease.

CLAIM 6: Allowing physicians to routinely test for AIDS will drive people at high risk of carrying HIV "underground" and result in the lack of provision of vital health care services to those who need it most.

REALITY: Due to the unprecedented prohibition of routine HIV testing, the vast majority of HIV carriers are *already* "underground," and unknowingly or knowingly are in danger of spreading a lethal infectious disease to others. Routine HIV testing in hospitals, STD clinics, TB clinics, and by private physicians would *help*, not hinder, the treatment of those with the disease. Individuals with HIV disease need to be diagnosed as early as possible so they can receive treatment *and* be instructed not to engage in activities which could transmit the disease.

CLAIM 7: Routine obligatory testing of patients for HIV disease would result in AIDS patients being "stigmatized" and unable to receive appropriate health care.

REALITY: In a study of homosexuals with HIV disease, 97% admitted they had *not* been denied medical care by physicians due to their infectious condition.[57] There are physicians, dentists and others health care professionals who specialize in the treatment of people with HIV disease. Physicians who are made aware that a patient has HIV disease may wish to refer them to infectious disease specialists just as they may refer patients with heart disease to cardiologists. Such referrals are common in medical practice and *appear* to be permitted under the ADA. (Physicians should nevertheless *always* seek legal counsel *prior* to establishing any policy regarding HIV-infected patients).

Moreover, it is incongruous to demand that physicians prescribe relevant treatment for patients who insist that the true nature of their disease is irrelevant.

CLAIM 8: Large scale mandatory HIV screening of patients (or health care workers) would be prohibitively expensive and yield many false positive results.

REALITY: The United States Army conducts mandatory HIV screening of all applicants and active duty personnel. Over a five year period (1985-1990), 4.66 million blood samples were tested for the presence of HIV disease using the ELISA test. Samples were collected from recruits, Army active duty, Army National Guard, Army Reserves, and the Coast Guard. Positive samples were subsequently analyzed using the Western Blot and other confirmatory tests.

Researchers from the Walter Reed Retroviral Research Group determined that the rate of false positive results over a five year period was approximately 1 out of 424,000 specimens tested. The five year average direct and indirect costs of the screening program was $4.55 per specimen tested – hardly a monumental sum, particularly when compared to the billions of dollars being spent on "AIDS research" and "AIDS education." The researchers concluded, "*A large scale, accurate and cost effective HIV screening program is feasible.*"[58]

RENOWNED HEART SURGEON REFUSES TO OPERATE

When asked why he refused to do coronary artery bypass surgery on two patients who tested positive for HIV, Milwaukee's Dr. W. Dudley Johnson, a coronary bypass pioneer, stated, "It is our policy not to do surgery [on AIDS virus carriers]." An assistant professor of surgery at the Medical College of Wisconsin, Dr. Johnson said he found it appalling that all surgeons do not insist on their patients being tested prior to surgery. He said *he already had high levels of antibodies to the hepatitis B virus, and "I would just as soon not have a high antibody level for AIDS."*[59] During prolonged heart surgery many health care workers can be exposed to the patient's blood.

COMPULSORY OPERATIONS COULD COST MANY LIVES

Opponents of mandatory HIV patient testing argue that exposure to HIV disease is simply an occupational hazard which health care workers must face. If a physician contracts AIDS, becomes demented and dies, "that just goes with the territory."

However, a physician who acquires HIV from a patient will not be able to provide vitally needed operations and treatment to thousands of others. The crux of the issue is: Does the palliative or non-existent benefit to a patient with a fatal infectious disease take priority over the grave danger to health care personnel?

When a doctor becomes infected with HIV, the following losses result:

1. He should no longer perform invasive procedures due to the risk of infecting patients.
2. He is subject to mental impairments which render him unfit to operate or otherwise practice medicine.
3. He will die a horrendous and untimely death.
4. Years of expensive, intense training and experience can no longer be a benefit to thousands of other patients who could have been helped.
5. His wife and children suffer the loss of a husband and father (or wife and mother if the doctor is female) and may be put at risk of infection.

This issue of operating on HIV-infected patients should be decided by individual physicians and dentists at risk of becoming mortally infected rather than arbitrarily dictated by politicians, bureaucrats and self-serving political special interest groups.

While it is unfortunate that individuals have contracted an infectious, fatal disease, it would be more tragic still if through political coercion more medical professionals lose their lives and are rendered incapable of providing surgical treatment to those who could have had their lives saved.

MORE HEALTH CARE WORKERS MAY BE INFECTED

Researchers from the University of California state ". . . *the possibility of seronegative health care workers who are latently infected cannot be excluded.*"[60] Some health care workers who have been infected with a minute dose of HIV may take longer to develop antibodies but are in reality infected with the virus. This is another reason why there should be increased testing of health care workers using sensitive tests which reveal the presence of the virus soon after infection occurs.

AIDS PATIENTS ANGRY AT BEING "STIGMATIZED"

AIDS advocacy groups have expressed indignation over the policy of placing AIDS patients in private isolation rooms with signs reading "BLOOD AND BODY FLUID PRECAUTIONS." They voiced resentment at having physicians and nurses wearing gowns, rubber smocks, face masks and eye goggles when treating them.

Excerpts from an article written by a homosexual hospitalized for AIDS reveal the mentality of those who contested the precautions being used by health care workers:

> . . . I was awoken by the sound of rustling plastic and opened my eyes to be confronted by a nurse in boots, plastic apron, hat, and rubber gloves. I wanted to die–there and then. When she returned 20 minutes later *I asked why she was dressed in this weird outfit and was told that she had the right to protect herself.* I replied that I also had a choice and I chose not to be cared for by an *ill-informed and insensitive nurse.* That salutary little experience was, fortunately, the only one I remember. I hasten to add that the hospital went to great lengths to educate its staff, and *this would never happen now. Moreover, my reaction proved to me that I had started fighting.*
> . . . *I had PCP, TB, CMV, herpes, and cryptosporidiosis. Jackpot!*[61]

The irate patient had *P. carinii* pneumonia, tuberculosis (which is readily transmitted by coughing, sneezing and breathing), CMV (which can cause severe birth defects if contracted by a woman shortly before or during pregnancy), herpes (which in AIDS patients appear as large ulcerating blisters on the face and rectal/genital area and can be transmitted to intact skin), and cryptosporidiosis (a contagious bowel disease which can result in 10-20 quarts of explosive, uncontrollable, infectious diarrhea per day). Besides AIDS, these other highly contagious infections warranted the strictest isolation measures to protect against contamination. Yet, the patient superciliously derided the poor nurse for trying to protect herself!

Among other factors, this contempt for being treated as carriers of a deadly contagious disease has been an impetus behind the crusade against universal testing. In deference to the demands of the AIDS lobby, health care workers and hospitals were told to treat *every* patient as though they had AIDS so that no one would have any idea of which patients carry the disease. In the article, the homosexual AIDS patient declares, "I hasten to add that the hospital went to great lengths to educate its staff, and "*this* [wearing of "stigmatizing" protective garments] *would never happen now.*"

Instead of allowing hospitals to routinely test patients for AIDS and place them in a separate unit or room, hospitals across the country have been compelled to spend untold millions of dollars on measures to treat every patient as though they have AIDS. In addition to the mammoth costs of treating AIDS, implementation of "universal precautions" has driven up the cost of health care.

SOUND MEDICAL PRACTICE TURNED TOPSY-TURVY

Recently enacted OSHA (Occupational Health and Safety Administration) regulations impose exorbitant ($50,000+) fines on medical and dental establishments and private businesses which do not comply with a slew of burdensome, costly and outlandish "infection control" policies and procedures. These Draconian "universal precautions" are supposedly designed to protect workers from hepatitis B and AIDS – diseases which the public has been told repeatedly are difficult to contract. In reality, these regulations allow those infected to remain anonymous while continuing to put others, including health care workers, at risk. Heavy-handed OSHA requirements are another means by which the AIDS lobby has circumvented the critical need of mandatory testing of patients and staff.

To practice routine hygiene when dealing with patients is prudent. There are 40 million people that come through hospitals annually *plus* millions of medical and dental patients treated in public and private facilities. To deny physicians, dentists, nurses and other health care professionals the right to know which patients actually have HIV disease and compel them to treat everyone as though they have AIDS is impractical, extraordinarily expensive and inimical to sound medical practice.

THE FOREMOST UNIVERSAL PRECAUTION

Compulsory testing of blood donors is the foremost universal precaution for preventing HIV transmission to transfusion recipients. Mandatory testing of patients should be the foremost "universal precaution" for curtailing HIV transmission to health care workers.

The New Jersey State Medical Society recently endorsed AIDS testing of all hospital patients. According to Dr. Robert Stackpole who wrote the proposal, *"Universal testing for HIV is long overdue."*[62]

MEDICAL ETHICS DEMAND MANDATORY TESTING

Martin S. Lewin, M.D., has written in *American Medical News*:

Medical ethics demand that a physician, more particularly a surgeon, infected with HIV either so inform patients or cease to have contact with them. *It is of equal importance that physicians know the HIV status of their patients....*

Because of the generally fatal nature of HIV infection, *it is mandatory not only that patients know of their possible exposure to HIV from their physician but also that each physician know of his possible exposure from his patient.* It is equally important to generate regulations on both points.[63]

CHAPTER TEN

THE THREAT OF "SAFE SEX"

We demand:
Federal encouragement and support for sex education courses, pre-
pared and taught by gay women and men, presenting homosexuality
as a valid, healthy preference and lifestyle as a viable alternative to
heterosexuality.
  – 1972 Gay Rights Platform[1]

Education concerning AIDS must start at the lowest grade possible as
part of any health and hygiene program. . . . There are a number of
people, primarily adolescents, that do not yet know they will be ho-
mosexual. . . . They must be reached and taught the risk behaviors
that expose them to infection with the AIDS virus. . . . There is no
doubt we need sex education in the schools and that it must include
[non-judgemental] information on heterosexual and homosexual
relationships.
  – Dr. C. Everett Koop, Surgeon General's Report on AIDS[2]

Teachers of first graders have an opportunity to give children a
healthy sense of identity at an early age. Classes should include refer-
ences to lesbians/gay people in all curricular areas. . . .
  – Contemporary curriculum for elementary schools[3]

In a classroom in the Dallas suburb of Plano, Texas, children sit
and watch with a mixture of embarrassment and fascination as the
teacher rolls a condom on and off a broom handle as part of a 13-
step demonstration for "safe sex." "Now you do it to each other,"
the teacher says smilingly. The boys tear open the condom packets
which have been handed out by the school. "That's right," the
teacher, still smiling, coos, "hand them to your partners. Inspect
the condom for any obvious pinholes. Now extend your finger, pre-
tending it is an erect penis. Have your partner gently roll the condom onto your finger." Some of the boys and girls, still exhibiting
vestiges of modesty, are obviously abashed. They hesitate. The
teacher perceiving their reluctance, takes control, "You may feel
uncomfortable with this, but it is a *life skill* you need to learn. Now

remember to roll the condom on gently, so as to avoid breakage."
There sit dozens of boys, with their middle fingers stretched out as
their distaff classmates roll condoms on. "Now remember," the
teacher cautions, "condoms can break without proper lubrication.
Take the tube of spermicidal jelly, squeeze the tube and smear the
jelly on the condom. The girls gently smear lubricating jelly over
the condom. "Now pretend your partner has ejaculated. *Gently* roll
the condom off his finger to avoid letting any of the sperm leak
out. When you have sex, you don't want to let any of the sperm
leak out and spill over into your vagina." The teacher then has the
students change roles, and the boys repeat the procedure using the
girls' fingers.

Similar hands-on demonstrations are being repeated across the
United States under the banner of AIDS awareness and prevention programs. Parents who object are subject to jibes and derision
from school officials such as:

– Your children are or soon will be sexually active.
– Don't try living in the dark ages. Times have changed.
– Your kids will have sex with whom they wish, when they wish,
  whether you like it or not.
– The question is not if they will become sexually active, but when
  they become sexually active will they have the skills necessary to
  avoid AIDS?
– In the age of AIDS, ignorance is not bliss; it can kill. Most parents don't feel comfortable talking about sexual reproduction
  and contraception with their children. It is the job of the schools
  to give the children the skills to cope with the real world.
– The former Surgeon General of the United States, Dr. C. Everett Koop, has urged the implementation of sex education programs to prevent AIDS.
– Education is the only means we have to fight AIDS.
– Parents who attempt to interfere with teaching children "safe
  sex" techniques can be considered accomplices in causing unwanted pregnancies, STDs and the spread of AIDS and death.

In the face of such a torrent of criticism, most parents give in
and allow their sons and daughters to participate in the "safe sex"
programs.

Before assessing the repercussions of explicit courses in "safe"
pre-marital sex and sodomy as a means of AIDS prevention, it is
critical to recognize that the notion "education is the only answer
to stopping AIDS" is a fundamentally flawed premise. The front
line of controlling the growth of a deadly sexually transmitted disease is not "education." Dr. Olav H. Alvig notes in the *American
Medical News*:

There is a sexually transmitted disease with a very long incubation period, that is life threatening, and incurable. AIDS? No, syphilis prior to 1945. It was defeated by routine epidemiologic techniques. Everyone was tested when hospitalized, married or inducted into the armed forces until the affected were identified, counseled and all contacts followed.[4]

Precedented effective public health measures* should not be glossed over as obsolete. Identification of infectious HIV carriers, contact tracing, and closing of the homosexual bathhouses and "sex shops" which are fountainheads of mass HIV dissemination are the foremost steps which need to be taken to combat the spread of AIDS.

HOMOSEXUAL BATHHOUSES DOING A BUSTLING BUSINESS

In a study of homosexual males who contracted AIDS, 50% admitted attending homosexual bathhouses.[5] The major function of these so-called bathhouses is to provide an inexpensive place where homosexual males can engage in frequent anonymous homosexual activities without fear of social or legal reprisal. The average patron may engage in homosexual acts with nearly a dozen or more participants.[6]

The bathhouses entice younger males by offering them discounts such as cheap locker rates. Younger males who contract HIV then spread it to unsuspecting partners, including young females. Contrary to popular belief, these sordid centers of mass contagion have not been shut down. Despite the deaths of thousands of homosexuals due to AIDS, the bathhouses remain in operation. In many areas, the baths have actually mushroomed, sometimes under the front of "health clubs for men," or as "sex shops." Contemporary homosexual travel guidebooks list the location of these and similar establishments across the United States and internationally.

When a restaurant is found to have unsanitary conditions responsible for causing repeated outbreaks of food poisoning or hepatitis, public health officials order the restaurant to be closed. It would be outrageous to leave the restaurant open and instead conduct "safe-eating" classes for school-children and distribute free stomach pumps.

In like manner, the failure to shut down the major breeding grounds of AIDS contagion and enact other disease control measures cannot be offset by instituting K-12 "safe sex" indoctrination workshops and distributing condoms.

*See Chapter 12

Foisting spurious "safe sex" programs on school-children while utterly neglecting the foremost effective disease control measures is a travesty of sound public health policy.

THE FAILURE OF "SAFE SEX" EDUCATION AMONG HIGH RISK GROUP MEMBERS

One way of assessing the validity of utilizing "safe sex" education to control the future spread of AIDS is to examine the results of similar campaigns among high risk group members. It would not be prudent to resort to measures which have proven ineffective and counterproductive. Those who don't remember the past are condemned to repeat it.

Over the past decade, homosexual males have been inundated with private and government sponsored books, pamphlets and workshops urging the adoption of various "risk-reduction" techniques to curtail the spread of HIV. Homosexual and non-homosexual tabloids, newspapers and periodicals have repeatedly run articles and ads describing in explicit detail the activities which can transmit HIV. Homosexual bathhouses have handed out "safe sex" kits to patrons.

These "educational efforts" have proven woefully ineffective in checking the spread of HIV disease in the targeted group. Evidence from around the world indicates that, despite massive "safe sex" campaigns, the impact on reducing the spread of HIV among homosexuals has been palliative at best.[7] By 1989, over 50% of homosexual males in Houston, Texas had contracted HIV disease.[8]

An apparent reduction in the rate of rectal/oral gonorrhea among homosexuals has been cited as evidence of "radical alterations in behavior," but this is not necessarily the case.[9] Between 1989-1990, after the expenditure of millions of dollars on extensive "AIDS education" efforts among homosexuals, the rate of gonorrhea in this group skyrocketed 400%.[10]

The notion of using a condom during rectal sodomy as "protected sex" is dangerous and misleading. A study of the use of condoms in HIV prevention efforts among homosexuals, which had received $2.2 million in federal grants, was suspended because the rate of HIV was so pervasive and the failure rate of condoms so high (during sodomy) that it would have caused more deaths than it prevented.[11] The lopsided emphasis on academic "risk-reduction techniques" rather than enactment of aggressive disease control measures has proven to be a public health disaster. Multitudes of homosexual/bisexual males have become infected, along with their unsuspecting female partners. Homosexual males who know they are HIV positive are more likely to continue engaging in "high-risk" behaviors.[12]

"SEX EDUCATION" SET THE STAGE FOR VD EPIDEMICS

In March of 1984, the U.S. Department of Education conducted hearings in seven cities regarding the Protection of Pupils Rights Amendment, also known as the Hatch Amendment. Testimonies of concerned parents, civic and church leaders and others were given. The major media and press virtually ignored the hearings. The book *Child Abuse in the Classroom* presents numerous transcripts from those hearings.[13] The following are several excerpts which vividly portray the type of indoctrination our nation's children are being subjected to:

– A parent of an eighth grader from Bellevue, Washington, testified that various questionnaires handed out to the children *presupposed* that all the children were already being promiscuous. "Of course, they constantly reminded the children to go to Planned Parenthood for their birth control.

"The parents have no idea the kids are being asked these things. There is one teacher in Bellevue who has all the boys say 'vagina'; he calls them individually and they have to all say this out loud in class. The boys say 'vagina' and the girls say 'penis'. One girl told me that she was so embarrassed that she could hardly bring out the word 'penis' because all these boys were sitting in the class. It just embarrassed her so. So he made her get up in front of the class and very loudly say it ten times."

"I FEEL WHAT THEY ARE ACCOMPLISHING IS TO EMBARRASS THEM, TO BREAK DOWN THEIR NATURAL SENSE OF MODESTY, TO JUST BREAK DOWN THEIR BARRIERS. . . . They say that they don't want the kids to have sex, but IF THEY BREAK DOWN THEIR NATURAL DEFENSES, THOSE KIDS ARE GOING TO HAVE SEX MORE EASILY."

– A parent from Lincoln City, Oregon, testified: "In my son's fifth grade Health class, all questions were answered without regard to a moral right or wrong. Homosexuality was presented as an alternative lifestyle. SEXUAL ACTIVITY AMONG FIFTH GRADERS WAS NOT DISCOURAGED since it was feared that the students might be embarrassed and not ask additional questions.

I was present when a plastic model of female genitalia with a tampon insert was passed around so they might understand how tampons fit. Birth control pills were passed around and examined. ANAL INTERCOURSE [sodomy] WAS DESCRIBED. AT NO TIME WAS THERE ANY MENTION OF ABSTINENCE AS A DESIRABLE ALTERNATIVE FOR 5TH GRADERS. The morality that was taught in the classroom that day was complete promiscuity."

– Another parent from the same area stated that his daughter had been punished for being removed from this type of program. Emotionally, she was openly chided and ridiculed by other children in the school, without intervention from her teachers; physically she was detained and threatened with a pink slip if she did not attend, causing her to lose "free time" during school, unlike the students who attended the programs.

– A father of three young boys from a town in Michigan delineated portions of a compulsory sex education curriculum for eighth graders which included the following questions:

One, do you know why your parents and/or religion have taught that intercourse should wait until marriage? Do you accept these ideas? If so, then would you be creating a lot of inner turmoil to go against your own beliefs?

Two, do you really feel comfortable and firm in your own beliefs? Try to imagine how you would feel about losing your virginity. Would it make you feel less valuable, less lovable, less good? If so, it is a bad bargain. [Note: this last line would be cited by education authorities as "encouraging abstinence." Read on.] . . .

Five, what does intercourse mean to you – a permanent commitment for life, fidelity for both partners, love?

Six, however you answered question five, does your current relationship meet those criteria? . . .

Seven, is your current relationship emotionally open and intimate? . . . You are much more likely to have a satisfying experience if the relationship is on that level before you have intercourse.

Eight, can you get effective contraception and will you both use it faithfully and correctly?

Nine, are you prepared to face a pregnancy should your contraception fail?

Ten, Do you have the opportunity for uninterrupted privacy, free from fear of being heard or intruded upon?"

When the school boards are confronted by parents' objections [to this type of indoctrination] they say, 'Well, your children have a choice.' But when my sister-in-law refused to consent to having my niece enrolled in this type of program, the school authorities made the girl compile book report upon book report, an unreasonable amount of book reports, to be done each week. *Not only that, she was separated from her schoolmates and completely isolated and made a social outcast, until enough pressure was exerted upon her mother that she finally consented for her daughter to become part of this sex education program.*

Is this not an attempt to change and subvert our children's way of thought and discredit parents who hold traditional values and beliefs?"

– From Phoenix, Arizona: "The need to protect pupils' rights is evident from 'health education' programs. One of the most objectionable sex questionnaires was published by the Federal Department of Health Education and Welfare [H.E.W.] in 1979. Consider some of the questions deemed to be appropriate for all adolescents of junior high age or older:

#12. How often do you normally masturbate (play with yourself sexually)?

#13. How often do you normally engage in light petting (playing with a girl's breasts)?

#14. How often do you normally engage in heavy petting (playing with a girl's vagina and the area around it)?

Also consider these questions on page 150 from the "Psychological Inventory":

#112. I think *sexual activities like hand stimulation and oral sex are pleasurable ways to enjoy sex and not worry about getting pregnant.* [Note: Mutual masturbation is now taught in AIDS education as "safe sex" or "outercourse." A latex "dental dam" is being recommended during oral sex.]

#119. For me, trying out different sexual activities is an important part of learning about what I enjoy.

This type of questioning has to be regulated under the Hatch Amendment."

PARENT GETS OBJECTIONABLE CURRICULUM REMOVED

Mary Park Hiles, a leader in the fight for children's and parents' rights, testified:

"My first introduction to how schools have changed occurred five years ago. *I saw a movie which was shown to 8th graders in the kindergarten through 12th grade Human Development curriculum in their Human Sexuality Unit. The movie was 20 minutes long and depicted nude masturbation in detail. It showed how men do it, women do it, why they do it and where it feels best. Teenage actors were used.*

I determined to find out what was behind this K-12 curriculum. A teacher called me and said she had a copy of the 13-year curriculum guide and said she would leave it in her top desk drawer. I could come in when she was out, take it, and use it any way I wanted. *I xeroxed 200 copies, spread it around the school, and both the program and the principal were removed from the school."*

These types of teaching are not isolated occurrences happening in a few radical-type fringe schools San Francisco and New York. They are being taught in school districts across the country, in rural and urban communities. Prior to and along with the advent of the AIDS epidemic, sex education and "values clarification" courses have been introduced in school systems throughout the United States and parts of Canada. Frequently, the children are not allowed to bring home the books and pamphlets they are instructed with at school; they are told that their parents "wouldn't understand" and might object.

IS TEACHING "SAFE SEX" BETTER THAN NOTHING?

"Safe sex" advocates argue that, notwithstanding the lack of public health measures, there are thousands of people who have been infected with HIV and are not aware of their condition. Many people, especially adolescents, are continuing to engage in pre-marital sex and risk exposure to a myriad of STDs including HIV, as well as possibly experiencing an unplanned pregnancy. Certainly, they contend, it would be better for a young girl not to become pregnant in the first place than to face the dilemma of whether to abort or give birth to an "unwanted child." It is appropriate, even moral, "safe sex" advocates assert, to instruct young people as to precautions which could help forestall these undesirable outcomes.

THE GOALS OF SEX EDUCATION

That there is a major problem of STDs and pre-marital pregnancy among teenagers cannot be denied. The issue is whether conventional sex instruction classes have curtailed or in fact, contributed to the problem of pre-marital sex among children and adolescents.

The following are brief excerpts from a cross-section of the premiere sex instruction textbooks which have been used across the country for a number of years.

The books *Boys and Sex* and *Girls and Sex* (New York: Delacorte Press, 1981) by Wardell Pomeroy, Ph.D, co-author of the Kinsey Reports, are extremely graphic in their explicit, glowing descriptions of heavy petting, foreplay and a variety of positions for sexual intercourse. *The books have been recommended reading for 6th grade children* (11-year-olds!) in the Milwaukee Public schools and elsewhere.

"LOVING" BESTIALITY

Pomeroy states: "I have known cases of farm boys who have had A LOVING SEXUAL RELATIONSHIP WITH AN ANIMAL and who felt good about their behavior until they got to college . . . where they were made to feel guilty" (pp. 171-172).

ALSO FROM *BOYS AND SEX*:

PREMARITAL INTERCOURSE DOES HAVE ITS DEFINITE VALUES AS A TRAINING GROUND for marriage or some other committed relationship. . . . In this sense, boys and girls who start having intercourse when they're adolescents, expecting to get married later on, will find that it's a big help in finding out whether they are really congenial or not; to make everyday-life comparisons again, IT'S LIKE TAKING A CAR OUT ON A TEST RUN before you buy it" (p. 117).

There are many possible positions [for intercourse], one is . . . . Another position is . . . . In still another position . . . . One advantage of these positions is . . . (p. 127).

FROM *GIRLS AND SEX:*

PETTING IS ALSO EXTREMELY USEFUL AS A LEARNING EXPERIENCE for later relationships, perhaps one that's better than intercourse itself. A boy ought to know how to stimulate a girl properly, and she ought to know what it's like to be stimulated. . . . THERE ARE MANY GIRLS WHO REGRET AFTER MARRIAGE THAT THEY DIDN'T HAVE PRE-MARITAL INTERCOURSE, because they've come to realize what a long, slow learning process it is after marriage. . . .

And from *Changing Bodies, Changing Lives: A Book for Teens on Sex and Relationships* (New York: Random House, 1980):

LESBIANISM AMONG 7-YEAR-OLDS

For you, "exploring sex" might mean kissing and hugging someone you're attracted to. . . . Later, it might mean giving each other orgasms, or even making love. . . . *Often this kind of sexual exploring is with a friend of your own sex.* Lisa remembered: *"I had my first sexual experience when I was seven years old. It was with my best friend.* We were constantly together. . . . Then one day we started fooling around and touching each other all over. For about a year, we'd sleep over at each other's houses and do this" (p. 85).

"EXPLORING SEX WITH SOMEONE OF YOUR OWN SEX"

We're also taught that a person is either all heterosexual or all homosexual, and for life. This isn't true, but it makes us afraid of any same-sex feelings we might have. MOST PEOPLE ARE NEITHER "ALL STRAIGHT" OR "ALL GAY" (p. 112).

Fear of gayness hurts straight people, too. Fear and prejudice go away quickest when you can meet some open homosexuals and know them as people. . . . *The rest of this chapter may be a way for you to "meet" some gay and lesbian teenagers indirectly and dispel some of the myths that contribute to the fear and discrimination against gay people* (pp. 112-114).

Barry, seventeen, is gay: "I REMEMBER MAKING OUT WITH A GUY FOR THE FIRST TIME. We used to play basketball in the lot down the street and then come back to my place for a soda. This one time we were clowning around with towels drying off each other's sweat, and we started leaning up against each other. IT WAS REAL EXCITING AND REAL TENDER. We hugged and kissed for a while, then we went for a walk to get used to what had happened" (p. 95).

LESBIANS MAKE LOVE [SIC] IN LOTS OF WAYS. Sometimes . . . [graphic, positive description of lesbian acts are given]. GAY MEN, TOO, HAVE MANY WAYS OF MAKING LOVE [SIC]. One may . . . [graphic, positive descriptions of oral and rectal sodomy are given] (p. 122).

You may think, as many people do, that WE SHOULD STOP THINKING VIRGINITY IS SO SPECIAL, and make our decisions about sex for other reasons (p. 99).

As the AIDS death toll mounted among homosexuals, it would seem reasonable for there to have been a semblance of recognition that homosexual sodomy was not the ideal alternative lifestyle that had been extolled. Yet in 1986, the book *Learning About Sex; The Contemporary Guide for Young Adults* by Gary F. Kelly (New York: Barron's) presented young people with the following pearls of wisdom:

SADO-MASOCHISM MAY BE VERY ACCEPTABLE AND SAFE for sexual partners who know each other's needs and have established agreements for what they want from each other (p. 61).

. . . A FAIR PERCENTAGE OF PEOPLE PROBABLY HAVE SOME SORT OF SEXUAL CONTACT WITH AN ANIMAL during their life-times, particularly boys who live on farms. THERE ARE NO INDICA-TIONS THAT SUCH ANIMAL CONTACTS ARE HARMFUL. (p. 61)

SOME PEOPLE ARE NOW SAYING THAT PARTNER-SHIPS–MARRIED OR UNMARRIED–SHOULD NOT BE EXCLU-SIVE. They believe that while a primary relationship is maintained with one person, the freedom for both partners to love and share sex with others should always be present. . . . There is no general statement that can be made here about the "best" or "healthiest" way to be . . . . *Swinging or mate swapping . . . happens between couples who are friends and gradually become involved sexually* (pp. 136-137).

HOMOSEXUALITY IS RECOGNIZED TO BE A VALID LIFE-STYLE which seems to be suitable for those who prefer to love and have sexual rela-tionships with their own sex. . . . Most human beings have the potential for both heterosexual and homosexual attraction, and that most of us learn to be heterosexual because our culture finds that pattern more acceptable (pp. 56, 58).

In the traditional marriage, however, it was sometimes impossible for the partners to be who they really were as individuals . . . but MOST GAY MEN AND WOMEN REPORT THAT THEY HAVE ALWAYS FELT THEM-SELVES TO BE AT AN ADVANTAGE IN FINDING TRUE EQUAL-ITY IN A RELATIONSHIP (p. 133).

Oral sexual contact means using the mouth or tongue to. . . . It is a common way of achieving orgasm for both males and females. . . . A majority of peo-ple find oral sexual contact to be pleasurable and acceptable (p. 71).

ANAL SEX REFERS TO THE INSERTION OF THE MALE [SIC] PENIS INTO THE ANUS OF HIS PARTNER. It is a form of sexual behavior that may be shared by male homosexuals and by heterosexual couples. . . . Unlike the vagina, the anus does not have its own source of lubrication, thus *great gentleness and care must be taken, and a lubricating substance is often neces-sary for insertion.* Because bacteria live in the rectum, THE PENIS SHOULD NOT BE INSERTED IN THE VAGINA OR MOUTH FOLLOWING ANAL INSERTION WITHOUT BEING WASHED FIRST [Note the graphic teaching of "safe" sodomy] (p. 72).

There are, of course, many other double standards for males and females, many of them as equally absurd. Take, for example, the idea that it is all right for girls to touch and kiss each other as ways of showing tenderness and affection, but that is not all right for boys (p. 73).

School-children are taught that anal sodomy-the number one means of HIV transmission in the United States – is merely an-other positive form of sexual expression; they only need to use a lubricant and wash off afterwards. Not surprisingly, this book received the highest accolades from leading sex educators: "*A must for all young people*," said Dr. Patricia Shiller, Founder, American Association of Sex Educators, Counselors, and Therapists. Dr. Mary S. Calderone, Co-founder and Former President, Sex Information and Education Council of the U.S. (SIECUS) asserted, "There isn't a person picking up this book who won't find something of special help and meaning in it." *Learning About Sex* was voted onto the Best Books for Young Adults List by the American Library Association.

PROSELYTIZING CHILDREN

Project Ten is a national project designed to encourage confused teenagers who feel they are homosexually inclined to accept their inclination as positive and to teach their peers to be more loving and tolerant toward them. The name "Project Ten" is based on the grossly inflated estimate that 10% of the population is homosexual – a claim that has been thoroughly debunked in the well-documented exposé, *Kinsey, Sex and Fraud*.[14]

Project Ten distributes *One Teenager in Ten*, a handbook presenting case histories ostensibly narrated by homosexual/lesbian teenagers who have "come out of the closet" – oftentimes through the help and seduction of a much older deviant counterpart.

"Amy," describes in sensuous, graphic detail various lesbian acts perpetrated on her at the age of 13 by her 23-year-old dance teacher. Writing of her introduction into lesbianism, the girl, barely into puberty, writes "I became a lesbian and a 'woman' that weekend!"

Elsewhere, "Rick," describes his warm feelings about undergoing receptive anal sodomy for the first time (at age 15) by an older drifter he just met: "He came back with a tube of KY stuck in his towel. . . . I felt like a bride on her honeymoon. . . . I was in love."[15]

In the foreword, *Publishers Weekly* describes the meanderings of the newly initiated teenage lesbians and homosexuals in glowing terms: "Heard here are courageous voices, voices of young people wise beyond their years."

SEX EDUCATORS HAVE A DISTINCT AGENDA

A publishing house in Boston has issued two colorfully illustrated books aimed at children ages two to five that portray homosexual and lesbian pairs as loving "families." *Daddy's Roommate* depicts a boy whose parents divorce. Daddy moves in with Frank. The men eat, shave, work, fight and sleep together. "But they always make up," and the boy's relationship with both males is described as warm and loving. *Heather has Two Mommies* follows a similar theme.[16]

As outrageous as the courses and texts just described may appear, they are representative of the views taught nationally in "values clarification" curricula which are insinuated throughout various courses – including home economics, hygiene, physical education, English and social studies.

Parents and other concerned citizens need to realize that there is a distinct ideological framework undergirding the groups which crusade for universal mandatory K-12 AIDS/sex "education." These groups believe that pre-marital sex is an integral, positive part of growing up. In their view, children and adolescents who do *not* engage in sexual experimentation will become repressed and suffer sexual dysfunction later in marriage or with "significant others" in adulthood. Parents and concerned others should not be surprised that rational arguments about the failure rate of condoms are falling on deaf ears.

The explicit indoctrination that is taking place in many of the nation's classrooms has had a definite impact; up to 50% of teenagers admit to engaging in pre-marital sex, many with more than one partner. One million teenage girls become pregnant each year and 2.5 million teens contract a venereal disease.

Now the self-styled "family planning" groups which have promoted the behaviors leading to the epidemic of VD and the vast number of teen pregnancies claim that they have the answer to curbing the transmission of AIDS among adolescents – condom education. Researchers report, however, that exposure to a sex instruction program which includes discussion of contraceptives increases the likelihood by up to 40% that a youngster will engage in pre-marital sex (fornication).[17]

Parents and teachers need to seriously question whether promoting the conventional copulate-before-marriage-or-suffer-pangs-of-remorse-for-missing-out approach used in typical sex-instruction curricula is really in the best interests of children. They may wish to consider a fresh progressive approach which boldly inculcates sound ethical values, self-restraint and abstinence.[18]

Dr. Melvin Anchell, renowned psychiatrist and authority on human sexuality, states:

> *The truth is that typical sex-education courses are almost perfect recipes for producing personality problems and even perversions later in life.*[19]

GIVE CONDOMS? GET SINGLE MOMS

Commerce City, Colorado – One of the nation's first high schools to give out condoms has been rewarded by a soaring birth rate among its students.

Adams City High's birth rate has climbed to 31% above the national average of 58.1 births per 1,000 students in the three years since it started handing out condoms. . . .

"Being pregnant at Adams City High used to be a social death sentence," reports *USA Today*'s Jana Mazanec. That "was before AIDS, safe sex and condoms became household words and teen pregnancy came out of the closet," she adds. . . .

Many people blame the increasing birth rate and the overall "acceptance" of pregnancy not only on condom distribution, but also on the controversial teen parenting program which the school offers. The program, which began in 1979, includes an on-campus nursery which takes care of the babies while the young mothers attend school [*Education Reporter*, No. 77, June 1992].

A SEX EDUCATION VICTIM'S TESTIMONY AND PLEA

East Detroit, Michigan: A mother of three children testified about the 10th grade Health and Composition classes at her local public high school: "A publication used in the health class entitled 'Sexual Intercourse' is, in effect, a virtual 'do it yourself' manual. The student is taken through foreplay, erections, when to have intercourse, positions for intercourse, orgasm. . . . This is the description that the publication asks the [adolescent] reader to consider when deciding whether or not to engage in sexual activity:

'There are two qualifications for joining in any kind of sexual activity–that an individual feels that it is right for him or her at that particular time with that particular person and that he or she is fully able to handle the sex, the love and the consequences.'

"I have a very personal testimony to share concerning Values Clarification and the effects it has on an individual, both short and long term. I was educated by the very system that I am testifying about. As a result of the indoctrination that I received as a student, I began abusing drugs and became sexually promiscuous. As a result, I became pregnant twice, and twice aborted my babies, the effects of which are still evident today. I was applauded by my teachers for my decision to abort and encouraged to share my experiences with my peers. When I was a senior in high school I was living with my boyfriend. Because of this I was invited to share in the Marriage Class at my school, and I discussed the personal and intimate details of that situation. It was only after I had nearly ruined my life that I began to reconsider what I had been taught in the public schools. By the grace of my Lord, Jesus Christ, I started to take positive changes in my life. Today, I have three children to raise, three children whom I wish to protect from the effects of this type of teaching. This is my personal mission for testifying before you today.

My suggestion, ladies and gentlemen, is that specific rules and penalties be adopted to prohibit this use of values-altering techniques practiced under the guise of education. Those rules should specifically name the techniques as Values Clarification, situation ethics, and methods used to accomplish their objectives.

Please stop this horrendous crime against the minds of our young people and the family institution. Our future as a country depends on it."[20]

Many parents are growing increasingly leery of the types of values their children are being instilled with in their local schools. It is no small wonder that private schools are experiencing a surge in enrollments and that the homeschool movement is a growing phenomenon.[21]

CHAPTER ELEVEN

THE
AMERICANS WITH DISABILITIES ACT:
A PANDORA'S BOX

In spite of the horror of the AIDS epidemic, in many ways the cause was advanced by it.
    – Cleve Jones, homosexual lobbyist, "Gay Rights Advancing Under the Banner of AIDS," *Wall Street Journal*[1]

We demand that the Federal Government amend all federal Civil Rights Acts, other legislation, and government controls to prohibit discrimination in employment, housing, public accommodations, and public services. . . .
    – National Gay Rights Platform

Private employers and privately operated establishments used by the general public as customers, clients or visitors . . . may not discriminate against individuals . . . being regarded as having a physical or mental impairment.
    – Americans with Disabilities Act

AIDS AS A WEAPON OF POLITICAL WARFARE

Don't call us AIDS victims. AIDS is not my weakness. AIDS is my strength.
    – Paul Diamond, a homosexual activist diagnosed with Kaposi's sarcoma[2]

As the AIDS epidemic expanded, homosexual advocacy groups quickly realized that the negative association of sodomy with a fatal communicable disease could reverse past political achievements. Without aggressive countermeasures, AIDS could impede their drive for a national law equating homosexuality with race, skin color and ethnicity. Homosexual groups had previously succeeded in pressuring the American Psychiatric and Psychological Associations into declaring that homosexuality was no longer a mental aberration.[3] It was therefore not possible for homosexual groups to claim that homosexuality was a mental impairment covered by handicap anti-discrimination laws.

Homosexual groups mapped an extraordinarily effective strategy to transform AIDS from being viewed as a deadly, communicable disease into a special politically protected "civil right" and a "handicap." Attention was diverted from the urgent necessity of public health measures to prevent AIDS carriers from disseminating contagion throughout the population. The focal point became protecting the rights of "AIDS victims" or "People with AIDS (PWAs)." It was repeatedly argued that precedented measures like reportability and contact tracing should not be used to protect the uninfected from a deadly infectious contagion; it was the "AIDS victims" which needed to be protected from the "insensitivity and irrational fears" of the public.

In cities and states with the highest numbers of AIDS cases, homosexual and AIDS advocacy groups succeeded in preventing HIV from being declared a sexually transmitted or communicable disease.[4] At the same time, they aggressively prodded local and state legislators into defining HIV infection/AIDS as a "disability" or a "handicap."

Public health measures to prevent the spread of deadly AIDS contagion were blocked. Instead, laws were enacted to heavily penalize private businesses, individuals and even physicians who attempted to treat AIDS as a communicable disease rather than as a specially protected "handicap." Although many homosexuals were infected with HIV disease, some were not, or did not want to let their condition be known. This necessitated other laws being passed and defined to include *all* homosexuals as members of a specially protected "handicapped" group.

LINGUISTIC SUBTERFUGE

Colorado Governor Roy Romer issued an executive order adding "persons *perceived to be at risk* from HIV infection" protected against discrimination under the state's human rights code.[5]

Since the vast majority of AIDS cases occurred among male homosexuals, measures like Romer's had the intended effect of providing *de facto* special civil rights status for homosexuals, *including those not known to be infected with AIDS*. All this was done without using politically charged terms such as "sexual preference" or "sexual orientation." Through carefully executed legislative subterfuge, AIDS, a fatal infectious disease overwhelmingly linked to promiscuous sodomy, had become a deadly wellspring of political power for the homosexual movement.

MANY STATES REFUSED TO CAPITULATE

Many state legislatures, however, refused to concur with the demands of the homosexual lobby to treat AIDS as a "handicap" rather than as a communicable disease. In Texas, for example, state legislators amended the state's handicapped law to specifically *exclude* HIV infection or AIDS from being considered a "disability." Homosexuals and transvestites were likewise excluded from being considered "disabled" under the state's Fair Housing Law.

Homosexual groups were frustrated by the unwillingness of many states and municipalities to grant *de facto* special civil rights status for homosexuals via HIV/AIDS legislation. They found it even more galling that in some cities and states, concerned pro-family citizens were increasingly successful in repealing homosexual preference legislation. These defeats added enormous impetus to the drive for a federal law which would impose the goals of the homosexual movement on all areas of the United States.

HIJACKING THE NOBLE CAUSE OF THE HANDICAPPED

Homosexual lobbyists, AIDS activists and their Congressional allies in Washington, D.C., realized that a federal law which overtly prohibited discrimination based on "sexual orientation" or "HIV infection" would be unpalatable to the majority of Americans and unlikely to pass.

Instead, they determined to use a national bill ostensibly designed to protect the rights of the handicapped to further their own political agenda.

The vehicle chosen was a bill called the "Americans with Disabilities Act (ADA)." The benevolent title of the Act touched the heartstrings; it sounded as American as apple pie, a positive, compassionate gesture to help the less fortunate.

When most people think of the term handicapped they think of people in wheelchairs, the blind, the severely retarded, persons with muscular dystrophy, etc. People have grown accustomed to wheelchair ramps and spaces designed for handicapped parking. A bill which only seemed to affirm the cause of the handicapped to better access to jobs and public facilities did not raise red flags in the minds of most of the public. Many in the media did not know, or did not care to present, the full sweeping demands imposed by the ADA.

Its sponsors touted the ADA as the "long overdue Emancipation Proclamation of the disabled community." Those daring to raise misgivings or concerns about what the ADA really entailed were portrayed as uncaring brutes who wanted to oppress the handicapped. To oppose the ADA was viewed as tantamount to kicking the crutches out from a crippled person, stealing a seeing-eye dog or wanting to maintain barriers against people in wheelchairs in the way black Americans used to be kept out of restaurants and stores.

A FINE-SOUNDING TITLE

The title of the bill, "The Americans with Disabilities Act (ADA)" gives such a noble, humanitarian impression that it would seem almost unthinkable that it could really have much wrong with it. When most Congressmen were approached by apprehensive business groups and pro-family organizations concerned about the extreme provisions of the bill, they indignantly maintained that the ADA was a splendid, compassionate piece of legislation which might at most might need a little "fine tuning."

The ADA was drafted with significant input by attorneys from the ACLU, various disabilities rights groups, militant AIDS advocacy groups and the aggressive support of Senator Ted Kennedy (D-Mass).

BUSH IGNITES SUPPORT FOR THE ADA

During his first presidential campaign, then candidate George Bush announced his support of the ADA along with calling for an end to discrimination against "People with AIDS." Bush's outspoken endorsement of the ADA ignited frenetic activity among the bill's supporters, particularly the AIDS lobby.

STACKED HEARINGS

Purported public hearings were held on the ADA. Only a very limited number of opponents were allowed to speak, with severe time constraints. They faced committees dominated by the bill's aggressive sponsors. Responsible spokespersons from the disabled community who opposed the measure as being counterproductive were said to not represent the "mainstream" views of the handicapped and were not allowed to speak. People in wheelchairs and blind people with seeing-eye dogs were packed into the committee hearing rooms. Wrenching testimonies were given by AIDS patients and other "people with disabilities" who claimed to have suffered untold mental anguish because of societal stereotyping and discrimination.

Under such emotionally charged circumstances, those who opposed the ADA were made to appear as heartless reactionaries who wanted to keep the handicapped confined in institutions and prevent them from becoming productive members of society.

Congressmen, senators, pro-family groups and members of the business community who attempted to raise rational, serious objections regarding the ADA's radical demands were drowned out by a hail of emotionalism and angry accusations of bigotry toward the handicapped.

John Sloan, president of the National Federation of Independent Businesses, wrote:

> It was a stampede. Someone spooked the herd, and it rolled over everything in its path, knocking aside logic, crushing common sense and flattening democratic legislative procedure.
>
> The herd, in this case, was the Senate [and later also the House]. What spooked it was the Americans with Disabilities Act, a bill supposedly designed to prevent discrimination against disabled citizens.
>
> Unfortunately, like a lot of legislation being written in Washington these days, what started out as a good idea could become bad public policy.
>
> On the surface, the Act appears to be a noble effort to improve access to public facilities and expand job opportunities for disabled people. In today's society that is a concept that should be accepted by everyone without hesitation. But this bill, in its present form, will have a decidedly negative impact on businesses, especially small independent businesses.[6]

HOW SOUND ESTABLISHED EMPLOYMENT PRINCIPLES DEALT WITH THE HANDICAPPED

It should be noted that prior to the clamor for enactment of the ADA, 48 states did have existing statutes on the books covering employment of the handicapped and accessibility of the handicapped to public buildings. Designated handicapped parking spaces, wheelchair ramps, specially designed bathrooms stalls in new restaurants, and other facilities had become commonplace. As most of the media reported it and the public was led to believe, the ADA was merely confirming positive changes in policies toward the handicapped which had already been taking place.

In regard to employment, virtually all states already had laws on the books barring discrimination against individuals with legitimate physical handicaps *which did not interfere with their ability to perform the job*. These were generally reasonable statutes which balanced the opportunity of the handicapped to be considered for employment with the right of employers to exercise appropriate discernment in their hiring practices.

EXAMPLES OF PRIOR BALANCED STATE LAWS

In Kansas, the state law prohibited discrimination against the handicapped in employment, stating:

> The term "physical handicap" means the physical condition of a person, whether congenital or acquired by accident, injury or disease which consti-

tutes a substantial disability, but IS UNRELATED TO SUCH PERSON'S ABILITY TO ENGAGE IN A PARTICULAR JOB OR OCCUPATION.[7]

In Kentucky, the law read:

Preemployment inquiry – Basis for rejection of applicant for employment or housing.

(1) Nothing in [the statute] shall be construed to prevent an employer from making any preemployment inquiry about the existence of an applicant's handicap and about the extent to which that handicap has been overcome by treatment, medication, appliances or other rehabilitation.

(2) Nothing contained [in the statute] shall be construed to prohibit the rejection of an applicant for employment . . . on the basis of:

(a) A physical handicap *which interferes with a person's ability to adequately perform assigned job duties;*

(b) Any handicap which is not medically demonstrable by medically accepted clinical or laboratory diagnostic techniques, including, but not limited to, alcoholism, drug addiction, and obesity or

(c) Any communicable disease, either carried by, or afflicting the applicant.[8]

Statutes like the above allowed employers – who provided the resources to finance the business and create the job in the first place – to determine if applicants had conditions which would interfere with their ability to perform the job. Communicable diseases were not covered as "handicaps" nor were alcoholism, drug addiction or obesity.

STATE STATUTES OVERTURNED

These types of balanced state statutes, however, were unacceptable to the radical civil rights attorneys and social activist politicians who proposed the ADA. They determined it was necessary to discard years of sensible state laws to safeguard the rights of individuals with legitimate physical handicaps. Instead they expanded the meaning of the word disability to encompass a limitless array of *thousands* of physical ailments – including communicable diseases – and *hundreds* of psychological disorders.

THE ADA: A MASTERPIECE OF LEGISLATIVE NEWSPEAK

The term "Newspeak" was first used in George Orwell's classic novel *1984*, a depiction of life under a totalitarian regime run by the archetypal dictator Big Brother. Newspeak refers to the state mandated transformation of the meaning and usage of language in order to advance its political and social agenda. Examples of Newspeak terms used in *1984* include:

WAR IS PEACE
FREEDOM IS SLAVERY
IGNORANCE IS STRENGTH

By redefining certain terms and eliminating others, Newspeak steers the public into a predetermined politically expedient mode of thinking.[9]

The writers of the ADA use a variety of slippery, positive sounding Newspeak-type words and phrases which have meanings and implications far beyond what a cursory reading of the Act would suggest.

In contrast to its benign-sounding title, the definitions and demands of the ADA are so outlandishly Orwellian and outrageously radical that at first blush they may seem fantastic and unbelievable. In the brief overview of the bill which follows, the language and interpretation of the ADA's implications are not being exaggerated or overstated. They are taken in context from the Act itself and from regulations subsequently issued by the Equal Employment Opportunity Commission (EEOC).

TRIVIALIZING THE CONCEPT OF DISABILITIES

According to a dictionary written prior to the ADA, the term "disability" means:

> 1. A disabled state or condition; incapacity. 2. Something that disables: a handicap. 3. A legal incapacity or disqualification.[10]

In standard English usage, when someone is disabled, *it means they have an incapacitating injury or illness which prevents or disqualifies them from working.* Disability insurance, for example, is specifically designed to provide an income for an individual who through organic illness or injury is rendered unable (dis-abled) to work.

Under the ADA, however, the term "disability" is defined to include:

- every individual who has a "physical impairment"
- every individual who has a "mental impairment"
- every individual who may or *may not presently have* such an impairment but who has a "record of" such impairment
- every individual *who does not actually have* a "physical or mental impairment" but who could be "regarded as" having such an impairment.
- every individual *who does not actually have* a "physical or mental impairment" but who has a "known relationship to or association with an individual with a known disability"

– any individual with a "physical or mental impairment" who has "reasonable grounds" for believing they are "about to be subjected to discrimination" *even if such "discrimination" has not actually occurred.*[11]

The writers of the ADA declare that 43,000,000 people have mental or physical impairments which are covered by the Act.[12] Added to that vast number is everyone who has a known "relationship with" at least one of the 43 million individuals covered by the ADA. If each of those 43 million has a relationship with only one other person, then 86 million people are potentially covered by the Act. Add to that number everyone who has a "record of" such impairments or "is regarded as having" such impairments, and it would be difficult to find many individuals who are *not* members of at least one of the ADA's sweeping new classes of individuals granted disability-related status. This trivializes the very concept of disabilities. *Moreover, all of the 43 million individuals now classified as disabled plus the millions of people in other "disability-related" categories covered under the ADA are potential plaintiffs in lawsuits* against private employers and businesses.

MENTAL AND PHYSICAL IMPAIRMENTS INTERPRETED

Mental or physical disabilities covered by the ADA are defined as conditions which:

... limit major life activities ... including caring for oneself, performing manual tasks, walking, seeing, hearing, speaking, breathing, learning and working. *This list is not exhaustive.* For example, other major life activities include, but are not limited to, sitting, standing, lifting, reaching.[13]

A *physical* impairment is defined as:

(a) a physiological disorder or condition, cosmetic disfigurement or anatomical loss that affects one or more of several body systems.[14]

The physiological conditions covered by this definition are virtually limitless. A review of *Cecil's Textbook of Medicine*, beginning with "abdominal angina" and ending with "zygomycosis," indicates that *over 20,000* physiological disorders and conditions could be considered as "physical impairments."

A *mental* impairment is defined to include:

(b) a mental or psychological disorder, including mental retardation, organic brain syndrome, emotional or mental illness and specific learning disabilities.[15]

The term "emotional or mental illness" incorporates several hundred mental conditions listed in the American Psychiatric Association's *Diagnostic and Statistical Manual of Mental Disorders.*[16]

MENTAL DISORDERS COVERED BY THE ADA

In the EEOC regulations issued to interpret the ADA, it is stated that "the definition of a mental impairment does not include common personality traits such as poor judgment or a quick temper *where these are not symptoms of a mental or psychological disorder.*"[17]

However, there are numerous mental or psychological disorders which *are* manifested not only by poor judgment or bad temper but by many other onerous, disruptive symptoms. If an individual demonstrates these symptoms as a result of "mental or psychological disorder," they are considered "disabled" under the ADA.

PSYCHOTICS AND SCHIZOPHRENICS COVERED

Psychotics and schizophrenics are also granted specially protected "disability" status under the ADA. Symptoms of psychosis include incoherence, delusions, hallucinations, paranoia and catatonic behavior.[18] Contrary to popular misconception, schizophrenia does not involve a multiple or "split" personality. It is characterized by recurring hallucinations, bizarre delusions and personality disintegration. A schizophrenic's ability to function in such areas as work, social relations and self-care is markedly impaired.[19]

Multiple personality disorder, portrayed in the films the *Three Faces of Eve* and *Sybil*, involves several distinct personalities within an individual and is also covered under the ADA.[20]

MENTAL DISORDERS CAN BE DEADLY IN THE WORKPLACE

When employers are prohibited from taking into account past or present psychiatric disorders or screening out psychotics the results can be disastrous.

CRANE OPERATOR WITH HISTORY OF MENTAL PROBLEMS IN FATAL ACCIDENT

SAN FRANCISCO, Nov. 30, 1989 – The operator of a crane that plummeted 16 floors, killing five people, twice tried to commit suicide during the previous nine months and was a chronic alcoholic, according to reports.

Lonnie Boggess, the 45-year-old crane operator who was among those killed, also *had been hospitalized for psychiatric observation twice* since

March, according to court documents obtained by McClatchey Newspapers. ...

Boggess' employer, Erection Co. of Kirkland, Washington, refused to comment. ...

When told of Boggess' past, including his two recent suicide attempts, Fire Chief Fred Postel said: "Oh no! You've got to be kidding!". . .

The contractor for the project said the accident apparently was triggered when the crane head rotated 180 degrees, causing the counterweight to crash into a section being inserted into the crane.

The contractor reported that the rotation occurred "for unknown reasons," causing the 240 ton [480,000 pounds] crane to crash onto a busy street in the heart of the city's financial district during rush hour, crushing a bus that it landed on top of. Besides Boggess, three ironworkers and a bus driver were killed and 21 people injured.

Boggess reportedly was seen slumped over the controls as the crane began its plunge, authorities said.

The accident occurred as workers were jacking up the crane from the 16th to the 20th floor.[21]

In Kentucky, a deranged former employee wounded 13 and killed 7 employees. He apparently was seeking vengeance for having been placed on long-term disability leave for his manic-depression. Coincidentally, a human rights commission had just previously ruled that the company was guilty of discrimination on the basis of "mental impairment" and should have accommodated him.[22]

Under the ADA employers face a grating catch-22. They are not allowed to screen out psychotic applicants when hiring. After they do hire them, they are not allowed to segregate or place them away from other employees – even if the normal employees are frightened or complain.[23]

L.H. Rockwell, Jr., President of the esteemed Ludwig von Mises Institute, notes:

The ADA also protects those who have trouble learning, reasoning, and remembering. If a supermarket manager refuses to hire a dimwit to ring the cash register he can be taken to court. A sales manager may prefer salesmen who can remember customers' names and preferences not to mention products, but discrimination against the memory impaired is not allowed.

Does a thousand-mile stare make you and your employees uneasy? You're out of luck, for this is no longer a chilling quirk but a certified disability.

Would you rather not hire a warehouseman with a history of drug use? If he's off crack this week he's on your payroll.

Say the applicant is a dyslexic with a history of drug addiction who not only has trouble reading, but can't learn or reason well thanks to minor brain damage. If he applies, you have to hire him and make necessary accommodations.[24]

The "mental impairments" covered by the ADA go far beyond obvious derangement. Any mental disorder which interferes with an individual's ability to work or function may be covered as a "disability."

ANTI-SOCIAL PERSONALITY DISORDERS

These "mental impairments" include:

Conduct Disorder: Manifested by behaviors such as: stealing, lying, deliberate fire-setting, breaking and entering, physical cruelty to animals, forcible rape, using weapons, initiating fights, and physical cruelty to people.[25]

Sadistic Personality Disorder: This disorder is manifested by a pervasive pattern of cruel, demeaning and aggressive behavior. Symptoms include: using physical cruelty or violence to dominate people, humiliating and demeaning people in the presence of others, getting other people to do what one wants through intimidation and terror, and fascination with violence, weapons, martial arts, injury, or torture.[26]

Intermittent Explosive Disorder: This "impulse control disorder" is manifested by *repeated explosive outbursts of violent rage which cause severe bodily harm to others* and/or destruction of property.[27]

BAD WORK ATTITUDE OR "MENTAL IMPAIRMENT"?

Under the ADA, there is a blurring of the distinction between what formerly were considered bad work attitudes and what are now defined as "mental impairments."

In less enlightened times, an individual who angrily refused to perform a job task to an employer's satisfaction and rudely insulted a supervisor for bringing up their poor performance would have been considered a prime candidate for dismissal. Individuals evincing these winsome qualities may now be able to qualify as having a federally protected "mental impairment" called "Passive Aggressive Personality Disorder." This "disabling" condition is characterized by:

A pervasive pattern of passive resistance to demands for adequate social and occupational performance . . . as indicated by at least five of the following:
1) procrastinates, i.e., puts off things that need to be done so that deadlines are not met
2) becomes sulky, irritable, or argumentative when asked to do something he or she does not want to do
3) seems to work deliberately slowly or to do a bad job on tasks that he or she really does not want to do
4) protests, without justification, that others make unreasonable demands on him or her
5) avoids obligations by claiming to have "forgotten"
6) believes that he or she is doing a much better job than others think he or she is doing

7) resents useful suggestions from others concerning how he or she could be more productive

8) obstructs the efforts of others by failing to do his or her share of the work

9) unreasonably criticizes or scorns people in positions of authority[28]

Hypochondria: What if an individual persistently claims to have a physical disorder which interferes with their ability to work, but extensive medical examination determines that the party has nothing physically wrong with them? Can they claim federal protection under the ADA? Apparently they can, if they are found to be suffering from a mental disorder called "Hypochondriacal Neurosis," which is defined to include:

> *Preoccupation with the fear of having, or the belief that one has, a serious disease, based on the person's interpretation of physical signs* or sensations as evidence of physical illness. . . .
>
> . . . *appropriate physical evaluation does not support the diagnosis of any physical disorder* that can account for the physical signs or sensations or the person's unwarranted interpretation of them.[29]

MALINGERING: THE ULTIMATE "DISABILITY"?

What if appropriate physical and psychological examinations determine an individual is unfortunate enough *not* to actually have a physical impairment or hypochondria but is in fact deliberately faking illness in order to obtain financial compensation without having to perform job tasks they consider "non-essential"? For these individuals, obtaining a classification under the "mental disorder" called Malingering could prove useful in making the employer provide "reasonable" accommodations:

MALINGERING (*DSM-III-R*, V65.20).
The essential feature of Malingering is *intentional production of false or grossly exaggerated physical or psychological symptoms* motivated by external incentives such as . . . avoiding work, obtaining financial compensation, evading criminal prosecution, obtaining drugs or securing better living conditions.[30]

In addition to the thousands of physical impairments covered by the ADA, employers and private business establishments must also provide "reasonable" accommodations for a legion of mental disorders.

ALL PRIVATE BUSINESSES ARE COVERED BY THE ADA

The hiring requirements of the ADA apply to all employers with 15 or more employees.[31] Religious organizations may give preference to members of their own faith and may require that employees abide by the religious tenets of their religious organization, but *must otherwise comply* with all the radical demands of the ADA.[32] Prior to the enactment of the ADA, a U.S. District Judge ruled that the Salvation Army had acted wrongly after the organization fired a woman who practiced witchcraft after she admitted using the agency copying machine to photocopy satanic rituals. The woman had filed a $1.25-million lawsuit against the Salvation Army.[33]

Virtually all *private* businesses *regardless of size or number of employees*, including private dentists' and doctors' offices, "mom and pop" stores, hospitals, etc., are defined as "public" accommodations under the ADA. They must provide what are called "reasonable" accommodations to all customers and visitors with mental and physical disabilities *upon demand*. This can include restructuring their places of business and providing other "auxiliary aids and services."[34]

All of these private businesses and stores are potential targets of lawsuits by disgruntled customers and visitors who claim to have been discriminated against because they have or are regarded as having "mental or physical impairments." Can a store, restaurant, library, etc., ask a malodorous psychotic vagrant who is incoherently muttering obscenities to leave the premises or ask them to sit in a section away from other patrons? The ADA states:

> *It shall be discriminatory* to afford an individual or class of individuals with disabilities . . . the opportunity to participate in or benefit from a good, service, facility, privilege, advantage or accommodation *that is not equal to that afforded to other individuals.*[35]

Institutions controlled by religious organizations such as churches and parochial schools, are not included in the definition of "public accommodations." Private schools which are not part of a religious group are considered "public" accommodations and subject to the provisions of the ADA.

TERMINATING AN EMPLOYER'S FREEDOM OF CHOICE

Prior to the ADA, it was up to an employer or manager to determine what tasks were required to be performed in a given job position and how and when they were to be done. If an employer defined a given position as a composite of several different duties, that is what the job required. An employee was not entitled to pick and choose the duties he or she liked, leave the rest undone and demand that the employer get someone else to do the tasks they did not feel like doing. They were required to accomplish all of the assigned duties of a job in the manner and time in which the employer wanted them performed.

COVERED INDIVIDUALS ONLY NEED PERFORM THE BARE "ESSENTIAL" FUNCTION OF A JOB

The employer's freedom of choice as to defining the requirements and method of performance of a given job has now been drastically curtailed.

Under the ADA, an employer can only request an individual with mental and/or physical disabilities to perform what are deemed to be the bare "essential functions" of a given job. Employers are *prohibited* from requiring individuals with mental and/or physical disabilities to perform any job tasks that are regarded as "non-essential" or "marginal" under the ADA.[36]

In the final analysis, federal bureaucrats or judges will decide whether or not an employer has properly called a given job function "essential" or has "discriminated" against an individual by requiring them to perform tasks of a given job which are "non-essential" or "marginal."

> The second factor in determining whether a function is essential is *the number of other employees* available to perform that job function *among whom the performance of that job function can be distributed.*[37]

If an employer contends that a given job position requires the performance of certain specific tasks which an individual with mental and/or physical impairment(s) is unable to perform, EEOC administrators or the courts may decide that the employer must "restructure" the job and redistribute various "marginal" functions of the job to other employees.

CAN CERTAIN JOB PRODUCTION LEVELS BE REQUIRED?

Maybe. If a party with a "mental or physical disability" alleges that an employer "intentionally selected the particular level of production to exclude individuals with disabilities," the employer may have to offer a "legitimate, nondiscriminatory reason" for its selection.[38] It will be up to federal bureaucrats or the courts to determine if the level of production required of a given job is appropriate or discriminates against the mentally and/or physically disabled.

The ADA concept of what constitutes the "essential" or "fundamental" function(s) of a job is open to broad ambiguous interpretation.

For example, a small business employer determines they need someone to fill the position of office manager. The employer asserts that the job requires an individual who is willing and able to perform a combination of all the following job tasks, including:

- analyzing business plans
- reviewing and placing written orders
- supervising the production of other employees
- using the telephone to speak with distributors and customers
- typing out reports and correspondence using a computer
- lifting boxes
- making periodic business trips

If an individual covered under the ADA applies for the position and claims they are only able to perform one or two "basic" aspects of the job, the employer must justify his contention that the other requirements of the job are "essential."

The EEOC administrator or jury hearing the case can decide that the "essential" function of the position is *really* merely "analyzing business plans." The employer would then be *compelled to redistribute* the other "non-essential" tasks of the position to other employees, unless he or she can *prove* that doing so would "impose an undue hardship on the operation of his business."

What the EEOC defines as the "essential function(s)" of a specific job title can vary from employer to employer. It is no longer left up to the employer to have the ultimate say in which of job tasks are an essential part of a given position. In the final analysis, it is up to the EEOC and the courts to define what are the intangible bare "essential" functions of any given job position on a *case-by-case basis*. When attempting to define job tasks, employers now face a tidal wave of semantic relativism imposed by Big Brother bureaucrats.

REVISIONIST EMPLOYMENT POLICY

Employers must also provide what the ADA calls "reasonable" accommodations. These so-called "reasonable" accommodations are designed to enable the individual with mental and/or physical disabilities *to perform the basic functions of a job which they could not otherwise accomplish*. This definition is a radical revisionist supplanting of previous state laws.[39]

WHAT DOES "REASONABLE" MEAN UNDER THE ADA?

The dictionary defines the word "reasonable" as:

2) Governed by or in accordance with reason or sound thinking. 3) Within the bounds of common sense. 4) Not excessive or extreme; fair; moderate; as in *reasonable prices*.[40]

According to the ADA, an individual with a mental and/or physical disability is "otherwise qualified" if he or she is qualified for a job, except that, because of the disability, he or she needs *reasonable* accommodation(s) to be able to perform the job's *essential* function.[41] "The determination of whether an individual is qualified for a particular position must be made on a *case-by-case basis* [by EEOC administrators or the courts]." "Reasonable" accommodations are defined by the ADA to include:

(A) making existing facilities used by employees readily accessible to and usable by individuals with disabilities and
(B) JOB RESTRUCTURING, part-time or modified work schedules, reassignment to a vacant position, acquisition or modification of equipment or devices, training materials or policies, the PROVISION OF QUALIFIED READERS OR INTERPRETERS, AND *OTHER SIMILAR ACCOMMODATIONS* for individuals with disabilities.

EEOC regulations state: ". . . JOB RESTRUCTURING MAY INVOLVE CHANGING WHEN OR HOW AN ESSENTIAL FUNCTION IS PERFORMED."[42]

"Reasonable accommodation" is not synonymous with but can include what is called "*supported employment*." Examples of supported employment include modified work training materials, *restructuring essential functions to enable an individual to perform a job*, or *hiring an outside professional ["job coach"]* to assist in job training.[43]

EMPLOYERS MUST PROVIDE "DAILY ATTENDANT CARE"

The term "daily attendant care" is generally used to describe the extensive level of care needed by mentally and physically disabled nursing home patients who cannot take care of themselves and require full-time aides to assist them in getting out of bed, walking, eating, using the bathroom, etc.

The ADA, however, requires *employers* to provide free "daily attendant care" on site in the *workplace* as a "reasonable" accommodation for individuals with incapacitating mental and physical conditions in order to enable them to perform what the EEOC deems to be the "essential" functions of a job. ". . . [I]T MAY BE A REASONABLE ACCOMMODATION TO PROVIDE PERSONAL ASSISTANTS [plural] TO HELP WITH SPECIFIED DUTIES RELATED TO THE JOB."[44]

In addition to having to restructure basic job functions, alter work policies and schedules, provide daily attendant care, readers and interpreters, job coaches, etc., for individuals with a host of incapacitating physical conditions, employers must similarly provide such "reasonable" accommodations in order to meet the demanding needs of dementia patients, psychotics, paranoids, schizophrenics and assorted neurotics.

Individuals covered under the ADA can legally *demand* changes in the *manner* and the *time* in which they perform the bare "essential functions" of a job. Employers *must* comply with and accommodate these demands unless they can *prove* to the satisfaction of EEOC administrators or juries that to do so would be "an undue hardship."

WHO PAYS FOR "REASONABLE" ACCOMMODATIONS?

All costs of these "reasonable" accommodations must be borne by the employer. The employer is absolutely *prohibited* from reducing the salary of the individual with disabilities in order to pay for their "reasonable accommodations." If the cost of the accommodations amounts to a significant percentage of the employee's salary or even exceeds the employee's salary, the employer must absorb the cost and provide the "reasonable" accommodations, unless they can *prove* that doing so would constitute "an undue burden."

WORKMEN'S COMP INQUIRIES PROHIBITED

Every employer covered under the ADA is federally prohibited from inquiring as to whether a job applicant has a mental and/or physical disability prior to offering them the position they desire. They also are prohibited from asking if an applicant has a history of disabilities or has filed claims under Workmen's Compensation with previous employers.

Nor can an employer inquire at the pre-offer stage about an applicant's worker's compensation history.[45]

These unprecedented constraints leave employers wide open to increased claims under Workmen's Compensation.

As many experienced employers have learned to their dismay, there are "professional claimants" who have a pattern of going from one employer to the next, working for a while and then claiming that a pre-existing or new injury or ailment is preventing them from continuing to work and claiming benefits under Workmen's Compensation (WC). The employer then must pay increased WC premiums.

EMPLOYERS: GUILTY UNTIL PROVEN OTHERWISE

Any time an employer has a job applicant who lets it be known that he or she is a member of a protected class under the ADA and the employer hires someone else who is not mentally or physically impaired, they are liable to have to defend their choice. The language of the Senate Committee hearings on the ADA suggests that when an employer has two applicants for a job, and one of them has known physical and/or mental impairments, the employer can be obliged to demonstrate a "non-discriminatory" reason for not hiring the individual with disabilities instead of the healthy applicant.*

For all practical purposes, an accused employer is considered guilty of "discrimination against the disabled" unless they can *prove* their reason for not hiring (or firing) a covered individual was not based on a discriminatory *attitude* or hiring practice. The *complete burden of proof is on the employer* to demonstrate why they hired someone who is mentally and physically normal and healthy instead of someone who is mentally and/or physically disabled.

The rationale that hiring an individual with physical and/or mental disabilities would drive up the cost of health insurance or Workmen's Compensation is unacceptable and discriminatory under the ADA.[46]

BUREAUCRATS AND JURIES WILL DECIDE

In each and every case in which a covered applicant or employee complains they have suffered unfair treatment, it is ultimately up to federal bureaucrats or the courts to decide, through scrutinizing the private employer's business and employment records, past and present profit/loss ratios, workplace environment, number of employees, etc., how and to what extent an accused employer should have "provided reasonable accommodations" for the individual's "physical and/or mental impairments."

A WRITTEN JOB DESCRIPTION IS NO GUARANTEE

Businesses can try to escape some of this by requiring certain abilities in a written job description. But they must be able to show, in a court of law, that the requirements are essential to the job.[47]

What may be deemed permissible for a given employer not to provide at a certain time of the year can be required a few months later.

An accommodation that poses an undue hardship for one employer at a particular time may not pose an undue hardship for another employer, or *even for the same employer* at another time.[48]

EMPLOYERS MUST PAY ALL COSTS OF LEGAL DEFENSE

All the costs of producing the extensive documentation needed to defend against charges of discrimination, past and present business and accounting records, accountants' and attorneys' fees, time off

---

*Radical disability rights activists refer to healthy people as "TABs," the "temporarily able-bodied."

from work to appear before federal EEOC administrators or in court, etc., are borne by the accused employer. These expenses can quickly mount into many thousands of dollars. Even if the federal bureaucrats reviewing the case agree that an employer has demonstrated he or she is not guilty of the charges, he or she must absorb the full onerous costs of their defense.

A BONANZA FOR ACCUSERS AND ATTORNEYS

As the ADA was being hastily propelled through Congress, its proponents reassured worried members of the business community that employers would not face expensive jury trials or exorbitant punitive ["punishing"] damages. Claims of discrimination against employers, ADA supporters maintained, would be handled by EEOC administrators. The U.S. Attorney General's office could also be called in to investigate claims of "flagrant" discrimination.[49]

Lo and behold, a little more than one year after the ADA was passed, Congress passed *another* bill entitled the "Civil Rights Act of 1991," in which EMPLOYERS CAN BE HAULED INTO COURT and, depending on their size, BE COMPELLED TO PAY UP TO $300,000 IN PUNITIVE DAMAGES for *each* complaining "disabled" party's:

> . . . future pecuniary [financial] losses, emotional pain, suffering, inconvenience, mental anguish, loss of enjoyment of life and other non-pecuniary losses.[50]

Under the ADA, private businesses defined as "public accommodations" which are found to be guilty of discrimination in provision of services and goods to individuals with "mental and/or physical impairments," face "*monetary damages* to persons aggrieved when requested by the Attorney General, *and* may, in order to "vindicate the public interest," be assessed *a civil penalty* of $50,000 for the first violation, and up to $100,000 for any subsequent violation.[51]

MAMMOTH AWARDS TO ACCUSERS

Jury Verdict Research, Inc., a private organization that monitors jury decisions throughout the country in cases involving claims of physical, emotional, and mental injury, reports that A FORMER EMPLOYEE CLAIMING WRONGFUL DISCHARGE HAS AN 86% CHANCE OF WINNING A CASE BROUGHT AGAINST A PRIVATE BUSINESS or industry. . . .

MOST WRONGFUL DISCHARGE CASES ARE BASED ON ALLEGATIONS OF EMOTIONAL DISTRESS or damaged reputation. In a study of cases within California, the Rand Corporation, a think-tank in Santa Monica, found that AWARDS TO EMPLOYEE-PLAINTIFFS [ACCUSERS] AVERAGED $650,000

Stephen A. Bokat, vice president and general counsel of the U.S. Chamber of Commerce, adds: *"Workplace litigation is causing unbelievable problems* for employers. You fully expect that every time you discharge an employee, or don't promote an employee, or demote an employee, you're going to get a lawsuit. That was not true even 10 years ago. . . .

The threat of litigation, according to the Rand study, can force business managers into such counterproductive activities as *accepting inadequate performance from individual workers, failing to meet changing business needs,* missing investment opportunities, and looking more to outside contractors for labor needs, regardless of whether that is the best course.

"The impact on small business can be especially dramatic," notes Moon, whose firm – Moon, Moss, and McGill – advises mostly small-business clients. *"The small-business man can least afford the extravagant legal fees and at the same time, can least afford to condone mediocre performance* while he gathers enough information and issues enough warnings to let somebody go."[52]

An employer accused under the ADA and the Civil Rights Act of 1991 has to defend himself against charges of having engaged in "discriminatory practices with malice or with reckless indifference to the federally protected rights of an aggrieved individual."

For an employer to attempt to defend him or herself against charges of maliciously and coldheartedly discriminating against the disabled would seem inherently counterproductive. An employer brought into court is likely to be asked by the plaintiff's attorney: "Why are you cruelly and insensitively refusing to provide "reasonable accommodations" for this unfortunate disabled individual who has now suffered untold emotional anguish?" This is tantamount to the classic interrogatory trap, "How long has it been since you stopped beating your wife?" The charge itself carries such an overwhelming presumption and implication of guilt, that the more one tries to defend himself, ("I do not maliciously discriminate against the disabled I discriminate for a good reason"), the guiltier they seem.

An employer who attempts to give rational arguments denying their ability to provide "reasonable accommodations" for the disabled individual(s) bringing charges, will be accused of being insensitive, unreasonable and discriminatory.

HOMOSEXUALITY NOT A "DISABILITY," BUT . . .

The definition of what constitutes a "mental impairment" under the ADA was so all-inclusive that then Senator Bill Armstrong (R-CO), saw the need to proffer an amendment, included in the final version of the Act, which states:

(a) HOMOSEXUALITY AND BISEXUALITY. – For purposes of the definition of "disability" homosexuality and bisexuality are not impairments and as such are not covered under this Act.

(b) CERTAIN CONDITIONS. – Under this Act, the term "disability" shall not include –

   (1) Transvestism, transsexualism, pedophilia [child molesting – a *DSM-III* "mental disorder"], exhibitionism, voyeurism, gender identity disorders not resulting from physical impairments, or other sexual behavior disorders;

   (2) Compulsive gambling, kleptomania [compulsive stealing], or pyromania [compulsive fire-setting];

   (3) Psychoactive substance use disorders resulting from *current* illegal use of drugs.[53]

The Armstrong amendment provides employers with critical protection from being forced to hire pyromaniacs, kleptomaniacs, child molesters, and active drug addicts. Under the amendment, it would *seem* that an employer might be able to refuse to hire an individual solely on the basis of their homosexuality, *if their reason has nothing whatsoever to do with that individual's increased risk of having HIV disease or other physical or mental impairments.*

However, the ADA has other provisions which effectively provide *de facto* specially protected homosexual civil rights status.

HIV CONSIDERED A "DISABILITY"

The ADA does not specifically mention HIV or AIDS. The EEOC regulations issued to interpret the Act make it clear that HIV/AIDS is covered as a "disability" under the ADA.[54]

In addition, to reflect current, preferred, ["politically correct"] terminology, the Commission has substituted the term "people who have AIDS" for the term "AIDS patients."[55]

HOMOSEXUALS "REGARDED AS" HAVING AIDS

An individual satisfies the third part of the "regarded as" definition of "disability" if the employer or other covered entity erroneously believes the individual has a substantially limiting impairment that the individual *actually does not have*. The situation could occur, for example, if an employer discharged an employee in response to a rumor that the employee is infected with *Human Immunodeficiency Virus [HIV]*. Even though the rumor is totally unfounded and *the individual has no impairment at all,* the individual is considered an individual with a disability because the employer *perceived* of this individual as being disabled. Thus, in this example, the employer, by discharging this employee, *is discriminating* on the basis of disability.[56]

An employee who himself "inadvertently" starts a rumor that he is HIV positive could also be "regarded as" being disabled.

LEGISLATING AN EMPLOYER'S THOUGHTS

EEOC Regulations state:

> [A]n individual meets the "regarded as" part of the definition of disability if he or she can show that a covered entity made an employment decision because of a *perception* of a disability based on *"myth, fear or stereotype."*

If an individual can show that an employer or other covered entity made an employment decision because of *perception* of disability based on "myth, fear or stereotype," the individual will satisfy the "regarded as" part of the definition of disability. *If the employer cannot articulate a non-discriminatory reason for the employment action, an inference can be drawn on the basis of "myth, fear or stereotype."*

A New Jersey court has ruled that male homosexuals per se are "regarded as" being "disabled" because their behavior puts them at risk of AIDS [228 N.J. Super. 370].

HOMOSEXUAL "LOVERS" OF AIDS CARRIERS

Under the ADA, all covered employers, including private schools, are prohibited from firing or declining to hire an individual because they have a known *relationship or association with* an individual with a disability.

> This provision is intended to protect any qualified individual, *whether or not that individual has a disability*, from discrimination because that person is known to have a *relationship with* an individual who has a known disability. THIS PROTECTION IS NOT LIMITED TO THOSE WHO HAVE A FAMILIAL RELATIONSHIP with an individual with a disability.[57]

This definition *includes* the homosexual sodomy partners of AIDS carriers and is a subtle *de facto* federal recognition of the concept of homosexual "marriage."

As soon as a homosexual job applicant or employee *lets it be known* that his male "roommate" has HIV/AIDS or that he "does volunteer work" with AIDS patients, he acquires special federally protected civil rights status. An employer who refuses to hire, attempts to discharge, fails to promote or otherwise practices "discrimination" *in any aspect of* the employment relationship toward a homosexual who has a known "relationship or association with people who have AIDS," can then be required to demonstrate *in court* that he did not do so because of a *"perception* of" a disability based on "subjective perceptions, irrational fears [e.g., "homophobia"], patronizing attitudes, or stereotypes."[58]

These provisions would appear to be a graphic fulfillment of the words of Paul Diamond:

Don't call us AIDS victims. AIDS is not my weakness. AIDS IS MY STRENGTH.[59]

ENCOURAGING HOMOSEXUALS TO "COME OUT"

Since the language of the ADA only provides protection for an individual whose "disability or association with an individual with a disability" is *known*, it can have the effect of encouraging homosexuals to "come out of the closet" so as to enjoy the protections afforded under the Act.

TUBERCULOSIS IS A PROTECTED "DISABILITY"

Tuberculosis is also considered as an "inherently substantially limiting impairment" under the ADA.[60]

> ... [S]uppose a municipality has an ordinance that prohibits individuals with tuberculosis from teaching school children. If an individual with dormant tuberculosis challenges a private [including religious] school's refusal to hire him because of the tuberculosis, the private school would *not* be able to rely on the city ordinance as a defense under the ADA.[61]

In other words, if a teacher has HIV/AIDS and is infected with TB, it would appear that a school cannot suspend, fire or refuse to hire the individual until *after* he or she has developed active, contagious tuberculosis, by which time he or she is likely to have exposed numerous students and other employees. Restaurants must likewise retain workers with AIDS unless they can prove that doing so poses a "direct threat" which cannot be met with "reasonable accommodation."

INVESTIGATIVE SQUADS TARGETING BUSINESSES

> Until the courts decide, businesses cannot be sure what compliance requires. That's why two-thirds of American companies have done nothing to prepare.
>
> To make up for that, government and private interest groups will use "testers." These actors, who will want to find out all the discrimination they can, will terrify small businesses. The smaller the business, the more ADA hurts.[62]

AN APPALLING NIGHTMARE

A clinical psychologist who formerly worked as an examiner for the U.S. Social Security Disability Determination Division, stated prior to the ADA's passage:

> For over 10 years, I regularly examined for Social Security people alleging to be disabled because of brain damage, emotional disturbances, retardation and mental illnesses. I consider myself reasonably competent to discuss certain forms of disabilities.

I am appalled at the nightmare the "Americans with Disabilities Act" will create. According to this Act, emotional and mental disturbances, which are self-induced in many cases, will be classified as disabilities similar to diabetes, or spina bifida, or a prolapsed mitral valve. As most honest mental health professionals know, many forms of disability, physical and psychological, include a crucial factor of character, of attitude, of willpower.

My clinical experience in my office leaves no doubt that many of the disability criteria presently used by Social Security *encourage* people to give in to the vicissitudes of life and *to be as sick as they can think they are sick.*

The ADA will set up a national reinforcement system to reward us for developing hypochondria and assorted neurotic aches and pains. As Saul Bellow wrote, "Hypochondriacs are their own terrorists."

The New Jersey Court decision [declaring homosexuals to be a protected "disabled" class because their behavior places them at risk of AIDS] has done incalculable harm. Homosexuality, particularly anal intercourse [sodomy], is a behavioral problem. Intravenous drug abuse is a behavioral problem.

If we turn our behavioral problems into disabilities, defended by law and supported by legal fines, we shall have taken one more fatal step toward the slag heap of history.

Economist L.H. Rockwell, Jr., points out, "A free market means allowing owners to hire, fire, promote and pay based on their assessment of an employee's contribution. But American businesses have lost that ability, setting us on the road to civil rights socialism. Even the Soviets recognized that people's abilities and attitudes affected their economic roles."[63]

CHAPTER TWELVE

ENDING THE DELUSION

Historians will look back in amazement at the opportunities that were missed to contain the transmission of AIDS before it spread to millions of people in the United States. . . .

We may be deluding ourselves in an effort to avoid unpleasant choices, trading off present discomfort for future upheaval. Eventually this disease may destroy many of the freedoms we now take for granted. The scope of the ultimate damage will depend on how long we delay instituting basic health measures to contain the spread of AIDS.

    – Dr. Joseph Feldschuh, M.D., *Safe Blood: Purifying the Nation's Blood Supply in the Age of AIDS*[1]

SECRECY LAW SHIELDS RAPIST WITH AIDS

Eleven rape victims whose attacker has the AIDS virus are not being allowed to know his identity in order to protect his privacy.

They cannot even be told officially that the man who raped them was the one who exposed them to the killer disease. . . .

Under California law anyone identifying an HIV carrier can get up to one year in jail or face a $10,000 fine. . . .

One Los Angeles rape victim was told to get tested by a health department notice pinned to her front door. She was simply told she had been in "contact" with a carrier. "In the 70s this was rape. In the 90s what this guy did to me was attempted murder," the victim said. . . .[2]

This atrocious case typifies the way the AIDS epidemic has been mishandled nationwide. With the exception of a few paltry state laws, *no practical effort has been made to prevent AIDS carriers from placing others at risk or warning people they have exposed of their danger.*

Anyone who thinks they are at risk can be tested anonymously outside the purview of public health authorities. Those who learn they are infectious HIV carriers are free to inform – or *not* inform – others whose lives they have placed in jeopardy.

The guardians of our nation's health have left it up to AIDS carriers, most of whom have contracted the disease through reckless and irresponsible behaviors (promiscuous sodomy, drug abuse and fornication) to be responsible enough to inform their partners – including unsuspecting spouses – of their lethal infectious condition.

SPOUSES OF AIDS CARRIERS NOT WARNED

Due to anonymous testing and highly restrictive HIV secrecy laws, health officials in many areas cannot even inform the endangered spouses of those infected with HIV that they are at risk.

AN EXPLODING NIGHTMARE

The consequences of this passive, "live and let die" policy have been disastrous. From the early 1980s when there were only a few dozen AIDS patients, the number of reported cases of AIDS has mushroomed into hundreds of thousands in the United States and millions worldwide. Untold numbers of people across the globe are unknowingly carrying HIV disease.

HOSPITALS UNDER SIEGE

In urban areas with a high density of AIDS cases, hospitals are imploding under the burden of AIDS patients, many of whom also have contagious forms of drug-resistant tuberculosis.[3] The stress caused by the rising number of AIDS patients in urban hospitals has resulted in AIDS patients being sent out to suburban and rural hospitals for care, thereby encouraging the dissemination of HIV and TB in low prevalence areas.

TIME TO DISPEL THE FOG OF UNCERTAINTY

How many people in the United States are currently infected with HIV disease? How far and how fast has the HIV epidemic spread into the heterosexual adolescent and adult populations? These are crucial questions to which public health officials can only offer rough guesses and politicized speculation. Incredibly, while the government has been pouring billions of taxpayer dollars into ostensibly "combatting AIDS," no one really knows precisely how many people are carrying the disease.

Since only individuals in the final stage of HIV disease classified as "AIDS" are reported to public health authorities, the current number of AIDS cases only reflects infections acquired years previously.

WHY "EDUCATION" WILL NOT HALT THE SPREAD OF AIDS

The "education-is-the-only-answer" approach has resulted in what can at best be described as a form of medical anarchy.

The wholesale unwillingness of legislators and public health officials to exercise standard disease control measures has aided and abetted the growth of the AIDS epidemic. This deadly passivity has been fueled by the drive of the homosexual movement to portray sodomy as a positive lifestyle and to obtain special "disabled" status for AIDS carriers.

CONTAINMENT OF OTHER INFECTIOUS DISEASES

Historically, the top priority in containing the spread of dangerous communicable diseases has been to prevent those infected from transmitting their contagion to people who are healthy.

In brief, various infectious diseases have been handled as follows:

Shigellosis (part of the "gay bowel" syndrome): strict isolation of those with active disease. Closing of restaurants known to be sources of infection.

Cholera: isolation of infectious individuals. Closing down of known sources of contagion such as a contaminated water pump, and avoidance of shellfish and other seafood harvested from contaminated water.

Yellow fever: isolation of those infected; eradication of mosquito breeding grounds.

Bubonic Plague: extermination of rats carrying infected fleas. Mandatory reporting of individuals with suspected plague to health authorities. Strict respiratory isolation of humans with plague-induced pneumonia (pneumonic plague). Avoidance of skin contact with buboes (boils).[4]

Smallpox: isolation of those infected from healthy individuals.

Tuberculosis: quarantine of individuals with active disease.

Curtailing the Spread of "Classic" Venereal Diseases: Prior to the discovery of antibiotics, syphilis was incurable. Over a lengthy period, syphilis caused dementia, heart disease, crippling joint disease, blindness and death. Individuals with syphilis or gonorrhea – conditions far less lethal than HIV – are not highly contagious but are routinely reported to health authorities and their contacts traced and tested.

RATIONAL STRATEGIES FOR CONTAINING AIDS AND TB

A rational humanitarian approach to combatting AIDS and its related contagions must encompass a broad range of practical measures:

1. Abolish anonymous HIV testing.

Due to the highly restrictive AIDS secrecy laws in many states, health authorities have been forced to conduct what is called "blind" testing. In blind testing, random HIV tests are run on anonymous specimens of blood drawn for other tests. When the anonymous samples test positive for AIDS antibodies, health authorities have no way of determining the identities of infectious virus carriers. These carriers remain unaware of their condition and unknowingly endanger the lives of others.

Anonymous Testing Breeds Walking Time Bombs

There are 11 people from the [homosexual] bars who have tested HIV-positive, five of them in the past week, who have not come for their test results. THESE PEOPLE ARE WALKING TIME BOMBS.
– Ross Walker, Vice President and HIV Manager of the Brady East STD Clinic in Milwaukee, Wisconsin. Testing, counseling and post-counseling at Brady STD Clinic are "completely anonymous," Walker stressed, and therapies are free.[5]

The individuals in the above case are infectious "walking time bombs" precisely because they were tested anonymously. No one knows who they are, where they are, or who their partners are or have been.

HIV Breaking Out Among Teenagers:
Health Officials Paralyzed

For the first time, TEENAGE GIRLS AND PEOPLE WITH NO HISTORY OF SEXUALLY TRANSMITTED DISEASE ARE TESTING POSITIVE FOR THE AIDS VIRUS AT SIGNIFICANT LEVELS at a central city health clinic, according to a four-year state study.

HIV is also spreading among high-risk populations of minority heterosexuals and individuals with venereal diseases, a trend that follows medical predictions.

However, it is THE RATE OF INFECTION AMONG TEENAGE GIRLS, WHICH IS THREE TIMES HIGHER THAN FOR TEENAGE BOYS, AND AMONG PEOPLE NOT PREVIOUSLY IN THE HIGH-RISK CATEGORY that have health officials and AIDS organizations leaders alarmed.

The January 1992 update by the Wisconsin AIDS/HIV Program, part of the State Division of Health, identifies these trends in the disease's progression based on a survey at a Milwaukee clinic serving predominantly black heterosexual patients.

The clinic treats people with sexually transmitted diseases, a population considered at greater risk for becoming infected with the human immunodeficiency virus, which causes AIDS. The clinic has been surveyed for four years.

HIV infection among teenage boys tested at the clinic went from zero percent in 1988 and 1989 to 0.5% [1 out of 200] in 1990 and 1991. Among girls, zero percent of those tested in 1988, 1989 and 1990 tested positive, while in 1991 1.6% were infected (roughly 1 out of 60 girls). For the teenage population as a whole, the increase in HIV infection grew from zero percent in 1988 and 1989 to 0.3% in 1990 and 0.9% in 1991.

Also, the update reports that the proportion of HIV-infected patients who have no history of sexually transmitted disease went from zero percent in 1988 to 27% in 1989, 32% in 1990 and 58% in 1991.

ALL THE HIV TESTS WERE PERFORMED BLINDLY. While the HIV tests were being tested anonymously for other reasons, their blood was also tested for HIV infection. THEY WERE NOT TOLD THE RESULTS AND THE STATE KEEPS NO RECORDS MATCHING TEST RESULTS WITH SPECIFIC INDIVIDUALS.[6]

Health officials are finding a chillingly high rate of HIV disease among teenagers but are unable to tell *a single one* of them that they are infectious. They literally do not have the foggiest notion of the identities of those carrying the virus! Health officials have no way of contacting the other people they have exposed (or who may have infected them in the first place) and warning them of their danger.

Health authorities across the United States are watching (albeit through "blind" studies) the HIV rate expand among teenagers, but remain effectively paralyzed when it comes to taking serious steps to stanch the flow of contagion to other young people.

Handing out condoms is a pathetic, counterproductive substitute for tough, aggressive HIV reportability and contact tracing. If there is to be any earnest effort to prevent the spread of AIDS in the adult and adolescent population, it is essential to stop conducting disease control "in the blind."

2.   Conduct sufficient large-scale mandatory testing to determine the true extent of AIDS spread in the overall population.

At present, health officials and politicians are approaching the AIDS crisis through a vague cloud of uncertainty. Dr. Robert Redfield of the Walter Reed Army Hospital estimates that millions of Americans are *unknowingly* carrying HIV disease.[7] When dealing with a fatal communicable disease which could annihilate vast numbers of people, it is critical to determine how far the infection has spread.

Mass Screening Yields Zero False Positives

AIDS advocacy groups allege that testing large numbers of people in low prevalence areas will yield a high number of false positive results and generate unnecessary panic. However, a survey of 250,000 blood donors in Minnesota who were screened for AIDS antibodies between March 1985 and April 1987 yielded zero percent (00.00%) false positives.[8]

HIV testing must be compulsory because those who are carrying the disease are likely to refuse HIV testing when it is optional. Between 1988 and 1989, officials from the Berkeley, California Department of Health and Human Services blindly tested 1008 specimens taken from STD patients for evidence of antibody to HIV. An overwhelming 81% of the seropositive specimens were from patients who declined confidential HIV testing.

The investigators concluded:

> . . . among STD patients there is an association between declining HIV testing and being HIV seropositive.[9]

Who Should Be Compulsorily Tested for AIDS?

Accurate, inexpensive, non-invasive urine and saliva tests could be utilized for various types of large scale testing.[10] Large scale mandatory AIDS screening should include:

All patients treated for STD. Health authorities estimate that 14 million cases of STD occur annually in the United States. In addition to herpes and syphilis, non-ulcerative STDs such as chlamydia and gonorrhea are associated with an increased risk of contracting HIV.[11]

Syphilis which has been previously treated can become reactivated during the course of HIV immunosuppression.[12] Individuals with HIV disease and syphilis may be at increased risk of transmitting syphilis (and other STDs) because their weakened immunity facilitates the proliferation of the infectious organisms.[13] Conversely, AIDS patients with secondary syphilis can test negative on the standard tests for syphilis.[14] HIV carriers with syphilis may not respond to standard antibiotic treatment.[15]

Without usage of other effective medications, HIV carriers are liable to develop devastating syphilis of the brain and spinal cord.[16] Mandatory HIV testing of venereal disease patients is critical not only for interrupting the spread of HIV and STD but also for providing appropriate treatment.

All patients treated for illicit drug abuse. Drug abuse is associated with high risk of HIV disease. HIV-infected drug abusers are at high risk of transmitting the disease to others.

Prisoners at local, state and federal correctional facilities. Criminal activity is associated with behaviors at heightened risk of acquisition of HIV disease. All adolescent and adult inmates should be tested.

The mainstreaming of HIV-infected prisoners with TB into the general prison population is largely responsible for the skyrocketing rate of TB among inmates.[17] Testing all prisoners for HIV would enable authorities to uncover inmates at high risk of tuberculosis.

AIDS-infectious prisoners have spread HIV to other inmates.[18] It is common for predatory inmates to forcibly sodomize younger, weaker prisoners. HIV-infected inmates desperately need to be segregated from the general jail/prison population because of the risk of transmission of HIV, tuberculosis, hepatitis and other infections to prisoners as well as correctional officers.

It needs to be underscored that violent criminals exhibit a callous disregard for human life and anger toward society. These individuals are liable to vent their pent-up rage on other inmates and prison workers. AIDS-infected criminals have nothing to lose by deliberately infecting others; they are already under a medical death sentence.

In one prison in the United States, inmates placed drops of AIDS-tainted blood in a guard's coffee. In Australia, a young prison guard was mortally infected when an inmate jammed a make-shift syringe filled with HIV-contaminated blood into his thigh.[19]

In an ironic turn of events, some attorneys associated with groups which fought the mandatory quarantine of TB carriers as a violation of their civil liberties are now reluctant to interview their incarcerated clients. The reason? The rate of TB in some correctional facilities has become so high that visitors are at risk.

Public high school and university students. Anecdotal horror stories abound regarding the spread of AIDS among American youth. Until large-scale mandatory testing is done in high schools and colleges, there is no way of evaluating the extent of HIV disease among U.S. teenagers. Even more importantly, without mandatory, non-anonymous testing, health officials remain unable to implement contact tracing and other methods to curtail the spread of HIV in the adolescent population.

Which Patients Should Be Tested?

Medical-surgical hospital inpatients and outpatients. Approximately 40 million people are hospitalized annually in the United States.[20] Mandatory HIV screening of this vast group would provide a critically needed understanding of how far the disease has spread in American society. *All HIV positive patients should be compulsorily screened for TB.* A new advanced TB test has been developed which provides rapid results in detecting the presence of active TB.

Patients admitted to hospitals, including emergency room patients. A rapid, economical, non-invasive urine or saliva test could be utilized for this purpose.

Patients of private physicians. Private physicians should be allowed and encouraged to conduct obligatory HIV screening of patients during routine physicals and in the course of medical treatment.

Gynecology patients. Women undergoing routine gynecological check-ups should also be tested for HIV. The prevalence of cervical cancer among women with HIV is as high as 40% but it may often go undetected by Pap smear in this group, according to Dr. Howard L. Minkoff, chief of maternal and child health, State University of New York, Downstate Medical Center. HIV infection also appears to be more common in women with pelvic inflammatory disease (PID) than in their non-infected counterparts, and PID may be much less responsive to standard antibiotic therapy. Yeast infections are also common in female HIV carriers.[21]

Dental patients. Since oral and dental problems are one of the early manifestations of HIV disease, authorizing and encouraging dentists, orthodontists and oral surgeons to routinely screen their patients for HIV would facilitate early detection of infectious carriers. There are rapid, accurate, low-cost saliva tests which could be easily used in the dental setting.[22] Dentists, orthodontists and oral surgeons should be permitted and encouraged to refer HIV-infectious patients to "Dental Care Centers of Excellence for People with HIV/AIDS." These separate facilities would be staffed by dental professionals trained to deal with the complex dental problems of patients with HIV disease.

All patients with known or suspected tuberculosis. Individuals with HIV disease are likely to test negative on the standard TB skin tests because of their impaired immune response (anergy), even in the presence of active contagious disease. Individuals with active TB pose a direct health threat to other patients, medical workers and the public at large.[23]

Psychiatric patients. Since HIV disease frequently is manifested by various mental and nervous disorders, testing these patients would help provide an accurate assessment of the extent of HIV-related dementia in the population.

3.   Individuals found to be carrying HIV disease should be confidentially reported to public health authorities and their past and present partners notified of their danger.

The first and foremost goal in combatting a deadly infectious disease should be preventing the spread of contagion to others. Until individuals carrying AIDS are brought under the scope of public health authorities and their contacts notified and tested, the disease will continue to spread unchecked. *HIV carriers should be required to keep in contact with public health officers and undergo periodic screening for evidence of TB.*

4.   Institution of routine compulsory HIV testing and TB screening in occupations where an individual could spread TB to the public, e.g., health care workers, food handlers, airline attendants, teachers and others.

Compulsory HIV testing would uncover individuals at high risk of manifesting active contagious tuberculosis. HIV testing should accompany TB screening because of anergy. The more sensitive DNA "fingerprinting" TB tests should be used with HIV carriers.

Flight Attendants and Food Handlers with TB

A flight attendant with HIV and TB who breathes infective microbes into the air which is recirculated in an airplane could infect hundreds of passengers and crew members on different flights before his or her condition is discovered. Food handlers, school teachers, and medical providers with active TB also can infect large numbers of people. High risk occupations warrant mandatory TB testing.

Rapid Test Could Help Curb Spread of TB

A new tuberculosis test that cuts diagnosis time from as long as four weeks to two days has proved accurate and easy enough for most laboratories to perform. The new test, described in the *American Review of Respiratory Disease*, uses polymerase chain reaction (PCR) to test sputum samples for a DNA sequence unique to M. tuberculosis. "Tuberculosis has become a public health nightmare with the problem of multidrug-resistant TB," said Lee Reichman, M.D., president of the American Lung Association in New York. "This test will make the diagnosis easier and more exacting. We can't treat it until we diagnose it."

The test can be used for testing individuals at high risk of TB such as HIV carriers and the close contacts of persons with contagious TB.[24]

5.   Institution of routine obligatory HIV testing in occupations where HIV-induced brain deterioration could pose an occupational hazard (see Chapter 2).

6.   Establishment of "TB Centers of Excellence" where individuals with contagious tuberculosis can receive advanced treatment.
Individuals with HIV disease are prone to developing aggressive forms of tuberculosis which do not respond to standard anti-TB therapies. These deadly multidrug-resistant strains of TB can be spread by airborne particles to the public at large, other patients and medical personnel. *Individuals with AIDS and active tuberculosis must be compulsorily quarantined in protective isolation units specially designed to prevent transmission of airborne contaminants.* They should be required to remain in these closely monitored treatment units until they are determined to be non-infectious. HIV carriers with TB should undergo mandatory screenings at regular intervals to determine if their TB has reactivated.

7.   Implementation of routine obligatory HIV screening of medical and dental workers involved in primary patient care.
The author's first book, *The AIDS Cover-Up?*, published in 1986, warned:

> As it stands now, a surgeon or dentist who knowingly is carrying the AIDS virus or has full-blown AIDS or ARC can still perform invasive surgical procedures without telling his patients of his condition. In light of the gravity of AIDS virus infection, *it would appear more ethical and in the best interests of the patients to allow them to have an informed choice in this regard.*[25]

If that recommendation had been implemented, the lives of Kimberly Bergalis and four other innocent victims of their AIDS-infected dentist could have been spared.

CDC: More Patients Will Become AIDS Victims

The CDC has estimated that over a hundred other hapless patients may have been infected by physicians and dentists.[26] According to Harold W. Jaffe, M.D., of the CDC's Division of HIV/AIDS, the Florida dentist's deadly legacy will not be the only case of HIV transmission from a dentist or doctor to a patient.

> We haven't found another case but *we assume that we eventually will find one.* And, given the inherent injury rate [in surgical and dental procedures], eventually another infected dentist or surgeon will expose a patient to his or her blood.[27]

In this age of unbridled enthusiasm for personal choice, it would seem consistent to require AIDS-infected medical and dental professionals to obtain written informed consent from their patients prior to performing invasive surgical procedures.

HIV-infected medical and dental professionals should be required to have their mental and physical status periodically examined by professional peer review panels.

8. Medical and dental professionals should be permitted to refer patients with HIV disease/AIDS to medical and dental treatment centers specifically designated for the treatment of infectious diseases.

Many AIDS patients carry secondary diseases (TB, various types of pneumonia, etc.) which pose a health threat to personnel and other patients in the waiting rooms. Routine "universal precautions" are not sufficient to adequately protect the lives of medical and dental personnel against HIV and secondary diseases. There are medical and dental procedures which result in the aerosolization of HIV-infective virions, creating a dangerous threat to personnel and other patients. It would be impractical and exorbitant to require all medical and dental offices to have separate rooms with negative air pressure and to treat every patient as though they had TB.

9. Amend the Americans with Disabilities Act (ADA) to exclude AIDS, tuberculosis and other communicable diseases from being considered federally protected "disabilities."

Dr. Richard Restak, a prominent East Coast neurologist, has noted:

> Throughout history, true humanitarianism has traditionally involved the compassionate but firm segregation of those afflicted with communicable diseases from those who are well. By carrying out such a policy, diseases have been contained.[28]

The ADA does precisely the opposite. It mandates the "mainstreaming" of communicable disease carriers throughout society. The ADA needs to be repealed outright or profoundly amended to protect the health of the public at large and to preserve the free enterprise system. Moreover, the language of the ADA is so broad and Orwellian that it trivializes the concept of "disability."

10. Imposition of criminal penalties for known AIDS carriers who persist in behaviors endangering the lives of others.

Individuals who knowingly transmit AIDS to other people are equivalent to criminal serial killers. One of the reasons for the early rapid growth of AIDS was that health officials did nothing to prevent known AIDS carriers from willfully spreading the disease to countless others. Historically, health officials have always been empowered to prevent infectious disease carriers from spreading contagion. Medical officials need the authority to protect the public from the Typhoid Mikes and Marys who knowingly and unknowingly are spreading AIDS.

11. Further develop and utilize tests for the early detection of HIV infection suitable for mass usage, such as in hospitals, STD clinics and blood banks.

The present AIDS antibody test may not show a positive test result for as long as 3 years after infection takes place.[29] This permits an unknown percentage of HIV-infected blood which falsely tests negative to slip into the general blood supply.[30] Heterosexuals with "silent" HIV infection may be a "source of uncontrolled spread of the virus."[31]

Rapid Test for HIV Developed

Scientists in Israel have developed an inexpensive, rapid and easy-to-use assay which tests directly for the presence of tiny amounts of the AIDS virus. *Since the method is a direct test for the presence of HIV rather than antibodies, it could drastically close the detection gap between HIV infection and formation of antibodies,* according to its co-developer, Dr. Alexander Honigman, Ph.D., a senior lecturer at the department of molecular genetics at the Hadassah Medical School. The method is "more relevant, more quantitative, faster, simpler and less expensive than existing methods," said Honigman's colleague, Zvi Bentwich, M.D., head of internal medicine at Kaplan Hospital in Rehovot. *The test detects one living cell infected with virus per 10 million cells,* said Honigman. Clinical studies of test are underway in Israel, the Karolinka Institute in Sweden, and McGill University's Jewish General Hospital.[32]

Mexico Using Saliva AIDS Test

Health authorities in Mexico have approved mass usage of a test which reveals the presence of AIDS antibodies in saliva. Medical officials gave their stamp of approval after conducting large scale testing on volunteers in various medical institutions. The saliva test called "Orasure" was designed by the Epitope Company in Oregon. The device resembles a toothbrush with a cotton swab at the end which is placed in the patient's mouth between the gums and cheek for two minutes. The test only costs about $3.00 (US) and is much safer for health care workers to perform and for laboratories to analyze.

12. Implementation of ongoing long-range studies of the potential of HIV transmission in settings of close personal contact.

National health officials are presently no longer conducting studies of the risk of non-sexual HIV transmission outside of the medical setting. They apparently have assumed the risk of "casual transmission" of AIDS is no longer worth studying. HIV is a protean lentivirus which mutates with ferocious rapidity. According to Dr. Gerald Myers, a molecular geneticist at the Los Alamos National Laboratory:

> The AIDS viruses now manifest themselves as a complex family tree, sprouting new genetic branches – and apparently very quickly at that.[33]

The world renowned Nobel Laureate, Dr. Joshua Lederberg, asserts:

> With so much at stake, *WE MUST INCREASE OUR VIGILANCE* regarding various modes of [HIV] transmission.[34]

13. Immigration authorities should require HIV and TB testing of all immigrants.

Foreigners who carry HIV disease should be returned to their respective countries. The public cost of funding treatment for AIDS is high enough without the additional undue burden of subsidizing expensive treatments for non-citizens. Furthermore, these infectious individuals are at risk of spreading AIDS and TB to the public.

14. Educational institutions should cease using noxious sex instruction and "AIDS education" courses which exacerbate the problems of pre-marital relations, out-of-wedlock pregnancies, abortions, venereal disease and emotional problems.

There is a vast interlocking industry of public and private family planning groups, corporations and government bureaucrats which has a vested financial interest in encouraging children and adolescents to engage in pre-marital sexual activity. Their lucrative income is based on providing counseling and welfare support for unwed mothers, abortion referral and provision services and treating the related psychological, financial and medical problems associated with promiscuity. These groups stand to lose money if there was a significant reduction in the rate of adolescent fornication.[35]

Progressive, constructive curricula are available which have been highly successful in positively changing the values and behaviors of young people in regards to pre-marital relations.[36]

15. Close all homosexual bathhouses.

Homosexual bathhouses are commercial establishments whose sole reason for existence is to facilitate *en masse* anonymous sodomitic encounters. Very early in the course of the AIDS epidemic, it was found that these bathhouses were major breeding grounds for AIDS and other malignant contagions. In his classic textbook, *The Homosexual Network*, Enrique Rueda writes:

> *The degree of promiscuity in the baths defies the imagination of those not familiar with homosexuality.* From the point of view of traditional values, they are probably some of the most destructive and degrading institutions in America today. *There is no indication, however, that any of the homosexual organizations have opposed or in any way showed interest in counteracting the effects of the baths.*[37]

Instead of appropriately being shut down, bathhouses and other hubs of mass contagion have, at the insistence of homosexual leaders, been semantically transformed into "educational centers."

For government and medical officials to allow the bathhouses to remain open makes a mockery of any purported claims to be "combatting AIDS."

16. Enact and enforce anti-sodomy laws.

As the anti-sodomy laws in various states were overturned, police were left powerless to shut down homosexual bathhouses, bars and sex shops which institutionalized promiscuous, anonymous sodomitic encounters. If the anti-sodomy laws had been left intact and used to shut down the bathhouses and other hubs of mass contagion, the lives of countless young homosexual males and their unsuspecting male and female partners could have been spared. Enforcing existing anti-sodomy laws and enacting new ones in the states without them would give law enforcement officials the ability to crack down on commercial establishments promoting the spread of AIDS and other infectious diseases.

STANDARD DISEASE CONTROL MEASURES ABANDONED

Precedented, effective means of disease control have been overwhelmingly ignored with regard to containing the spread of AIDS.

At the behest of homosexual and AIDS advocacy groups, most legislators and public health officials have resisted any form of mandatory testing, contact tracing, quarantine, or closing of homosexual bathhouses. AIDS advocacy groups allege that such measures constitute an "invasion of privacy" and an infringement of the civil rights of HIV carriers and high risk group members.

Most politicians and health officials have opted for promoting the illusory notion that "education" is the ultimate solution for halting the spread of AIDS.

A PROFOUND PATHOLOGY

What much of the public fails to realize when trying to make sense of the AIDS epidemic is that America's AIDS policy has been dictated by individuals who are suffering from a profound psychopathology. At the University of Texas at Arlington, in 1990–a decade into the AIDS epidemic–male heterosexual students complained that they were finding homosexual students sodomizing one another in the men's bathrooms. The homosexuals had carved "glory holes" in the steel partitions between the toilet stalls and were using them for anonymous sodomy. University police bolted steel plates on either side of the walls over the opening. The homosexuals, apparently using crow bars, repeatedly pried loose the steel plates and continued to be found engaging in anonymous sodomy between the partitions. The University's student newspaper, *The Shorthorn*, contained a front page photo of one of the glory holes. The jagged metal aperture was lined with toilet paper to help prevent injury among its users.[38]

This type of compulsive, self-destructive behavior will not be changed by "education."

A TIME FOR COURAGE

In the report *AIDS in the World 1992*, the International AIDS Center at Harvard University predicts that as many as 110 million people worldwide will have contracted HIV disease by the year 2000.

Dr. Johnathan Mann, Director of the Center, and former chief of the World Health Organization's global AIDS program, asserted:

> The World's vulnerability to the spread of AIDS is increasing not decreasing. The pandemic is spreading to new areas and new communities. The disease has not peaked in any country and will reach every country by the end of the century because governments and international organizations lack effective means to control it.

Governments do not lack the effective *means* to control the spread of AIDS. They only need the *courage* to enact tough uncompromising measures to stop it. They must cease and desist from allowing the purveyors of AIDS and TB to dictate public policy to the uninfected members of society.

EPILOGUE

BREAKING THE DEADLY SILENCE

SILENCE = DEATH
— Slogan of ACT-UP (AIDS Coalition to Unleash Power)

OVERCOMING THE STOCKHOLM SYNDROME

The "Stockholm Syndrome" is a phenomenon in which a set of positive feelings develop between hostage and captor. The term was coined after a 1974 incident in Stockholm, Sweden, where two criminals held four persons hostage in a bank vault for five days. Later, the ex-hostages sided with their captors, and two female hostages even became engaged to their former captors.

According to psychiatrists, the sympathy results from the mental trauma of being held in a helpless state. "Once a hostage really believes his life is in jeopardy, then for each moment that he's not killed, he feels a great and irrational gratitude to the hostage taker," says Dr. Charles Bahn of John Jay College of Criminal Justice in New York.

"The hostage is suddenly placed in an infantile situation," explains psychiatrist Dr. Frank Ochberg, an expert on hostage psychology and Director of Michigan's Department of Mental Health. "The hostage literally can't eat, can't move, can't use the toilet facilities, sometimes can't even talk, without permission. This is demeaning and frightening—throwing a person back to a set of emotions that are very primitive. These same infantile emotions are also the precursor to affection and love. It's what a one-year-old infant would feel toward a parent who, as the powerful being, takes away the terror of infancy. *Hostages don't recognize that their feelings are primitive. They usually describe their emotions in adult terms such as trust, compassion, or love.* . . . In the Stockholm Syndrome, part of the reason why terrorists reciprocate positive feelings toward hostages is that they themselves are in danger and depend on their hostages for safety."

Dr. Ochberg, who serves as a consultant to the Federal Bureau of Investigation (FBI) and the Secret Service, points out that once the hostage situation has been resolved, it may take awhile for the hostages to recover from the syndrome: "*The hostage can continue to have strong feelings about the hostage taker after captivity, and*

247

these emotions can color their interpretation of the terrorists' cause. This sympathetic feeling will eventually go away. . . . It's something primitive that is difficult to shake with reason." He adds that "hostages don't make good witnesses for the prosecution."[1]

Dissociative mental disorders may occur in people who have been subjected to periods of prolonged and intense coercive persuasion (e.g., brainwashing, thought reform, or indoctrination while held captive by terrorists or cultists). The predominant feature is a dissociative symptom, i.e., a disturbance or alteration in the normally integrative functions of identity, memory, or consciousness.[2] The case of Patricia Hurst who was kidnapped and raped by terrorists and then robbed banks on their behalf is an example of the mind-altering effects of the Stockholm Syndrome.

POLITICIANS AND HEALTH OFFICIALS REFLECT THE STOCKHOLM SYNDROME

The response of the political establishment to the AIDS epidemic bears striking resemblances to the Stockholm Syndrome. Dr. Edward Annis, former president of the American Medical Association, states:

> Gay-rights organizations have pressured legislators to place innumerable obstacles in the path of public health officials and private practitioners. RULES AND REGULATIONS HAVE BEEN DESIGNED TO CONTROL THE VAST NUMBER OF PEOPLE WHO ARE NOT INFECTED WITH AIDS, RATHER THAN TO INHIBIT THE ACTIONS OF THOSE WHO HAVE THE POTENTIAL TO SPREAD THE DISEASE.
>
> Some laws call for sanctions against doctors who divulge a diagnosis of AIDS to anyone but the patient, restricting such disclosures even to physicians to whom the patient is referred.[3]

Instead of enacting appropriate measures to protect the public, many politicians have identified with the cause of those spreading mass contagion.

Leading medical authorities have also proven susceptible to the Stockholm Syndrome and dissociative disorders. Dr. John Seale explains:

> *Many senior doctors in charge of numerous Aids patients develop profoundly neurotic attitudes which enable them to cope with their job by selective denial of reality.* In support of their patients for whom they can do little medically, they fiercely defend their rights of confidentiality, and freedom of association, *totally ignoring public health responsibilities to ensure that others are not infected.* They are regularly consulted by Government and the Media and other doctors on how to control the epidemic.[4]

BLOOD TERRORISM CONTINUES
In 1983, before the screening test for AIDS antibodies had been developed, Robert Schwab, a homosexual activist dying of AIDS and late president of the Texas Human Rights Foundation, angrily asserted:

> There has come the idea that if research money [for AIDS] is not forth-coming at a certain level by a certain date, all gay males should give blood ... whatsoever action is required to get national attention is valid. *If that includes blood terrorism, so be it.*[5]

In 1989, a study was presented in the *New England Journal of Medicine* which found that a shocking 87% of homosexual males who were infected with the AIDS virus failed to develop a level of antibodies detectable by the standard blood screening test for up to three years or longer.[6] Homosexual advocacy groups used these findings to argue that patient testing would endanger the lives of health care workers by giving them a false sense of security. At the same time, *they continued to fight for the right of homosexuals to donate blood* and succeeded in getting blood drives conducted in San Francisco's Castro district—the area with the highest density of AIDS cases in North America. Homosexual tabloids insisted that blood banks in high risk areas continue to solicit blood donations from their readers and threatened to sue them for discrimination if they stopped advertising.[7]

COURAGEOUS SURGEON THREATENED
Dr. Lorraine Day, then Chief of Orthopedic Surgery at San Francisco General Hospital, challenged the wisdom of the blood drive. "I don't want my patients, or any other patients, to receive HIV-contaminated blood," she said. As a result, she was viciously threatened by homosexual groups and assailed in the media for her "bigotry." Local and national health officials chastised Dr. Day for her "insensitivity" and sympathetically sided with the homosexuals. A la Stockholm Syndrome, they claimed it was time to "destigmatize" a group which had *suffered* so much discrimination.[8]

No mention was made of the anguish of the thousands of innocent blood transfusion recipients who had become infected with AIDS. No mention was made of the suffering of their spouses and children to whom they had unwittingly passed the virus. Celebrity AIDS victims like Ryan White, Arthur Ashe and others have been heralded by the media as proof that AIDS is not mainly a consequence of sodomy—anybody can get AIDS. In reality, *the vast majority of all AIDS-tainted blood transfusions in the United States can be traced to homosexual donors.*

Prior to the development of the AIDS antibody test, health officials were well aware that hepatitis B was pandemic among homosexuals. They knew that the hepatitis core antigen test could be used as a surrogate test for AIDS. Use of the surrogate test would have screened out 88% of AIDS-infected donors and saved many lives.[9] Health officials did not require blood banks to use the test. The lack of forthrightness by health officials and blood banks combined with the recalcitrance of male homosexuals produced a virological genocide of the hemophiliac population. Dr. Joseph Feldschuh states:

> It is important to recall that 50% *of* the entire hemophiliac population in the United States became infected with the AIDS virus when the blood banking industry [and public health establishment] was reassuring the public that there was nothing to worry about. At the present time, THIS TRAGEDY MAY BE IN THE PROCESS OF BEING REPEATED, BUT ON A FAR GREATER SCALE.[10]

SEXUAL TERRORISM

In an effort to appease homosexual groups, standard disease control methods have been largely abandoned by legislators and health officials and are rarely mentioned in the media. As a consequence, much of the public is not aware of the basic measures which should be used to curtail the spread of a deadly communicable disease such as AIDS. Dr. Annis comments:

> In protecting the rights of people who have AIDS and who refuse to change their behavior, THE GOVERNMENT ENCOURAGES THE SPREAD OF THE VIRUS to their unsuspecting sexual partners.[11]

Instead of being protected, the general public is being told to treat every sexual partner–even spouses–as though they are potential contagion carriers.

CLAMORING FOR A CONTRACEPTIVE DELUGE

Instead of demanding mandatory AIDS testing, contact tracing, closing bathhouses, quarantine of willful HIV/TB spreaders, etc., much of the public has been enticed into the clamor for a nationwide contraceptive deluge on adults, adolescents, and children alike. In clamoring for more explicit "safe sex" instruction, many people in society have fallen prey to the Stockholm Syndrome.

The hostages–in this case the deluded, fearful public at large–are siding with the cause of sexual terrorists, i.e., radical AIDS carrier groups who demand the right to spread the disease with impunity. Parents are being co-opted by sex-educrats and homosexual groups who want all children indoctrinated in the pansexual ethic.

WILTED FLOWER CHILDREN

In an increasing number of schools, it is the parents themselves who are demanding that children be taught graphic how-to lessons in pre-marital relations and condom usage. Some parents want to throw out progressive, effective programs which promote abstinence and moral restraint. They prefer the effete "if it feels good, do it" curricula of yesteryear.

Many of these parents are wilted flower children of the 60s and 70s who fornicated and cohabited with abandon. These aging roués and waning sirens have never recognized their own behavior as wrong. As long as their children are experimenting with pre-marital relations, they can justify their own past and present amoral lifestyles by telling themselves that "fornicating is just a normal part of growing up." Conversely, *their consciences are condemned by the moral purity and innocence of their own and others' children.*[12] These corrupt parents bitterly rail against the idea of children being taught chastity is the best policy.

The emotional, physical and spiritual best interests of children are being discarded by a generation of adults who do not have the moral wherewithal to guide and protect them.

AIRBORNE TERRORISM

Since the onset of the AIDS epidemic, health officials have propounded the notion that AIDS cannot be transmitted by "casual contact." Any form of "discrimination" towards AIDS carriers was said to be based on ignorance and paranoia. The greatest threat, or so the public was told, was not AIDS, it was AIDS hysteria, or the "fear of AIDS (FAIDS)." In light of the exploding epidemic of deadly airborne tuberculosis among HIV carriers, these reassurances have proven hollow.

According to Lee B. Reichman, M.D., MPH, professor of medicine and director, pulmonary division, University of Medicine and Dentistry of New Jersey, NJ Medical School:

> *It would seem now that there is plenty to fear. TB is back.* The advent of AIDS has led to coinfection by the HIV virus and *M. tuberculosis* as a worldwide problem.

While public health officials were reassuring the public ("you won't catch AIDS from your dentist, through the air," etc.) they had unmistakable early warning signs that tuberculosis was burgeoning among HIV carriers and posed a serious threat to the general population.[13] It was also readily apparent that many HIV carriers with active tuberculosis were refusing to comply with the extensive treatment regimens necessary to render them non-infectious to others.

Health officials maintained a deadly silence regarding the growth of tuberculosis until fatal outbreaks of the disease in hospitals, prisons and elsewhere drew media attention.

WHY TUBERCULOSIS IS OUT OF CONTROL

National health officials are now openly expressing dismay that "TB is out of control in this country," as though the galloping growth of the deadly disease was some kind of new phenomenon that suddenly crept up overnight. That clearly is not the case. Blaming the drug companies for the monumental growth of TB in the United States is a red herring. *The reason that tuberculosis is out of control is because the AIDS epidemic has been allowed to run out of control.* New TB cases have reached record numbers in this country because HIV carriers with active tuberculosis have not been compulsorily quarantined and their intimate and casual contacts tracked down and tested for TB.

Deadly drug-resistant forms of TB are raging out of control because the TB parasite has built up resistance among HIV carriers who do not comply with treatment.

Now that TB has been allowed to spread extensively, health officials and politicians are issuing the same type of specious admonitions they have for AIDS. "TB isn't just a problem among AIDS patients, it's *everybody's* problem. TB doesn't discriminate, anybody can get TB."

And, if they wait long enough and allow TB to reach epidemic proportions similar to AIDS, the claim will be made that there are so many people with TB it would be impractical and unworkable to impose any form of quarantine and would infringe on the civil liberties of people with contagious TB as well.

THE FEASIBILITY OF A SAFE BREATHING CAMPAIGN

In addition to the civil liberties issue, a major argument used against quarantining AIDS carriers is that AIDS is spread by well-defined risk behaviors; people can therefore voluntarily choose not to engage in those behaviors putting them at risk.

AIDS-related pulmonary tuberculosis is a different matter. In spite of popular media impressions to the contrary, having sexual relations is *not* necessary in order to exist. Breathing *is* an essential life function. One can choose not to have sex relations with someone (or anyone) and choose not to use drugs, but one simply *must* breathe in order to survive. A "safe breathing" campaign–"Get to know your breathing partners first and inspect their lungs for lesions; unless you are in a monogamous breathing relationship always put on your gas mask first and wear it from start to finish,"–would not be terribly efficacious. TB microbes are invisible to the naked eye and most people don't carry a current picture of their chest x-ray in their wallet.

It may be unpalatable to some die-hard civil libertarians and AIDS activist groups, but the way you prevent the spread of TB is to make certain that individuals with active contagious disease are not freely mingling with the public.

HUMANITARIANISM VERSUS LEGAL TERRORISM

Dr. Richard Restak, a prominent East Coast neurologist, has noted:

> Only sentimentalists refuse to make any distinction between the victims of a scourge and those not presently infected. . . .
> *The threat of AIDS demands from us all a discrimination based on our instinct for survival against a peril, that if not somehow controlled, can destroy this society.* . . .[14]

With respect to AIDS, the effective humanitarian approach to communicable disease containment has been turned into a topsy-turvy Orwellian nightmare. Under the so-called Americans with Disabilities Act (ADA), employers and "public accommodations" which attempt to "discriminate" against infectious AIDS carriers face the horrendous prospect of backbreaking litigation. The *healthy* uninfected members of society who try to protect themselves and others from the carriers of a deadly infectious disease face a host of devastating repercussions.

ANTI-HETEROSEXUAL TERRORISM

Prior to the enactment of the ADA, *The Gay Community News* printed an article by Michael Swift, a self-proclaimed "Gay Revolutionary" who vowed:

> We shall sodomize your sons, emblems of your feeble masculinity. . . .
> All laws banning homosexual activity will be revoked.
> If you dare to cry faggot, fairy, queer at us, we will stab you in your cowardly hearts and defile your dead puny bodies.
> THERE WILL BE NO COMPROMISES.
> ALL CHURCHES WHO CONDEMN US WILL BE CLOSED.
> . . . we [homosexuals] are fueled with the *ferocious* bitterness of the oppressed. . . . We too are capable of firing guns and manning the barricades of the ultimate revolution.
> TREMBLE, HETERO SWINE, WHEN WE APPEAR BEFORE YOU WITHOUT OUR MASKS.

These heterophobic ravings acquire deadly serious import under the ADA and the Civil Rights Act of 1991. Unenlightened churches, businesses and schools which dare to "discriminate" against or verbally "harass" AIDS-carrying homosexuals, or uninfected homosexuals who are "regarded as" being at risk of AIDS, face a terrifying onslaught of litigation and up to a $300,000 fine. When a daycare worker or schoolteacher—including one in a private school—announces that his homosexual "lover" has AIDS, he has *let it be known* that he "has a *relationship with* a person with a disability."[15] Heterosexuals have reason to tremble.

MEDICAL TERRORISM

Hospitals which try to protect vulnerable patients from AIDS-infectious health care workers—who are prone to dementia and various contagious secondary diseases—are now subject to disastrous federal penalties.

Under the Bush Administration's Department of Health and Human Services, the Westchester County Medical Center in Valhalla, N.Y., was ordered to forfeit over *one hundred million dollars* in Medicare/Medicaid reimbursement funds unless it hired an AIDS-infected pharmacist *without placing restrictions* on his duties. "This is an important precedent," said Michael J. Astrue, the Department's General Counsel. "It is the first civil rights enforcement action based on HIV discrimination by any federal agency . . . [it sends a message that] the federal government *will not tolerate discriminatory activity* for the disabled in general, and *specifically for individuals with HIV."*

In contrast, Barry Bowman, a spokesman for the Medical Center, expressed the hospital's concern regarding the potential transmission of HIV to patients:

> We still believe there is a possibility that *a pharmacist preparing intravenous medication could inadvertently undergo a needle stick and transmit his infection to a patient receiving that medication, because they receive it directly into the bloodstream.* Even if you are using universal precautions, that doesn't guarantee that needle sticks won't occur."

He said the loss of the federal funds would have a crippling effect on the medical center, which operates on a budget of about $200 million per year. "This is an extremely harsh penalty," Mr. Bowman said, pointing out that the 1,000 bed hospital serves poor people in a seven-county region north of New York City.[16]

RELIGIOUS GROUPS AND THE STOCKHOLM SYNDROME

Under the banner of an emotion-laden "compassion" many religious leaders and organizations have been subsumed into the homosexual agenda. Various professing evangelical ministries, magazines, denominations and para-church organizations have acted like ecclesiastical keystone cops in their madcap scramble to prove that they are not guilty of the unpardonable sin of "homophobia." One popular speaker on the religious talk show circuit actually argues that AIDS is God's judgment on the "homophobia" of the Church – a claim that has gone unchallenged by sympathetic interviewers and audiences.[17] A national charismatic magazine had a picture of a mother proffering her newborn infant close to the face of an AIDS patient with HIV-related pneumonia in an effort to show her "compassion."

The term "homophobia" is a politically charged epithet. It reflects the revisionist psychiatric concept that homosexuals are not psychologically disordered individuals.[18] *Heterosexuals* who maintain an intense revulsion toward sexual perversion are now said to be suffering from a *phobia*, an irrational, neurotic fear. In the view of the homosexual lobby, heterosexuals who display "homophobia" are emotionally sick and need to receive desensitivity training or therapy.[19] *Every time religious groups and others claim to oppose "homophobia" they are – wittingly or unwittingly – espousing homosexual ideology.*

Many religious groups and leaders have joined the politically correct chorus of voices which claim that "discrimination" toward AIDS carriers is the number one obstacle in trying to combat AIDS. In so doing they have become what Stalin called "useful idiots." *They played directly into the hands of homosexual groups who fought to have their deadly sodomy-induced disease transformed into a weapon of political warfare.*[20] While various religionists were zealously trying to demonstrate their "compassion," the homosexual/AIDS advocacy lobby succeeded in getting federal, state and local laws passed designed to cripple private and religious organizations opposed to their agenda.

THE BRAVE NEW WORLD OF AIDS "RESEARCH"

I don't think these kids are dead, but would I take the organs out? Yes.
– Art Caplan, director of the Center for Bio-Medical Ethics at the University of Minnesota[21]

In his chilling, eyewitness documentary, *The Theory and Practice of Hell*, Eugene Kogon, a former prisoner at Buchenwald concentration camp, describes how Nazi doctors used prisoners as human guinea pigs to conduct grisly scientific "research." With the full knowledge, consent and support of Nazi government officials, physicians and scientists dissected – without anesthesia – countless men, women, children and babies under the guise of helping humanity find a cure for various ailments.[22] Since the victims were destined to be put to death anyway, utilizing them in research experiments to advance the cause of science was viewed as a noble, vital undertaking.

Contemporary scientists have used a similar rationale for conducting grotesque human/animal vivisection experiments in the name of "AIDS research." The vaunted procedures consist of dissecting live aborted infants. The babies are removed from inside the womb through means which leave their bodies intact (suction abortion is very destructive and mutilated body parts don't work). Their internal organs are then transplanted into rodents. In a press report describing the procedure, Doctors Mike McCune and Irving Weissman at Stanford University said they gave 300 mice temporary human immunity by implanting them with human "stem cells." "With the consent [sic] of abortion patients, the scientists took liver, thymus and lymph cells [from the aborted babies] then injected the liver cells into the mice and surgically implanted the thymus and lymph cells into the rodents."[23] The researchers succeeded in "making a human mouse," said Dr. David Katz, president of the Medical Biology Institute a research center in La Jolla, California. Dr. Donald E. Mossier and colleagues at the Institute and Veterans Administration have published a study in the British Medical Journal *Nature* describing their "success" in reconstituting a fully functioning human immune system in mice with severe immune deficiency. One of the major uses of the human/animal vivisection experiments will be "AIDS research." "The potential of this for AIDS research is really extraordinary," exulted Dr. Anthony Fauci, director of the National Institute of Allergy and Infectious Diseases, "this is going to be a red-hot new field."[24] Other leading scientists are now advocating the usage of "human" mice for "AIDS research" on a vast scale.[25]

Mainline churches have maintained a deathly silence regarding the wholesale vivisection of infants in AIDS experiments. They prefer to remain in vogue by championing the cause of politically correct HIV "victims."[26]

REACHING OUT TO AIDS PATIENTS

Some popular religious leaders have made an analogy between Christ's healing people with leprosy and contemporary believers compassionately reaching out to AIDS sufferers.

HOW LEPROSY IS SPREAD

Leprosy, also called Hansen's disease, is a devastating, communicable illness which causes grievous disfiguring of the face, destruction of nerves and loss of various parts of the body such as the nose, fingers, and toes.

Traditionally, it had been thought that leprosy transmission involved contact with the skin of a person with active leprosy. According to the *Cecil Textbook of Medicine*:

> In endemic areas, THE RISK OF ACQUIRING LEPROSY AMONG HOUSEHOLD CONTACTS OF LEPROMATOUS CASES IS ABOUT EIGHT TIMES (800%) HIGHER THAN IN NORMAL HOUSEHOLDS.

Although not common, large numbers of leprosy-causing organisms can be shed from the ulcerated skin of leprosy carriers. In contrast,

> THE NASAL SECRETIONS OF THOSE WITH LEPROMATOUS DISEASE CONTAIN UP TO 200 MILLION M. LEPRAE [LEPROSY-CAUSING BACTERIA] IN A SINGLE NOSE BLOW. Thus, a major portal of entry [for leprosy organisms] may be the respiratory tract [i.e., through inhaling infectious microbes]. . . . BITING INSECTS MAY PROVIDE ANOTHER MEANS OF TRANSMISSION. . . .[27]

Prior to the discovery of antibiotics a few decades ago, leprosy, like TB, was incurable. "It is probable that leprosy is transmitted mainly by the respiratory route [through breathing], as with tuberculosis."[28] Hence, *the strict segregation of infectious leprosy carriers from close family members was medically warranted.*[29] The isolation of persons with contagious leprosy was not based on "ignorance, hysteria, bigotry and paranoia." As with TB, drug-resistant strains of leprosy have also appeared. A number of reports of leprosy in AIDS patients have been published.[30] AIDS may accelerate the spread of leprosy in endemic areas.[31] Conversely, leprosy may heighten the transmission of retroviruses.[32]

It needs to be underscored that while the Lord Jesus Christ healed individuals with leprosy, He did not abrogate the millenia-old preventive health guidelines regarding infectious disease.[33] He pointedly instructed the lepers who were healed to have their healings officially verified and undergo ceremonial cleansing.[34] The Biblical guidelines for sanitation and control of communicable disease are based on sound health principles. Proper disposal of human waste is a cornerstone of sound hygiene.[35] Protection of the healthy from those carrying contagious disease is the *sine qua non* of contagion control. It is not "unchristian" or "unloving" to proscribe someone with AIDS and active TB from singing in a choir or working in the nursery.

NO "PEOPLE WITH LEPROSY" BANNERS

The analogy between lepers in the New Testament and modern AIDS carriers in the U.S. has some serious inconsistencies. The lepers healed in the New Testament had not contracted the disease through orgiastic sodomy. They did not militantly display "People With Leprosy" banners in local St. Patrick's Day parades. They did not superciliously demand the right to keep their disease a secret and engage in behaviors exposing other people.[36] They were not calling for horrendous fines and prison terms for healthy people who tried to avoid contamination. They were not trying to break the financial back of religious institutions supporting traditional biblical morality.

TRUE COMPASSION VERSUS THE STOCKHOLM SYNDROME

Notwithstanding the ignoble social agenda of the AIDS lobby, it can be a noble, altruistic endeavor for some persons* to care for the physical, emotional and spiritual needs of those suffering with HIV disease. Intense suffering and impending death have a way of encouraging some people to think about eternal verities.

Contemporary homosexual magazines are replete with ads for bathhouses, bars, etc., side-by-side those of groups which promote the "mercy-killing" of terminally ill AIDS patients. It is far better for AIDS patients to speak with persons who will provide truly loving, compassionate counsel rather than to take advice from peers who encourage physical and spiritual suicide.

AIDS sufferers experience a wide gamut of emotions, particularly as HIV dementia sets in. Some AIDS patients are angry and resentful toward God for "letting this happen" to them, especially if they did not contract the disease through "high risk behavior." Others feel God cannot forgive them for the sordid behaviors through which they contracted AIDS. Some may feel little remorse over their past actions and view AIDS as a part of their *karma*. They may show animosity toward caregivers who do not express approval and acceptance of their "lifestyle." Patience, meekness and unflinching boldness are called for in dealing with the spiritual needs of AIDS sufferers. Man's extremity can be God's opportunity.

Jesus Christ, the Lord of Glory, was brutally whipped, beaten, and a crown of sharp thorns derisively shoved on His head. As He

---

*Pregnant women and women trying to conceive a child should avoid working with AIDS patients due to the risk of contracting HIV, TB, hepatitis, toxoplasmosis, CMV, parvovirus B19, and other infections which can have devastating effects on their babies.

hung in agony on the cross with bloodied sweat dripping into His eyes and blood seeping from the wounds in His hands and feet, *both* the criminals crucified on either side of Him cast blasphemous, mocking insults in His teeth.[37]

Then, as one of the felons felt death approaching and listened to the words of Jesus, he turned from his rebellion and placed his hope in the Savior.[38] The words of Christ, "I am the resurrection and the life: he that believes in Me, though he were dead, yet shall he live,"[39] apply to all people in all circumstances. While it is contaminated blood that has spawned the AIDS epidemic, it is the holy, precious blood of Christ, as of a Lamb without blemish and without spot, that provides the means of wholeness.[40] "By the blood of Thy covenant I have sent forth prisoners out of the pit wherein is no water."[41]

COMPASSION AND SANITY

Persons who care for AIDS patients should do so voluntarily and be fully apprised of the grave risks involved. Providing loving care for AIDS patients does not preclude taking stringent precautions against HIV, hepatitis, incurable TB and other AIDS-related infections. A compassionate response to AIDS includes implementation of tough disease control measures in order to save the lives of people who are uninfected. Genuine compassion need not be sundered from medical sanity.

THE DECEPTIVE PANACEA OF "SAFE SEX"

A number of decades ago in the island of Jamaica, the rat population grew to such an extent that they destroyed the crops. Jamaica introduced the mongoose, a carnivorous species of the coon, which looks like an elongated squirrel. The mongoose has three breeding seasons a year; there are twelve to fifteen offspring in each brood and they are deadly enemies of rats. The result was that the rats disappeared and there was nothing more for the mongoose to feed upon; so they attacked the snakes, and the frogs, and the lizards that fed upon insects. The results were that the insects increased and stripped the gardens, eating up the peas and the lettuce. The mongoose then proceeded to attack the sheep, the cats, the puppies, and the calves and the geese. Jamaica then had to spend a small fortune to get rid of the mongoose.

The "safe sex" panacea to the AIDS epidemic is analogous to the Jamaican mongoose solution. By shredding the natural sense of modesty and reserve of children and young people regarding intimate matters, it unleashes the same unbridled, dehumanizing libertinism responsible for the explosive growth of venereal disease in the first place. *"Safe sex" trivializes the meaning of human sexuality into brute animal gratification shrouded in latex.* It promotes the dangerous illusion that fornication and sodomy are intrinsically worthwhile pursuits as long as people avoid contracting AIDS. When intimate sexual expression is cut loose from its mooring in the institution of marriage, the result is untoward emotional and familial havoc.

By utterly divorcing the unitive and genitive aspects of human sexuality, "safe sex" promotes a sterile, self-indulgent licentiousness devoid of life and lasting meaning.

WHO SULLIED SEX?

For decades, sexual liberationists claimed that people needed to be liberated from the repressive Judeo-Christian ethic. They taught that everyone should be free to experience their own sexuality in any manner whatsoever with anyone that was willing.

Vast multitudes of people bought that line of reasoning but the result was not quite the erotic Elysium they had anticipated. At least 30 million Americans have incurable genital herpes, 14 million are infected with incurable genital wart virus which has been linked with cervical and penile cancers, four million new cases of chlamydia and one to two million cases of gonorrhea occur annually in the United States–diseases which have rendered multitudes of women and men permanently sterile.

Hundreds of thousands of people have been officially reported as having developed end-stage AIDS and untold millions more unknowingly carry HIV disease. In the minds of many, instead of being aligned with connubial bliss and the procreation of new life, human sexuality is now associated with personal misery, disease and death.

In light of these devastating repercussions, the Judeo-Christian teaching that intimate sexual expression should be confined within the bonds of a monogamous, faithful, lifelong commitment–that quaint institution known as marriage–appears not to be so oppressive after all.

THE CRITICAL MASS OF CONTAGION

Some scientists have suggested that when enough people have developed the combination of pulmonary AIDS and tuberculosis, a "critical mass" of contagion will be reached.[42] Analogous to the chain reaction meltdown of a nuclear reactor, the AIDS epidemic could burst forth out of its usual modes of transmission and be disseminated to vast numbers of the general population.

There is evidence that this "critical mass" process has already begun in Africa.[43]

Larry Kramer, the outspoken HIV-infected homosexual who founded ACT-UP, has written:

> When I first became aware of the disease, there were only 41 cases in the United States, now there are 12 million people infected with AIDS around the world: within the next eight years this figure could rise to 40 million. From 41 to 40 million should be enough not only to cause a level of panic but also to make everyone ask: how is this plague spreading so quickly?
>
> *I wonder if—despite everything we are being led to believe—AIDS is spread in ways we don't yet know about.* These figures are growing with such alarming rapidity that I wonder if AIDS is transmitted in ways other than sex, dirty needles and infected blood. . . .
>
> But what is there out there that we don't know about? Are not 40 million infected people trying to tell us that something else—another means of transmission, say—might be going on?[44]

THE PINK TRIANGLE

The international emblem of the homosexual movement is the pink triangle. The movement claims that the pink triangle was the identifying marker which homosexuals were forced to wear in the Nazi concentration camps. The slogan "SILENCE = DEATH" is usually superimposed on the triangle. It signifies that unless they militantly speak out, AIDS could result in homosexuals being similarly stigmatized and that many more will die.

THE REALITY OF HITLER'S RISE TO POWER

The Institute for Media Education has done an extensive analysis of the pervasiveness of homosexuality in the Nazi movement.

> The notion of Hitler's persecution of homosexuals is based on his assault against "fems" not "butch" homosexual Nazi supermen. MANY OF HITLER'S "INNER CIRCLE," AND THE KEY MEN WHO RECRUITED FOR THE PARTY AND WHO LED THE PARTY, INCLUDING THE MOST BRUTAL MILITARY BRIGADES, THE STORM TROOPERS, AND THE INFANTRY SCHOOL—WERE HOMOSEXUALS: including Ernst Roehm, Rudolf Hess and Gerhard Rossbach, while the infamous Goring was also said to be a transvestite.
>
> Captain Ernst Roehm served as a military adviser to the chief of Bolivian forces. Returning to Germany he was made "head of the Storm Troopers." However, his qualities as a leader were vitiated by strong homosexual desires which he indulged with brazen openness. He surrounded himself with dissolute young men whose frequent orgies did the party's reputation no good.
>
> Captain Roehm was so well known as a homosexual that articles in the press about him and his doctor lover were widely read by the public. Walter Langer, writing in *The Mind of Adolph Hitler*, noted that Rudolph Hess was

generally known as "Fraulein Anna." There were also many other [homosexuals close to Hitler] and it was supposed, for this reason that Hitler too belonged to this category.

Roehm made no attempt to hide his homosexual activities . . . Hitler said. The only criterion for membership in the party was that the applicant be "Unconditionally obedient and faithfully devoted to me."

Late in Hitler's rule Ernst Roehm was executed. However, this follows Roehm's growth in power and the possibility that he would use his Storm Troopers – many of whom would be homosexual, to overtake Hitler. Hitler attempted dozens of times to correct Roehm's many challenges to Hitler's authority. Roehm died because Hitler could no longer depend on him, and not because of Roehm's homosexual liaisons.

The German libertarian sexologist, Wilheim Reich, writing on Hitler's rise to power, observed:

The male supremacy of the Platonic era is entirely homosexual. . . . The same principle governs the fascist ideology of the male strata of [Nazi] leaders (Bluher, Roehm, etc.). . . .[45]

Dr. Edmund Bergler, a world renowned psychiatrist who wrote extensively on the subject of homosexuality, asserted:

[The] claim that homosexuals are always on the side of democratic thinking is especially amusing: one remembers only too well Roehm and his homosexual storm troopers, purged by that other gangster Hitler, when they threatened his power in 1936.

IT IS ALSO WELL KNOWN THAT THE *CAPOS* IN HITLER'S CONCENTRATIONS CAMPS WERE ONLY TOO FREQUENTLY RE-CRUITED FROM THE RANKS OF HOMOSEXUAL CRIMINALS. (Capos were overseers drawn from the ranks of prisoners.) I had firsthand information on this point from a patient who had spent six years in the infamous camp at Dachau.[46]

ACT-UP STUDIES HITLER

The average gay man or woman could not immediately relate to our subversive tactics, drawn largely from the voluminous *Mein Kampf* ["My Battle" by Adolf Hitler], which some of us studied as a working model. . . . And we justified our methods with the consolation that they were unfortunately necessary in order to precipitate a higher good for our people: "Let us do evil that good may come."

But now, nearly two years later, I recognize the error in this line of thinking. . . . If we allow our organization to take on this absolutist bent . . . we will be acting up in a "Queer Nation" not worth living in. Or, perhaps more tragic, not worth fighting for.
– Eric M. Polland, a former member of ACT-UP/D.C.[47]

POLITICALLY CORRECT STORM TROOPERS

In the classic 1960s film, *The Cardinal*, Nazi brown shirts invade a Catholic church, brutalize the clergy and parishioners and shower consecrated communion wafers on the floor. The scenario appears to be repeating itself in the form of militant homosexual advocacy groups who invade and desecrate churches and overrun medical conferences.

When New York City Health Commissioner, Dr. Stephen Joseph, attempted to address the Fifth International Conference on AIDS in Montreal, calling for sound public health measures to control the epidemic, he was shouted down by enraged homosexual militants calling *him* a "liar and a murderer." The Stockholm Syndrome prevailed among the conference attenders; no one moved to stop the vociferous demonstrators from interrupting (usually with their standard Orwellian chant of "SHAME! SHAME! SHAME!") the speeches of Dr. Joseph or anyone else whom they considered "politically incorrect." Dr. Stanley Monteith, a prominent California orthopedic surgeon, has faced similar verbal assaults when advocating effective health measures at various AIDS conferences.[48]

TIME TO END THE DEADLY SILENCE

Some pressing issues remain: how many more martyrs like Kimberly Bergalis will have to be sacrificed on the altar of political expediency before the rights of the healthy and uninfected population are taken into account? How many more teenagers and adults must contract HIV before health officials stop conducting health policy "in the blind" and enact tough, effective means of disease control? How many more medical and dental workers will have to contract AIDS from patients before *their* rights are protected? How many children, women and men have to acquire deadly forms of tuberculosis before AIDS and TB are treated as communicable diseases rather than as politically protected "disabilities?"

Dr. Annis comments:

> Gay-rights activists and their sympathizers have demanded that the government spend whatever it takes to find a "silver bullet" that would make sodomy, bisexual promiscuity and drug abuse acceptable and safe.
>
> No such discovery is on the horizon. . . .
>
> But *many carriers – apparently unwilling to modify their behaviors – defiantly continue to infect others.*[49]

It is time to tear down the wall of politically correct silence regarding AIDS. Now is the time for the lay and medical communities to rise up and insist that truly humanitarian steps be taken to stop the spread of AIDS and its related contagions throughout society.

Silence equals death.

PART I

DEMENTIA IS COMMON
IN HIV DISEASE

Dementia is common in patients with AIDS.
– The respected journal *Science*[1]

The central nervous system of nearly every HIV-positive patient becomes affected by the AIDS virus itself or by one of the associated diseases during the course of the illness.
– German physicians[2]

If people who've been infected with the AIDS virus don't get killed by immunosuppression, they'll die from chronic dementia, pre-senile dementia.
– Dr. Richard Tedder, a leading British virologist, depicts dementia as part of a fatal two-edged sword confronting individuals infected with HIV[3]

A progressive dementing illness is among the most common and devastating manifestations of infection by the retrovirus that causes AIDS.
– Researchers from Barcelona, Spain[4]

The nervous system is profoundly affected by acquired immunodeficiency syndrome. . . . Human immunodeficiency virus can directly infect the brain, producing a dementia. It [HIV] can also cause aseptic meningitis, spinal vacuolar myelopathy, distal symmetric peripheral neuropathy or inflammatory demyelinating polyradiculoneuropathy. Neurologic disorders due to other infectious agents are also common in AIDS patients.
– Physicians from Northwestern University Medical School Chicago, Illinois[5]

Neurological manifestations are common in HIV-infected individuals. Autopsy data suggest that the brain may be affected in as many as 80% of cases.
– British researchers from the Middlesex Hospital Medical School in London[6]

Neurologic complications and cerebrospinal fluid (CSF) abnormalities are common in AIDS.[7]
– Researchers from Abbott Laboratories, North Chicago, Illinois

A large number of AIDS patients show evidence of neurologic involvement, known as AIDS-related subacute encephalopathy [brain deterioration], which has been correlated with the presence of HIV in the brain.
– Researchers from the UCLA School of Medicine, Los Angeles, California[8]

Central nervous system (CNS) involvement occurs frequently in patients with the acquired immunodeficiency syndrome (AIDS).
 – Italian researchers from the Department of Neurology, University of Padova[9]

Human immunodeficiency virus (HIV), the etiologic agent of AIDS, was found to infect and replicate in human brain cells . . . direct infection of glial/neuronal cells by HIV may contribute to the CNS dysfunction frequently observed in HIV infected individuals.
 – Retrovirus Diseases Branch, Centers for Disease Control in Atlanta, Georgia[10]

Disorders of the nervous system frequently complicate Acquired Immune Deficiency Syndrome (AIDS). They may be related to the development of opportunistic agents (toxoplasmosis, cryptococcossis, cytomegalovirus, JC Virus), or primary CNS lymphoma. There is also a constellation of neurologic disorders which may result from direct Human Immunodeficiency Virus (HIV) replication in the CNS and HIV has been found in brain and CSF of numerous patients suffering from AIDS.
 – French researchers from the Division de Radiobiologie et Radioprotection Centre de Recherches du Service de Sante des Armees Clamart, France[11]

HIV establishes a chronic infection in the central nervous system (CNS) of AIDS patients.
 – Researchers from the University of California, San Diego School of Medicine, Department of Pathology[12]

Mental changes are common in patients with acquired immunodeficiency syndrome (AIDS). . . . The most frequent form of dementia in patients with AIDS is of a subcortical type. Impaired memory or reduced psychomotor speed, or both, are common in patients without global intellectual deterioration.
 – Neurologists from Amsterdam[13]

Mental symptoms are common in patients with AIDS. Optimal management involves the identification and treatment of underlying mental disorders rather than symptomatic treatment alone. Organic mental disorders are very frequent in AIDS. . . . There is a high probability that such common symptoms as agitation, irritability, and insomnia will be caused by an organic mental disorder.
 – Researchers from the Division of Behavioral Medicine and Consultation Psychiatry, Mount Sinai School of Medicine, New York[14]

Patients with AIDS constantly challenge clinicians with the diversity of diseases that are seen, but also in the many ways they present. Neurological presentations are common in AIDS patients. . . . These neurological complications are the second most frequent cause of death in AIDS patients. Nurses must have a solid knowledge base regarding AIDS and its neurologic manifestations.
 – The journal *Critical Care Nursing Clinics of North America*[15]

Infection with human immunodeficiency virus Type-1 (HIV-1), the causative agent of AIDS, can be associated with central nervous system as well as immune system disease. Advanced AIDS can be complicated by a dementia. Short of frank

dementia, many AIDS patients manifest neuropsychological (NP) impairment including disturbance in speeded information processing, abstraction, learning, and recall.
- Researchers from the University of California, San Diego School of Medicine[16]

Neuropsychiatric problems have assumed an increasingly prominent role in HIV-infected individuals. Disease occurs at all levels of the central and peripheral nervous systems by a variety of mechanisms. The AIDS dementia complex is the prototypical example of "direct" effects of HIV on the neuraxis, while infections such as toxoplasmosis and cryptococcal meningitis are complications of HIV-induced immunosuppression.
- Researchers from the AIDS Clinic, University of California, San Francisco[17]

Patients with the acquired immunodeficiency syndrome (AIDS) are subject to a spectrum of central nervous system (CNS) disorders. Recent evidence implicates the human T-cell lymphotropic virus type III (now called HIV) in the pathogenesis of some of these illnesses.
- Pathologists from the University of Rochester, NY back in 1986[18]

A wide variety of neurologic conditions associated with the acquired immunodeficiency syndrome (AIDS) have been attributed to human immunodeficiency virus (HIV) infection of the central nervous system (CNS).
- Researchers from the Department of Pathology, George Washington University Medical Center, Washington, D.C.[19]

The first case of AIDS positively identified in a non-foreigner in Taiwan was a 25-year-old unmarried male who had practiced homosexuality for ten years. The patient began to have abdominal pain accompanied with loose stools and weight loss in June 1985, followed by fever, cough, headache, dizziness, and loss of memory. Facial hyperpigmentation and extensive oroesophageal candidiasis were noted. . . .
    Human immunodeficiency virus (HIV) antibodies were positive by ELISA and Western blot, and the virus was isolated from the blood. At autopsy, disseminated cytomegalovirus infection, extensive CNS toxoplasmosis and early lesions of Kaposi's sarcoma were demonstrated. The detection of HIV in the adrenal medulla supports the consensus that the virus is neurotropic [infects cells in the brain and nervous system].
- The *Asian Pacific Journal of Allergy and Immunology*[20]

Cerebral infection with human immunodeficiency virus can result in the development of symptoms covering a wide spectrum of psychiatric disorders including adjustment disorders, affective disorders, delirium and dementia. The rapid and insidious nature of the disease requires an approach that relies on differential diagnosis, thorough psychiatric and neurological examination and, when indicated, additional tests such as EEG, LP, CT or MRI. The treatment of psychiatric symptoms is based on traditional pharmacological principles, although at lower doses due to the patients' propensity to develop delirium.
- Swiss scientists[21]

Patients showing organic personality disorders mostly resemble each other to such a degree as to form a separate group. We suggest to name this group according to the most prominent psychopathology as "AIDS-lethargy". This status is characterised by a specific apathy, tiredness and indolence of the patients combined with the lack of emotional participation related to their own destiny. AIDS-lethargy is the first manifestation in appearance of the HIV infection of the brain itself. Another sequel of the brain infection is AIDS dementia which can be classified as "subcortical dementia" and differs from the more current forms of dementia clinically. Affected are mainly neuropsychologic functions like arousal, attention, mood and motivation, whereas the hallmarks of cortical involvement – aphasia, agnosia and apraxia – are not present.
  – German researchers[22]

Recent evidence has demonstrated that human T-lymphotropic retroviruses are present in the brain of patients with acquired immunodeficiency syndrome (AIDS). Studies by neuropathological, ultrastructural and nucleic acid hybridization techniques indicate that these human retroviruses are neurotropic as well as lymphotropic. Striking similarities to the animal retroviruses of the lentivirus subfamily provide a rationale to implicate these human retroviruses (lentiviruses) in the pathogenesis of AIDS encephalopathy.
  – Researchers from the UMD-NJ Medical School, Newark, New Jersey and
    the National Institutes of Health, Bethesda, Maryland[23]

PART II

DEMENTIA OCCURS EARLY
IN HIV INFECTION

The AIDS dementia complex may be the earliest and, at times, the only evidence of HIV infection. . . .
  – Researchers from the Department of Neurology, Memorial Sloan-Kettering Cancer Center in New York[24]

HIV is neurotropic [infects cells in the brain and nervous system] and may enter the central nervous system early in the course of infection. Neurologic disease may be the only clinical manifestation of HIV infection.
  – Researchers from the Department of Neurology, Massachusetts General
    Hospital[25]

We have shown previously (*NEJM* 1990;323:864-870) that   67% OF ASYMPTOMATIC HIV-SEROPOSITIVES HAVE ABNORMALITIES IN ELECTROPHYSIOLOGIC TESTS. . . . This small but carefully controlled study did not produce data suggesting that AZT corrects early neurologic abnormalities in asymptomatic HIV-seropositives.
  – Neurologists and infectious disease specialists from Geneva, Switzerland[26]

AIDS patients show a very high rate of cognitive impairment. . . . A high percentage of them perform pathologically on timed psychomotor tasks. . . . 62% of AIDS and 34% of asymptomatic seropositives . . . are cognitively impaired.

. . . Psychomotor slowing, low verbal fluency, decreased attention and poor monitoring information (for problem solving, learning and recall) with relative preservation of vocabulary and visual-spatial reasoning suggest a "subcortical pattern" of cognitive impairment, even in the absence of other signs of CNS damage.
  – AIDS Specialists from Rome, Italy[27]

Up-to-date subtle methods demonstrate significant [cognitive] changes in early stages of HIV-infection.
  – German Researchers[28]

Psychiatric symptoms and neuropsychological deficits occur in all stages of HIV-infection. . . .
  – Psychiatrists from the University of Munich, Germany[29]

Neuropsychiatric impairment (NPI) is present early in the course of asymptomatic HIV infection.
  – Researchers from Uniformed Services, University of the Health Services, Bethesda, Maryland[30]

The asymptomatic HIV-positive patients showed a significantly longer mean reaction time. . . . Asymptomatic HIV-infected patients are slower and have a greater variability in speed on a simple test for reaction time.
  – The National Hospital, Oslo, Norway[31]

It has become apparent that the HIV itself is responsible for a significant percentage of neurological disease in the HIV-seropositive individual. The onset may be subtle and may occur before the onset of frank immunosuppression ["AIDS"].
  – Physicians from the Department of Radiology, NYU Medical Center/Bellevue Hospital Center, New York[32]

Following its early entry into the central nervous system (CNS), HIV-1 alters cerebral cell architecture and may subsequently affect higher cognitive functions.
  – Researchers from the Division of Intramural Research, Researchers from the National Institute of Mental Health, Bethesda, Maryland[33]

The neuropsychologic sequelae of acquired immunodeficiency syndrome and human immunodeficiency virus were studied by comparing the results of a neuropsychologic test battery administered to the following three groups of Danish homosexual men: 20 patients with acquired immunodeficiency syndrome, 20 asymptomatic subjects who tested positive for the human immunodeficiency virus, and a matched control group of 20 subjects who tested negative for the human immunodeficiency virus. The group with acquired immunodeficiency syndrome performed significantly worse than the control subjects on the tests measuring concentration, memory, and psychomotor speed. The group with human immunodeficiency virus performed significantly worse than the control subjects on the tests measuring verbal memory and psychomotor speed. On the other tests, their results varied. The study supports the hypothesis that not only patients with acquired immunodeficiency syndrome but also asymptomatic subjects with human immunodeficiency virus may be neuropsychologically impaired early in the course of the disease.

- Psychologists from the Institute of Clinical Psychology, University of Copenhagen, Denmark[34]

A group of 86 HIV-pts. (CDC stages from II to IV) were cross-sectionally studied with neuropsychological and neurophysiological methods. The percentage of abnormalities detected even among pre-AIDS stages is very high (from 25 to 50% of the cases). . . .

- Researchers from the Neuro-AIDS Unit at the University of Pavia in Italy[35]

NOW FOR A LITTLE CONDOM SENSE

ARE CONDOMS THE ANSWER?

The place was the World Congress of Sexiologie in Heidelberg. The speaker was Dr. Theresa Crenshaw. "If you had available the partner of your dreams," she asked, "and knew the person carried HIV, how many of you would have sex depending on a condom for protection?" She scanned the audience of 800 sexologists, most of whom recommended condoms to their clients. No one raised their hand. After a long delay, she saw one hand timidly raised in the back of the room. She was irate. She told them "it was irresponsible to give advice to others that they would not follow themselves." Commenting later, she explained, "Putting a mere balloon between a healthy body and a deadly disease is not safe."[1]

What exactly did those sexologists know? Why would they refuse "safe sex"? Perhaps they knew that a study done in Florida of heterosexual couples showed that 30% had caught HIV from their spouse even though they knew their mates were HIV positive and conscientiously used condoms.[2] Perhaps they knew that the one large scale test of the effectiveness of condoms in preventing the spread of AIDS was cancelled because the federal government was worried that "condoms may be incapable of providing protection to study participants."[3] Perhaps they knew that in 1987 the Department of Health and Human Services released a report stating "there are no clinical data supporting the value of condoms" in preventing HIV.[4] Perhaps they knew that the AIDS virus is 450 times smaller than the sperm,[5] that the FDA has no performance standards for condoms,[6] and that surgical gloves three times thicker than condoms have leaked blood.[7]

How well would a condom protect a Philadelphia teen from HIV? No one knows. We do know one out of every five adolescents using condoms is pregnant at the end of a year.[8] But a boy can only get a girl pregnant one week a month. An HIV positive partner can pass the virus 365 days a year.

All the "safe sex" message does is perpetuate risky behavior. As condom expert Malcom Potts said: "Telling a person who engages in high-risk behavior to use a condom is 'like telling someone who is driving drunk to use a seat belt.'"[9]

Billions of dollars have been poured into sex education programs in hopes that they would reduce teen pregnancy rates. After twenty years of these programs it's time to look at the results. Researchers report that:

> Exposure to a sex education program that includes discussion of contraceptives increases the likelihood by up to 40% that a youngster will become sexually active.[10]

> Sex education courses may increase the students' knowledge of contraceptives but they do not increase their use of them.[11]

Faced with these results, sex educators are urging that contraceptives be distributed in the schools–most often through a school-based clinic. Their reasoning is kids may be too lazy to go to the trouble to get contraceptives themselves, but perhaps if we hand them to them free they will use them.

Researchers from *Pediatrics*, however, dismissed studies from the only clinics reporting success from such tactics as flawed.[12] In fact, Douglas Kirby, "director of research of the Center for Population Options, an organization dedicated to sex education and school clinics," in a 1988 report on the "Effectiveness of School-Based Clinics," said:

> At the Center for Population Options, we have been engaging in a research project for several years on the impact of school-based clinics. . . . We find basically that there is no measurable . . . I want to underline that word and put it in boldface . . . there is no measurable impact upon the use of birth control, nor upon pregnancy rates or birth rates.[13]

The January/February [1991] issue of *Family Planning Perspectives* further confirms the failure of this approach: a recent study of six urban school-based clinics shows that distributing contraceptives did not reduce the pregnancy rate and may have actually increased it. In addition, 4-5 percent of students using the clinic said they would have refrained from sexual intercourse if there had been no clinic in the school.[14]

In short, providing contraceptives in schools does not increase adolescents' use of them but does increase sexual activity. All such a policy does is increase the number of students at risk for pregnancy, HIV and other sexually transmitted diseases. [Reprinted from The Parents' Coalition for Responsible Sex Education, March 1991.]

NOTES

OVERVIEW
A DEADLY IRONY

1. Cited in *American Medical News*, 20 November 1987.

2. "110 Million AIDS Carriers by the Year 2000," *International Healthwatch Report*," June 1992.

3. Liz Tucci, "AIDS-Patients," Associated Press, 15 July 91.

4. Edward R. Annis, "No Disease Should Be Placed on a Pedestal," *Private Practice*, January 1989.

5. G. Antonio, *The AIDS Cover-Up?* (San Francisco: Ignatius Press, 1986), p. 128.

6. *Fort Worth Star Telegram, 30 July 1985.*

7. L. Montagnier, "Lymphadenopathy-Associated Virus: From Molecular Biology to Pathogenicity," *Ann of Int Med* 1985;103:689-693.

8. "Reported Cases of AIDS-like or Immunodeficiency Symptoms Among Individuals Testing HIV Antibody Negative: Implications for Hemophilia," Hemophilia Information Exchange, 31 July 1992, National Hemophilia Foundation, NYC; CDC, *Mortality and Morbidity Weekly Report (MMWR)* "Unexplained CD4+ Lymphocyte Depletion in Persons without Evident HIV Infection – United States," 31 July 1992; G. Crowley, "Is a New AIDS Virus Emerging?" *Newsweek*, 27 July 1992.

9. D. Mildvan et al., "A Study of HIV-2 in an HIV-1 Seronegative High Risk Population in New York City," IV International Conference on AIDS, Stockholm, 1988, Vol. 2, p. 371, No. 7788. Researchers from Beth Israel Medical Center in NYC and Genetic Systems Corp., Seattle, WA, reported: "*Objective:* In a large at-risk population *followed since 1984*, we identified a subgroup with either clinical manifestations compatible with HIV infection or excessive exposure history, but who were found to be HIV-1 seronegative. *Methods:* SAMPLES COLLECTED IN 1986-87, were retested for HIV-1 and screened for HIV-2 . . . FORTY-SIX [46] PATIENTS WERE STUDIED: 2 homosexual males, 42 IV drug users, 1 African male with ARC; and one multiply transfused heterosexual female with ARC. *Results:* ALL SERA WERE FOUND TO BE NON-REACTIVE FOR HIV-1 AND HIV-2. *Conclusions:* These data suggest that THE CAUSE OF THE CLINICAL SYNDROME IN THIS GROUP OF PATIENTS IS NEITHER HIV-1 OR HIV-2. . . ." The samples were collected between 1986-1987, indicating that the problem of covert AIDS existed *at least five to six years* before it was brought to light by the medical establishment or the media. It is noteworthy that at the time, almost all the cases were among AIDS high risk group members; one case involved a transfusion recipient. Of the "new" covert AIDS cases being reported, almost half have been in people with no known risk factors.

10. "Undetectable AIDS: An Ominous Turn," *International Healthwatch Report*, August 1992; see also: J. Moore, "AIDS Minus HIV?" *Lancet*, 22 August 1992, p. 484.

11. B. Spire, J. Sire et al., "Sequence Analysis of a Highly Cytopathic Strain of HIV 1: Correlation Between Biological and Genomic Variability," V International Conference on AIDS, Montreal, 1989, p. 628.

12. "New HIV Found," *Orange County Register*, 1992, date not available.

13. W.E. Simon, *A Time for Truth* (New York: Berkley Books, 1979), p. 59.

14. "High Rate of TB Infection Found Among Hospital Doctors," *Medical World News*, June 1992, p. 31.

15. "Atlanta Plans Fight Against TB Surge," *Medical Tribune*, 11 June 1992.

16. Joseph Feldschuh, M.D., *Safe Blood: Purifying the Nation's Blood Supply in the Age of AIDS* (New York: The Free Press, 1990), p. 107. This book is indispensable for physicians and laymen who desire accurate information about the hazards of blood transfusions and how to guard against receiving contaminated blood. Dr. Feldschuh states: "In high risk areas like New York, AIDS is still not classified as a communicable or sexually transmitted disease. In 1987, the New York State Society of Obstetricians and Gynecologists [along with the N.Y. State Surgeons Society, the Society of Orthopedic Surgeons and the Medical Society of New York] sued the State Health Department to change this classification, but they lost the case in court. While there are serious civil rights issued involved, such considerations must be weighed against public health concerns."

17. "Prominent Doctors Groups Demand Mandatory AIDS Testing and Reporting," *International Healthwatch Report*, July 1988. Dr. Levitan asserted that designating AIDS a communicable disease would enable New York to more aggressively fight the disease.

CHAPTER ONE
WHY RAGE WILL NOT PRODUCE A CURE OR VACCINE

1. *Los Angeles Times*, 20 June 1990

2. B. Minutaglio, "Buying Time" *Dallas Life Magazine*, 9 August 1992.

3. Judith A. Johnson, "AIDS and Other Diseases: Federal Spending and Morbidity and Mortality Statistics," *CRS Report for Congress*, Congressional Research Service, The Library of Congress, April 18, 1991.

4. S. Mattheny et al., "Sources of Payment for Selected Services of HIV-Infected Patients in 21 U.S. Cities," VI International Conference on AIDS, San Francisco, 1990, Vol. 2, p. 288.

5. F.J. Hellinger, "Forecasting the Medical Care Cost of the HIV Epidemic in the United States: 1991-1994," VII International Conference on AIDS, Florence, 1991, Vol. 2, p. 21.

6. "Model Suggests 100% of HIV-Infected May Progress to AIDS," *Medical World News*, 8 February, 1988.

7. Graham Hancock and Enver Carim, *AIDS The Deadly Epidemic*, (London: Victor Gollancz Ltd., 1986), p. 141.

8. William T. O'Connor, *AIDS: The Alarming Reality* (P.O. Box 808, Vacaville, CA 95696: The HIVE Foundation, 1988), p. 5 citing T. Folks et al., "Induction of HTLV-III/LAV from a Nonvirus-producing T-cell Line: Implications for Latency," *Science* 1986;231:600-602. Dr. O'Connor explains: "When a person is infected [with HIV], the virus enters a cell and takes over the cellular mechanisms responsible for the production of human DNA, forcing the creation of the virus' genetic material which is then incorporated into the chromosomes of the infected person."

9. R.C. Gallo and F. Wong-Staal, "A Human T-Lymphocyte Retrovirus (HTLV-III) as the Cause of the Acquired Immunodeficiency Syndrome," *Annals of Internal Medicine* 1985;103:679. Dr. Robert Gallo states: *"Integrated viral genes are duplicated with the normal cellular genes so all progeny ["offspring"] of the originally infected cell will contain viral genes."* See also: Seymour Bakerman, M.D., Ph.D., *Understanding AIDS* (Greenville, NC: Interpretive Laboratory Data, Inc., 1988), p. 43-44, P.O. Box 7066, Greenville, NC 27835.

10. Bo Oberg, "Antiviral Therapy," IV International Conference on AIDS, Stockholm, 1988, Vol. 1, p. 108.

11. J.A. Levy, "Human Immunodeficiency Viruses and the Pathogenesis of AIDS," *JAMA* 1989;261;20;2997-3006.

12. G. Cordier, J.L. Cadore et al., "In Vivo Activation of Alveolar Macrophages and Lymphocytes in Spontaneous Interstitial Lung Disease Due to the Visna-Maedi Virus in Sheep," V International Conference on AIDS, Montreal, 1989, p. 603; Lois Ann Salzmann, *Animal Models of Retroviral Infection and Their Relationship to AIDS.* (Orlando, Florida: Academic Press, 1986).

13. J. Seale, "Aids Virus Infection: Prognosis and Transmission," *J Roy Soc Med* 1985;78:613-615.

14. D. Thompson, "A Losing Battle With AIDS," *Time*, 2 July 1990, pp. 42-43.

15. Lawrence K. Altman, "Studies Give New Clues on Action of AIDS Virus," *New York Times*, 14 December 1989.

16. "'Latency' of HIV Repudiated," *Medical Tribune*, 3 October 1991, pp. 1, 20.

17. O.F. Rudolf, M.A. Koch et al., "Immunological Detection of HIV-Infected Peripheral Blood Lymphocytes," III International Conference on AIDS, Wash., D.C., 1987, No. THP.4. Using the PCR "genetic fingerprinting" technique, scientists have detected a very high percentage (greater than 10%) of certain blood cells (PBMC) containing HIV sequence in seropositive individuals. See also: K. Hsia, E. La Blanc et al., "HIV DNA Is Present in a High Percentage of Peripheral Blood Mononuclear Cells in Infected Individuals," V International Conference on AIDS, Montreal, 1989, p. 614.

18. A.G. Fettner and W.A. Check, *The Truth About AIDS* (New York: Holt Rinehart Winston, 1985), p. 179.

19. R. Golubjatnikov et al., "Homosexual Promiscuity and the Fear of AIDS," *Lancet*, 17 September 1983, p. 681; W. Winkelstein et al., "Sexual Practices and Risk of Infection by the Human Immunodeficiency Virus," *JAMA* 1987;257:321-325.

20. G. Antonio, op. cit., p. 27.

21. A.R. Moss et al., "Three Year Progression to Clinical AIDS in Seropositive Men: The San Francisco General Hospital Study," III International Conference on AIDS, Wash., D.C. 1987, No. TP.53; M.T. Schechter et al., "Progression to AIDS in a Cohort of Homosexual Men: Results at 5 Years," IV International Conference on AIDS, Stockholm, 1988, Vol. 1, No. 4098; N.A. Hessol et al., "The Natural History of HIV Infection in a Cohort of Homosexual and Bisexual Men; A Decade of Follow-Up," IV International Conference on AIDS, Stockholm, 1988, No. Vol. 1, 4096; J.E. Kaplan et al., "Evidence for Increasing Risk of Developing AIDS in Men with HIV-Associated

Lymphadenopathy Syndrome–A 6-Year Follow-Up," IV International Conference on AIDS, Stockholm, 1988, Vol. 1, No. 4099; A. Lifson et al., "The Natural History of HIV Infection in a Cohort of Homosexual and Bisexual Men: Clinical Manifestations, 1978-1989," V International Conference on AIDS, Montreal, 1989, p. 60; A.R. Moss, "Progression to AIDS in the San Francisco Hospital Cohort Study," V International Conference on AIDS, Montreal, 1989, p. 60.

22. "Model Suggests 100% of HIV-Infected May Progress to AIDS," op. cit.

23. M.A. Wainberg et al., "Rapid Generation of AZT-Resistant Strains of HIV-1 After Low-Dose Therapy and by In Vitro Selection," VII International Conference on AIDS, Florence, 1991, Vol. 1, p. 79.

24. S. Buchbinder et al., "HIV Disease and the Impact of Prophylactic Therapies (PROP) in the San Francisco City Clinic Cohort: A 13-Year Follow-Up," VII International Conference on AIDS, Florence, 1991, Vol. 2, p. 33.

25. N. Hessol et al., "Impact of HIV Infection on Mortality and Accuracy of AIDS Reporting on Death Certificates," VII International Conference on AIDS, Florence, 1991, Vol. 2, p. 298.

26. P.A. Volberding, "Keeping Up-To-Date with Zidovudine," Patient Care, 14 November 1990, pp. 127-138.

27. A. Venet, V. Le Gros et al., "Asymptomatic HIV-Seropositive Subjects Are Not Healthy Carriers," IV International Conference on AIDS, Stockholm, 1988, Vol. 2, No. 7769.

28. R.D.F. Kunze, P. Trinkler et al., "Immunological Abnormalities in Different Clinical Stages of HIV-1 Infection," IV International Conference on AIDS, Stockholm, 1988, Vol. 1, No. 2131.

29. B. Vandvik, F. Chiodi et al., "Intrathecal HIV Antibody Synthesis in HIV Infection," IV International Conference on AIDS, Stockholm, 1988, Vol. 1, No. 2147.

30. A. Sonnerborg, B. Johansson et al., "Detection of HIV-1 DNA and Infectious Virus in Cerebrospinal Fluid," VII International Conference on AIDS, Florence, 1991, Vol. 2, p. 29.

31. J. Feldschuh, op. cit., p. 110 citing "'Healthy HIV Seropositive' Said to Be a Misnomer," Internal Medicine News, 15-31 January 1989.

32. G. Antonio, op. cit., pp. 10-20.

33. Cecil Textbook of Medicine, 18th edition, James B. Wyngaarden and Lloyd H. Smith, Jr., Editors, (Philadelphia: W. B. Saunders Co., 1988), p. 1800.

34. H.C. Lane and A. Fauci, "Immunologic Reconstitution in the Acquired Immunodeficiency Syndrome," Ann of Int Med 1985;103:714-718.

35. G.W. Hoffmann and M.D. Grant, "Hypothesis: AIDS Is an Autoimmune Disease Caused by HIV Plus Allogeneic Cells," V International Conference on AIDS, Montreal, 1989, p. 613; P. Bonara, L. Maggioni et al., "Anti-Lymphocyte Antibodies and Progression of Disease in HIV-Infected Patients," VII International Conference on AIDS, Florence, 1991, Vol. 2, p. 149; F. Tumietto, P. Costigliola et al., "Anti-Lymphocyte Auto-Antibodies: Evaluation and Correlation with Different Stages of HIV Infection," VII International Conference on AIDS, Florence, 1991, Vol. 2, p. 149; R.B. Stricker, T.M. McHugh et al., "An AIDS-Related Cytotoxic Autoantibody Reacts with a Specific Antigen on Stimulated CD4+ T Cells," Nature 1987;327:710-713; B.E. Kloster, R.H. Tomar et al., "Lymphocytotoxic Antibodies in the Acquired Immunodeficiency Syndrome," Clin Immunopathol 1984;30:330-335; B. Dorsett, W.E. Cronin et al., "Anti-Lymphocyte Antibodies in Patients with the Acquired Immunodeficiency Syndrome," Am J Med 1985;78:621-626; D.D. Kiprov, R.E. Anderson et al., "Anti-Lymphocyte Antibodies and Seropositivity for Retroviruses in Groups at High Risk for AIDS," N Engl J Med 1985;312:1517.

36. F. Tumietto, P. Costigliola et al., "Anti-Lymphocyte Auto-Antibodies: Evaluation and Correlation with Different Stages of HIV Infection," VII International Conference on AIDS, Florence, 1991, Vol. 2, p. 149.

37. M.D. Grant, M.S. Weaver, and G.W. Hoffmann. "Autoantibodies Against Collagen in AIDS: Correlation with Risk Factors and Disease Progression," V International Conference on AIDS, Montreal, p. 576.

38. Jay Levy, "Human Immunodeficiency Viruses and the Pathogenesis of AIDS," JAMA 1989;261:2997-3006.

39. Maria M.E. de Bracco, L Sterin-Borda and E. Borda, "Antibodies Against Neurotransmitter Receptors in HIV-Infected Individuals," VI International Conference on AIDS, San Francisco, 1990, Vol. 2, p. 343.

40. C. Andrzejewski, J. Benton et al., "Autoreactivity in Patients with HIV," V International Conference on AIDS, Montreal, 1989, p. 436; J.F. Quaranta, M. De Matteis et al., "Incidence of Autoantibodies in HIV Infection," V International Conference on AIDS, Montreal, 1989, p. 476; P. Costigiola, E. Ricchi et al., "HIV Infection and Red Cell Autoantibodies," IV International Conference on AIDS, Stockholm, 1988, Vol. 2, No. 2504.

41. G. Hancock and E. Carim, op. cit., p. 140.

42. P. Piot, "The Natural History and Clinical Manifestations of HIV-Infection," III International Conference on AIDS, Wash., D.C., 1987, No. M.2.3.

43. G. Antonio, op. cit., p. 138; C. Cheng-Mayer, J.T. Rutka et al., "The Human Immunodeficiency Virus (HIV) Can Productively Infect Cultured Human Brain Cells," *Proc Natl Aca Sci USA* 1987;84:3256-3530.

44. G. Hancock and E. Carim, op. cit., p. 28.

45. C. Kalama et al., "Natural History of Central Nervous System (CNS) Impairment in HIV Infection," V International Conference on AIDS, Montreal, 1989, p. 452; S.M. De La Monte et al., "Acute Meningitis During HIV Seroconversion," VII International Conference on AIDS, Florence, 1991, Vol. 1, p. 210.

46. T.M. Lacorte et al., "Neuropsychological Study of the AIDS Dementia Complex," VII International Conference on AIDS, Florence, 1991, Vol. 1, p. 204.

47. R.M. Levy et al., "Neuroepidemiology of Acquired Immunodeficiency Syndrome," cited in M.L. Rosenblum, R.M. Levy and D.E. Bredesen, Editors, *AIDS and the Nervous System* (New York: Raven Press, 1988), pp. 13-27.

48. E.F. Terwwilliger et al., "Mechanisms of Infectivity and Replications of HIV-1 and Implications for Therapy," *Ann Emerg Med* March 1990;19:233-241.

49. G. Hancock and E. Carim, op. cit., p. 143.

50. I.P. Everall et al., "Neuronal Loss in the Frontal Cortex in HIV Infected Individuals," VII International Conference on AIDS, Florence, 1991, Vol. 1, p. 63.

51. J. Day, I. Grant et al., "Neuropsychiatric Follow-Up of Subjects on AZT Licensing Trial: San Diego Cohort," V International Conference on AIDS, Montreal, 1989, p. 448.

52. M.L. Rosenblum et al., op. cit., 395 pages.

53. R.M. Levy and D.E. Bredesen, "Central Nervous System Dysfunction in Acquired Immunodeficiency Syndrome," in M.L. Rosenblum et al., op. cit., p. 29. The authors state: "HIV has as a target both the immune system and the nervous system."

54. H. Budka, "Productive Infection By HIV of the Human Central Nervous System (CNS) Tissues," V International Conference on AIDS, Montreal, 1989, p. 457.

55. A. Vital, C. Vital et al., "Morphological Findings on Peripheral Nerve Biopsies in 15 Patients with HIV Infection," VII International Conference on AIDS, Florence, 1991, Vol. 1, p. 183.

56. D.R. Cornblath, J.C. McArthur et al., "Painful Sensory Neuropathy (PSN) in Patients with AIDS," III International Conference on AIDS, Wash., D.C., 1987, p. 85. This process may represent a degeneration in the dorsal root ganglion cells from *direct HIV infection*.

57. A. Moglia, C. Zandrini et al., "Peripheral Neuropathy in AIDS: Possible Role of AZT Treatment?" VII International Conference on AIDS, Florence, 1991, Vol. 1, p. 210.

58. B.P. Mulhall, I. Jennings, "Autonomic Neuropathy in HIV Infection," IV International Conference on AIDS, Stockholm, 1988, Vol. 1, No. 4090; J.L. Gastaut, J. Pouget et al., "HIV-1 Infection and Autonomic Nervous System," VII International Conference on AIDS, Florence 1991, Vol. 1, p. 186; R. Malessa, P. Ohrman, "Peripheral Autonomic Surface Potential (PASP) as a Marker of Autonomic Nervous System Dysfunction in HIV-Seropositives," VII International Conference on AIDS, Florence, 1991, Vol. 1, p. 193; A. Vital, C. Vital et al., "Morphological Findings on Peripheral Nerve Biopsies in 15 Patients with HIV Infection," VII International Conference on AIDS, Florence, 1991, Vol. 1, p. 183.

59. J. Ashok, G. Sutherland et al., "HIV Heart Muscle Disease-The Edinburgh Experience," VII International Conference on AIDS, Florence, 1991, Vol., 1, p. 275.

60. G.L. Simon, A.M. Ross et al., "Clinically Silent Cardiac Abnormalities in Patients with HIV Infection," IV International Conference on AIDS, Stockholm, 1988, Vol. 1, No. 7093; Ignatius Fong, A. Elzawi et al., "Cardiac Abnormalities in HIV-Infected Patients," VII International Conference on AIDS, Florence, Vol. 1, p. 282.

61. A. Hershkowitz, S. Willoughby et al., "HIV-Associated Cardiomyopathy: Evidence for Autoimmunity," VI International Conference on AIDS, San Francisco, 1990, Vol. 2, p. 205.

62. C. Gadol et al., "Congestive Cardiomyopathy in Association with Acquired Immunodeficiency Syndrome in Children," III International Conference on AIDS, Wash., D.C. 1987, p. 90.

63. "AIDS Giving Rise to Cardiac Problems," *JAMA* 1990;263;16:2149.

64. S. Reichert, C. Visser et al., "Echocardiographic Abnormalities in AIDS," V International Conference on AIDS, Montreal, 1989, p. 268.

65. D.W. Anderson, R. Virmani et al., "Cardiac Pathology and Cardiovascular Cause of Death in Patients Dying with the Acquired Immunodeficiency Syndrome," III International Conference on AIDS, Wash., D.C., 1987, p. 9; V. Joshi, J. Talberg, C. Alberto et al., "Cardiologic Findings in Autopsies of AIDS Patients," V International Conference on AIDS, Montreal, 1989, p. 486.

66. D.W. Anderson, R. Virmani et al., "Cardiac Pathology and Cardiovascular Cause of Death in Patients Dying with the Acquired Immunodeficiency Syndrome," III International Conference on AIDS, Wash., D.C., 1987, p. 9; S.E. Lipshultz, S. Chanock et al., "Cardiac Manifestation of Pediatric Human Immunodeficiency Virus Infection," IV International Conference on AIDS, Stockholm, 1988, Vol. 1, No. 7089; W.S. Chung, R.B. Himelman, et al., "Cardiac Abnormalities in HIV Infection," IV

NOTES   277

International Conference on AIDS, Stockholm, 1988, Vol. 1, No. 7092; Ignatius Fong, A. Elzawi et al., "Cardiac Abnormalities in HIV-Infected Patients," VII International Conference on AIDS, Florence, 1991, Vol. 1, p. 282; L. Caggese, A. Manter et al., "Cardiac Involvement in HIV Infection," VII International Conference on AIDS, Florence, 1991, Vol. 1, p. 283.

67. L. Resnick et al., "Detection of HTLV-III/LAV-Specific IgG and Antigen in Bronchoalveolar Lavage Fluid from Two Patients with Lymphocytic Interstitial Pneumonitis Associated with AIDS-related Complex," *Am J Med* 1987;82:553-556.

68. W. Travis, C. Fox et al., "Lymphoid Pneumonitis in 50 Adult HIV-infected Patients: Lymphocytic Interstitial Pneumonitis Versus Nonspecific Interstitial Pneumonitis," VII International Conference on AIDS, 1991, Florence, Vol. 2, p. 65.

69. S. Z. Salhuddin, R.M. Rose, J.E. Groopman, P.D. Markham, R.C. Gallo, "Human T Lymphyotropic Virus Type III Infection of Human Alveolar Macrophages," *Blood* 1986;68;1:281-284.

70. *MMWR*, 1 April 1988, Vol. 37, No. S-4.

71. J.K. Maesaka, F.P. Siegal et al., "Renal Tubular Nephropathy in AIDS Causing Volume Depletion and Malnutrition," III International Conference on AIDS, Wash., D.C., 1987, p. 87.

72. H. Busch, S. Riechman et al., "Mikroalbuminaria as an Early Sign for AIDS Associated Nephropathy (AAN)," VII International Conference on AIDS, Florence, 1991, Vol. 1, p. 274; W. Umana, P.L. Kimmel et al., "Microalbumin Excretion in HIV-Infected Patients," VII International Conference on AIDS, Florence, 1991, Vol. 1, No. M.B. 2383.

73. W. Cronin, M. Shevchuk et al., "The Prevalence of HIV Positivity in Kidneys of AIDS Patients," VI International Conference on AIDS, San Francisco, 1990, Vol. 2, p. 212.

74. T.K.S. Rao et al., "Nephropathy: As the Initial (Only?) Sign of Human Immunodeficiency Virus Disease," IV International Conference on AIDS, Stockholm, 1988, Vol. 1, No. 7098; F. Raffi; A. Testa et al., "Schonlein - Henoch Purpura and Glomerulonephritis as the Initial Manifestation of HIV Infection," VII International Conference on AIDS, Florence, 1991, Vol. 1, p. 279.

75. N J. Marques, O.R. Santos et al., "Nephropathy As the Initial Sign of AIDS," V International Conference on AIDS, Montreal, 1989, p. 268.

76. T.K.S. Rao et al., "Acquired Immunodeficiency Syndrome (AIDS) Associated Renal Disease: A Longitudinal Analysis," III International Conference on AIDS, Wash., D.C., 1987, p. 36.

77. B. Lutz, B. Francis et al., "Heat Related Disorders and HIV Infection," VII International Conference on AIDS, Florence, 1991, Vol. 1, No. M.B. 2426.

78. M.A. Hasan et al., "High HIV Seroprevalence in Patients with Chronic Renal Failure," VII International Conference on AIDS, Florence, 1991, Vol. 1, p. 279.

79. J.L. Jian et al., "Infection of HIV-1 Proviral RNA and Viral RNA in Urine Pellets from HIV-1 Seropositive Individuals," VI International Conference on AIDS, San Francisco, 1990, Vol. 2, p. 164.

80. Y. Cao et al., "Detection of HIV-1 in the Liver of AIDS Patients," VI International Conference on AIDS, San Francisco, 1990, Vol. 2, p. 152.

81. A.M. Steffan et al., "Productive Infection of Primary Cultures of Human Hepatic Endothelial Cells (EC) By Human Immunodeficiency Virus (HIV)," V International Conference on AIDS, Montreal, 1989, p. 686; M.P. Schmitt et al., "Human Immunodeficiency Virus (HIV) Multiplies in Primary Cultures of Human Kupffer Cells," V International Conference on AIDS, Montreal, 1989, p. 686.

82. A. Hatzakis, A. Karafoulidou et al., "Hepatomegaly and HIV Infection," VII International Conference on AIDS, Florence, 1991, Vol. 1, p. 229.

83. E. Kahn et al., "Giant Cell Transformation of the Liver in Pediatric AIDS," V International Conference on AIDS, Montreal, 1989, p. 494 citing Witzblen, *Hum Pathol* 1988;19:603.

84. P. Detruchis et al., "Liver Lymphomas in HIV Infection," IV International Conference on AIDS, Stockholm, 1988, Vol. 2, No. 7603.

85. A. Pesce, H. Vinti et al., "Spontaneous Rupture of Spleen in an HIV Seropositive Thrombocytopenic Patient," V International Conference on AIDS, Montreal, 1989, p. 484.

86. F. Bricaiare et al., "Pancreatic Disturbances and AIDS," III International Conference on AIDS, Wash., D.C., 1987, p. 187.

87. M. Shelton, L. Woods, et al., "Pancreato-Biliary Disease in Pediatric AIDS," VII International Conference on AIDS, Florence, 1991, Vol. 2, p. 184; S. Dowell, E. Holt, et al., "Pancreatitis Associated with HIV Infection," V International Conference on AIDS, Montreal, 1989, p. 260; A. Bernal, G. Piot et al., "Acute Pancreatitis in Patients with AIDS," V International Conference on AIDS, Montreal, 1989, p. 260; F. Bricaiare et al., "Pancreatic Disturbances and AIDS," III International Conference on AIDS, Wash., D.C., 1987, p. 187.

88. M. Chase, "Six AIDS Patients Die in Trial of DDI, Experimental Drug Being Widely Used," *Wall St. Journal*, 12 March 1990.

89. J-M. Hiza, G. Kaplan et al., "Articular Manifestations in HIV-Infected Patients," IV International Conference on AIDS, Stockholm, 1988, Vol. 2, No. 7515.

90. R.H. Wirthington, P. Cornes et al., "Isolation of Human Immunodeficiency Virus from Synovial Fluid of a Patient with Reactive Arthritis," Br Med J 1987;294(6570):484.

91. L.H. Calabrese, A. Myers, D. Kelley, "Rheumatic Symptomatology in Patients Infected with the Human Immunodeficiency Virus (HIV): Prevalence and Relationship to Clinical and Laboratory Studies," V International Conference on AIDS, Montreal, 1989, p. 265; Ian F. Rowe, S.M. Forster et al., "Joint, Bone and Muscle Lesions and HIV Infection," V International Conference on AIDS, Montreal, 1989, p. 265.

92. S. Gafa, F. Vezzani et al., "Effect of Zidovudine on HIV Related Arthritis," V International Conference on AIDS, Montreal, 1989, p. 282; M. Galeazzi, T. Tuzi et al., "Rheumatoid Arthritis and Human T Cell Lymphotropic Viruses," Arthritis Rheum 1986;29(12)1533-4; F. Oberlin, V. Leblond, J.P. Camus et al., "Reactional Arthritis in 2 Homosexuals with Positive HIV Serology," Presse Med 1987;16(7):355.

93. R. Olivier, D. Fassin, et al., "Prevalence of Rheumatic Manifestations in AIDS," VII International Conference on AIDS, Florence, 1991, Vol. 1, p. 284.

94. B. Rio, J.M. Tourani et al., "HIV-Related Cytopenia," IV International Conference on AIDS, Stockholm, 1988, Vol. 2, No. 7516.

95. T.M. Folks, S. Kessler et al., "Infection and Replication of Human Immunodeficiency Virus-1 (HIV) in Purified CD4 Negative Precursor Cells from Normal Human Bone Marrow," IV International Conference on AIDS, Stockholm, 1988, Vol. 1, No. 2067.

96. A. Freedman, F. Gibson et al., "In Vitro HIV-1 Infection of Human Bone Marrow Eosinophils," VII International Conference on AIDS, Florence, 1991, Vol. 1, p. 92.

97. VII International Conference on AIDS, Florence, 1991, Vol. 2, p. 215, W.B.2134.

98. W.O. Harrison, S.W. Berg et al., "Asymptomatic Myositis in HIV Antibody-Positive Men," III International Conference on AIDS, Wash., D.C., 1987, p. 88; I.F. Rowe, S.M. Forester et al., "Joint, Bone, and Muscle Lesions and HIV Infection," V International Conference on AIDS, Florence, 1991, Vol. 1., p. 258; J. R. Trujillo, E. Gomez-Lucia et al., "Retroviral Effects on Muscle Cells," VII International Conference on AIDS, Florence, 1991, Vol. 1., p. 257.

99. M. Dalakas et al., "AIDS and the Nervous System," JAMA 1989;261(16)2396-2399.

100. C. Conlon, S.B. Lucas et al., "HIV Enteropathy in Lusaka, Zambia: A Clinical, Microbiological, Histological and Functional Study," V International Conference on AIDS, Montreal, 1989, p. 261.; D. Church, L. Sutherland et al., "Gastrointestinal (GI) Structure and Mucosal Function in HIV Positive Patients," V International Conference on AIDS, Montreal, 1989, p .262.

101. T. Uchida et al., "Signet Cell Carcinoma of the Stomach in a Patient with Acquired Immunodeficiency Syndrome: A Case Report," Japanese Journal of Clinical Oncology 1989;19:75-78; D.H. Frager et al., "Squamous Cell Carcinoma of the Esophagus in Patients with Acquired Immunodeficiency Syndrome," Gastrointestinal Radiology 1988;13:358-360.

102. S. Fleming, K. M. MacDonald et al., "Direct In-Vitro Infection of Human Small Intestine and Colon with HIV," VII International Conference on AIDS, Florence, 1991, Vol. 1, p. 63.

103. L. Deirdre et al., "Gastrointestinal Tissue Cultures for Human Immunodeficiency Virus in HIV-Infected/AIDS Patients," VI International Conference on AIDS, San Francisco, 1990, Vol. 2, p. 152.

104. G. Ramirez, L.R. Braathen et al., "In Vitro Infection of Human Epidermal Langerhans Cells with HIV," in Histopathology of the Immune System, (New York: Plenum Books, 1989).

105. L.R. Braathen et al., "Langerhans Cells as a Primary Target for HIV Infection," Lancet, 7 November 1987, p. 1094.

106. M. Cuisini, R. Zerboni et al., "Muco-cutaneous Manifestations in HIV Positive Patients," III International Conference on AIDS, Wash., D.C., 1987, p. 89.

107. G. Ramirez, L.R. Braathen et al., "Latent Infection of Epidermal Langerhans Cells in HIV-Positives?" IV International Conference on AIDS, Stockholm, 1989, No. 2089; J. Ramsauer, P. Racz et al., "Langerhans Cells in the Pathogenesis of the HIV Infection," IV International Conference on AIDS, Stockholm, 1989, No. 2090.

108. E. Tschachler, V. Groh et al., "The Skin Represents a Site of Virus Replication During Infection with Human Immunodeficiency Virus (HIV)," III International Conference on AIDS, Wash., D.C. 1987, p. 80; G. Zambruno, L. Mori et al., "HIV-1: Proviral DNA Is Present in Epidermal Langerhans Cells of HIV-Infected Patients: Detection Using the Polymerase Chain Reaction," VII International Conference on AIDS, Florence, 1991, Vol. 2, p. 60.

109. J. Wallace, J. Oliver et al., "Primary HIV-1 Infection with Virus Demonstrated in Histocytes of Skin Rash," V International Conference on AIDS, Montreal, 1989, p. 252; I. Gilson, J. Barnett, et al., "Basal Cell Carcinoma in HIV Disease," V International Conference on AIDS, Montreal, 1989, p. 252; see also: Skin Manifestations of AIDS by Neal S. Penneys, (Hagerstown, MD: J.B. Lippincott Co., 1990), contains 250 illustrations of the skin lesions associated with HIV disease.

110. "Researchers: Sunlight Accelerates Growth of AIDS Virus," (UPI) Los Angeles, 5 May 1988.

111. "Report Links Ozone Resistance, HIV," *Dallas Morning News*, 15 February 1992.

112. A. Minnella, E. Pizzigallo et al., "Retinal Manifestation in HIV Patients," V International Conference on AIDS, Montreal, 1989, p. 260; A. Minnella, A. Antinori et al., "A Study of Retinal Cotton Wool Spots in HIV Patients," V International Conference on AIDS, Montreal, 1989, p. 260.

113. M. Chiama, M. Blini et al., "Opthalmic Problems in Pediatric Patients with HIV Infection," VII International Conference on AIDS, Florence, 1991, Vol. 1, p. 282; C. Perro, S. Geier et al., "Cognitive Deficits and Ocular Microangiopathic Syndrome (OMS)," VII International Conference on AIDS, Florence, 1991, Vol. 1, p. 210; J. Verdejo, J. Sanz, et al., "Ocular Manifestations of Acquired Immunodeficiency Syndrome," VII International Conference on AIDS, Florence, 1991, Vol. 1, p. 274.

114. T. Tervo et al., "Recovery of HTLV-III from Contact Lenses," *Lancet*, 15 February 1986, pp. 379-380; R. Gallo et al., "HTLV-III in the Conjunctival Epithelium of a Patient with AIDS," *Am J Ophthalmology* 1985;100:507-509, cf., G. Antonio, op. cit., p. 109; S. Liotet et al., "Anti-HIV antibodies in tears of patients with AIDS," *Fortschritte Der Opthalmologie* 1987;84:340-341; R.J. Pomerantz et al., "Infection of the Retina by Human Immunodeficiency Virus Type I," *N Engl J Med* 24 December 1987;317:1643-1647.

115. C. Graziosi et al., "Lymphoid Tissues Function as 'Reservoirs' for HIV Infection," VII International Conference on AIDS, Florence, 1991, Vol. 1, p. 63.

116. L. Barzan et al., "Nasopharyngeal Lymphatic Tissue in Patients Infected with Human Immunodeficiency Virus: A Prospective Clinicopathologic Study," *Arch Otolaryngol Head Neck Surg* 1990;116:928-931.

117. M. De Silva et al. "Detection of HIV-Related Protein in Testes and Prostates of Patients with AIDS," *Am J Clin Pathol* 1990;93:196-201.

118. B. Elem et al., "Haematuria Frequency Syndrome in Patients with Positive HIV Serology," *Br J Urol* 1991;67:146-149.

119. Peter Nara, "AIDS Viruses of Animals and Man, Nonliving Parasites of the Immune System," *Los Alamos Science*, No. 18; 1989;56-89.

120. M. Saag, J. Gibbons et al., "Extensive Heterogeneity of HIV Genomes *In Vivo*," III International Conference on AIDS, Wash., D.C. 1987, p. 107.

121. "AIDS-Associated Virus Yields Data to Intensifying Scientific Study," *JAMA*, 22/29 November 1985, pp. 2865-2866.

122. F.E. McCutcheon, B.L.P. Ungar et al., "Genetic Relationships Among International HIV-1 Isolates," VII International Conference on AIDS, Florence, 1991, Vol. 2, p. 63.

123. W.E. Robinson et al., "Antibody-Dependent Enhancement of Human Immunodeficiency Virus Type 1 Infection," *Lancet* 1988;1;790-794; T. Joualt et al., "HIV Infection of Monocyte Cells: Role of Antibody-Mediated Virus Binding to Fc-Gamma Receptors," *AIDS* 1989;3:125-133.

124. Peter Nara, op. cit., pp. 77-85.

125. Jay A. Levy, "Human Immunodeficiency Viruses and the Pathogenesis of AIDS," *JAMA*;1989;261(20):2997-3006).

126. E.A. Ojo-Amaize et al., "Antibodies to Human Immunodeficiency Virus in Human Sera Induce Cell-Mediated Lysis of HIV-Infected Cells," *J Immunol* 1987;139:2458-2463; J. Homsy et al., "Antibody-Dependent Enhancement of HIV Infection," *Lancet* 1988;1:1285-1286; A. Takeda et al., "Antibody-Enhanced Infection by HIV-1 via Fc Receptor-Mediated Entry," *Science* 1988;242:580-583.

127. Peter Nara, op. cit., pp. 55-84. The scientists state: "Certain antiviral antibodies produced during lentiviral infection serve no useful biological purpose and therefore seem to perpetuate rather than eliminate infection in the host. . . . *In the case of HIV, coating of the virus by nonneutralizing antibody may lead to engulfment by and subsequent infection of the macrophage. . . . *The immune activation induced by a successful vaccine is controlled by the immune system's activator and suppressor networks. With time the induced protective state falls to levels of non-protection, but the state is permanently programmed into the immune system's memory network. Reinfection of the host cells with the real pathogenic viral agent causes release of chemical signals that rapidly recruit and deploy appropriate memory cells. These cells produce antibodies, T4 cells, and T8 cells that eliminate the virus before it can spread to a critical number of susceptible target cells and cause significant life-threatening disease. [Antibodies and killer T8 lymphocytes in AIDS patients are capable of *attacking* their own normal, uninfected T4 cells]."

128. J.A. Levy, "The Human Immunodeficiency Viruses: Detection and Pathogenesis," in J.A. Levy, ed. *AIDS Pathogenesis and Treatment* (New York: Marcel Dekker, Inc., 1989), pp. 159-230.

129. G.W. Hoffmann and M.D. Grant, "Hypothesis: AIDS Is an Autoimmune Disease Caused by HIV Plus Allogeneic Cells," V International Conference on AIDS, Montreal, p. 613.

130. "AIDS Mutates Quickly," *Dallas Morning News*, 4 September 1987, p. 3A.

131. "Vaccine for AIDS Called Doubtful," *Dallas Morning News*, 12 September 1992, p. 7A.

132. Lawrence K. Altman, "Advances In Treatment Change Face of AIDS," *New York Times*, 12 June 1990.

133. J. Seale, *J Roy Soc Med* 1986;77:121.

134. M. Waldholz, "Stymied Science," *The Wall Street Journal*, 26 May 1992, pp. A1, A6.

135. Ibid.

CHAPTER TWO
THE DEVASTATING IMPACT OF HIV BRAIN DETERIORATION

1. "Neuropsychiatric Manifestations of AIDS-Spectrum Disorders," *Hospital and Community Psychiatry* 1986; 37:135-142.

2. G. Hancock and E. Carim, op. cit., p. 13.

3. Erica E. Goode and Joanne Silberner, "AIDS: Attacking the Brain," *U.S. News and World Report*, 7 September 1987:48-49.

4. J. Goudsmit et al., "Pathogenesis of HIV and Its Implications for Serodiagnosis and Monitoring of Antiviral Therapy," *J Virol Methods* 1987 August;17:19-34; P.L. Lantos et al., "Neuropathology of the Brain in HIV Infection," *Lancet*, 11 February 1989:309-311.

5. B.C. Einspruch, reviewing *Behavioral Aspects of AIDS*, edited by D.G. Ostrow, (New York: Plenum Medical Book Co., 1990), 414 pp. in *JAMA*, 13 November 1991;266:2624.

6. I.J. Koralnik, A. Beaumanoir et al., "A Controlled Study of Early Neurologic Abnormalities in Men with Asymptomatic Human Immunodeficiency Virus Infection," *New Engl J Med* 1990;323(13)864-870.

7. M.M. Beckham, "Neurologic Manifestations of AIDS." *Crit Care Nurs Clin North Am* 1990;2:29-32.

8. G.M. Shaw et al., "HTLV-III Infection in Brains of Children and Adults with AIDS," *Science* 1985;227:177-182.

9. *Washington Times*, 28 July 1987.

10. "HIV Infection Classification," *Mortality and Morbidity Weekly Report*, 25 December 1987.

11. R.W. Price, J. Sidtis, M. Rosenblum, "The AIDS Dementia Complex: Some Current Questions," *Annals of Neurology*, 1988;23 Suppl: S27-33; see also: R.W. Price et al, "The AIDS Dementia Complex," in M.L. Rosenblum et al., op. cit., p. 209.

12. D.A. Rottenberg et al., "The Metabolic Pathology of the AIDS Dementia Complex," *Ann Neurol* 1987;22:700-6; see also: W.F. Tsoi, "Psychological and Psychiatric Aspects of HIV Infection," *Singapore Med J* 1990;31:198-201; P. Scherer, "A SIDA ataca o cerebro [AIDS Attacks the Brain]," *Servir* 1990;38:220-7 (Published in Portuguese).

13. H. Hollander "Neurologic and Psychiatric Manifestations of HIV Disease," *J Gen Intern Med* 1991;6(1 Suppl):S24-31; see also: C. Joyce "Evidence for Direct Effect of HIV on Brain," *Nurs Stand* 1990;5:16.

14. R.M. Levy et al., "Neurologic Complications of HIV Infection," *Am Fam Physician* 1990 Feb;41(2):517-36.

15. H.A. Minardi, "When the Brain is the Target: Support in Neurological Manifestations of HIV/AIDS," *Prof Nurse* 1990;5:298-302.

16. M. Maj, "Psychiatric Aspects of HIV-1 Infection and AIDS," *Psychol Med* 1990 Aug;20(3):547-563.

17. Mark L. Rosenblum, Robert M. Levy and Dale E. Bredesen, eds., *AIDS and the Nervous System* (New York: Raven Press, 1988).

18. *The American Heritage Dictionary of the English Language*, William Morris, ed., (Boston: Houghton Mifflin Co., 1979), p. 350.

19. *Dorland's Illustrated Medical Dictionary*, Elizabeth J. Taylor, ed., (Philadelphia: W.B. Saunders Co., 1988), p. 442.

20. C. Silvano, R. Brustia et al., "AIDS in Presenile Age; Frequency of AIDS-Dementia Symptoms," VII International Conference on AIDS, Florence, 1991, Vol. 1, p. 184.

21. R.D. Dix & D.E. Bredesen, "Opportunistic Viral Infections in Acquired Immunodeficiency Syndrome;" V.G. Pons, R.A. Jacobs and H. Hollander, "Nonviral Infections of the Central Nervous System in Patients with Acquired Immunodeficiency Syndrome," in M.L. Rosenblum, et al., op. cit., pp. 221-262;263-284.

22. Confabulation, also referred to as fabrication, involves the unconscious filling in of gaps in memory with fabricated facts and experiences. This is commonly seen in organic amnesia. It differs

from lying in that the patient has no intention to deceive and believes the fabricated memories to be real [*Dorland's Illustrated Medical Dictionary*, op. cit., p. 372].

23. *Annals of Neurology* 1983;14:403-418.

24. G.M. Shaw et al., op. cit.

25. *Annals of Neurology* 1983;14:403-418.

26. J. Levy et al., "Isolation of AIDS-Associated Retroviruses from Cerebrospinal Fluid and Brain of Patients with Neurological Symptoms," *Lancet*, 14 September 1985:586-588.

27. *New Eng J Med* 1985;313:1493-1497;1498-1504.

28. R.W. Price et al., "The AIDS Dementia Complex: Some Current Questions," *Ann Neurol* 1988;23(suppl):S27-S33; R.M. Levy et al., "Neurological Manifestations of the Acquired Immunodeficiency Syndrome (AIDS): Experience at UCSF and Review of the Literature," *J Neurosurg* 1985;62:475-495; S. Gartner et al., "Virus Isolation From and Identification of HTLV-III/LAV-Producing Cells in Brain Tissue from a Patient with AIDS," *JAMA* 1986;256:2365-2371; T. Pumarola-Sune et al., "HIV Antigen in the Brains of Patients with AIDS Dementia Complex," *Ann Neurol* 1987;21:490-496.

29. A. Fauci, *Science*, 5 February 1988;239:617-622.

30. Transcript from NOVA, No. 1314, "Can AIDS Be Stopped?" p. 5, WGBH Educational Foundation, Boston, Massachusetts, 1986.

31. *Postgraduate Medicine* 1986;81:72-79.

32. E.L. Kramer, J.J. Sanger, "Brain Imaging in Acquired Immunodeficiency Syndrome Dementia Complex," *Seminars in Nuclear Medicine* 1990 Oct;20(4):353-63.

33. S. Lunn, M. Skydsbjerg et al., "A Preliminary Report on the Neuropsychologic Sequelae of Human Immunodeficiency Virus," *Archives of General Psychiatry* 1991 Feb;48(2):139-42.

34. "Neuropsychiatric Manifestations of AIDS-Spectrum Disorders," op. cit.

35. R. Anand et al., "Preliminary Molecular Characterization of a Human Immunodeficiency Virus (HIV-1) Associated with Neuropathology," *Ann Neurol* 1988 23 Suppl:S62-65. "A human immunodeficiency virus (HIV-1) was isolated from the brain of a patient with progressive dementia but no obvious immunosuppression."

36. S. Lunn et al., "A Preliminary Report on the Neuropsychologic Sequelae of HIV," *Arch Gen Psychiatry* 1991 Feb;48:139-142.

37. N. Diederich, A. Karenberg, U.H. Peters, [Psychopathologic Pictures in HIV Infection: AIDS Lethargy and AIDS Dementia] *Fortschritte Der Neurologie, Psychiatrie Und Iherr Grenzbebiete-fortschr Neurol Psychiatr* 1988 Jun; 56(6):173-85 (Published in German).

38. L. Resnick, J.R. Berger, et al., "Early Penetration of the Blood-Brain-Barrier by HIV," *Neurology* 1988 Jan; 38(1):9-14.

39. W. Luer et al., "The Cerebrospinal Fluid Diagnosis of HIV-Encephalitis," III International Conference, Wash., D.C., 1987, No. TP.157.

40. D.H. Gabuzda, M.S. Hirsch, "Neurologic Manifestations of Infection with Human Immunodeficiency Virus. Clinical Features and Pathogenesis," *Annals of Internal Medicine* 1987 September:107(3):383-91).

41. M.L. Rosenblum et al, "Overview of AIDS in the Central Nervous System" in M.L. Rosenblum et al., op cit., p. 7.

42. I. Grant et al., "Progressive Neuropsychological Deficit in HIV Infection," III International Conference on AIDS, Wash., D.C. 1987, No. MP.145.

43. Ibid.

44. A. Sonnerborg et al., "Quantitative Detection of Brain Aberrations in HIV Type 1-Infected Individuals by Magnetic Resonance Imaging," *J Infect Dis* 1990;162:1245-51.

45. B.A. Navia, R.W. Price, "The AIDS Dementia Complex as the Presenting or Sole Manifestation of HIV Infection," *Arch Neurol* 1987;44:65-69.

46. "Neuropsychiatric Manifestations of AIDS Spectrum Disorders," op. cit.; P.B. Carrieri et al., "Psychiatric Disorders as First Symptom in AIDS Patients," *Acta Neurol* 1990 April;12:143-146; W.W. Weddington, "Organic Mental Disorders Caused by HIV," *Am J Psychiatry* 1991 Feb;148:275-276; M.A. Cohen et al., "Firesetting by Patients with AIDS," *Ann Intern Med*, 1 March 1990;112:386-387.

47. "Neuropsychiatric Manifestations of AIDS-Spectrum Disorders," op. cit.; see also S.W. Perry, "Organic Mental Disorders Caused by HIV: Update on Early Diagnosis and Treatment," *Am J Psychiatry* 1990 Jun;147(6):696-710.

48. M. Ricci et al., "Neuropsychiatric Manifestations of Early HIV Disease," IV International Conference on AIDS, Stockholm, 1988, Vol. 2, No. 8558.

49. See Appendix A, Part I.

50. C.S. Thomas et al., "HTLV-III and Psychiatric Disturbance," *Lancet*, 17 August 1985, pp. 395-396.

51. G.H. Jones, C.L. Kelly, J.A. Davies, "HIV and Onset of Schizophrenia," *Lancet*, 25 April 1987, p. 982 citing B.A. Navia, B.D. Jordan, R.W. Price "The AIDS Dementia Complex: 1. Clinical Features," *Ann Neurol* 1986;19:517-524.

52. A. Beckett, "Neuropsychiatric Manifestations of HIV Infection," *New Dir Ment Health Serv*, Winter 1990 (48):33-42.

53. J.L. Fabian, "Psychiatric Morbidity in Patients Hospitalized for AIDS: Experience in a Quebec Hospital," *Canadian Journal of Psychiatry*, October 1990 35(7):581-4.

54. M.M. Derix et al., "Mental Changes in Patients with AIDS," *Clin Neurol Neurosurg* 1990;92(3):215-22.

55. S. Snyder et al., "Evaluation and Treatment of Mental Disorders in Patients with AIDS," *Compr Ther* 1990;16:34-41.

56. R.E. Prier, J.G. McNeil et al., "Inpatient Psychiatric Morbidity of HIV-Infected Soldiers," *Hosp Community Psychiatry* June 1991 42(6):619-23.

57. R. Malouf et al., "The Spectrum of Altered Mentation in AIDS and ARC," V International Conference on AIDS, Montreal, 1989, p. 447.

58. "AIDS Dentist Said to Plot Infections," *Washington Times*, 11 June 1992.

59. *Dorland's Illustrated Medical Dictionary*, op. cit., p. 1476.

60. "Neuropsychiatric Manifestations of AIDS-Spectrum Disorders," op. cit.

61. Ibid.

62. *Dorland's Illustrated Medical Dictionary*, op. cit., p. 1492.

63. "Neuropsychiatric Manifestations of AIDS-Spectrum Disorders," op. cit.

64. *Dorland's Illustrated Medical Dictionary*, op. cit., p. 1385.

65. Ibid., p. 714.

66. "Neuropsychiatric Manifestations of AIDS-Spectrum Disorders," op. cit.

67. K. Kieburtz et al., "Manic Syndrome in AIDS," *Am J Psychiatry*, August 1991;148:1068-1070.

68. *American Psychiatric Association: Diagnostic and Statistical Manual of Mental Disorders*, Third Edition, Revised, [*DSM-III-R*] (Wash., D.C.: American Psychiatric Association, 1987).

69. K. Kieburtz et al., op. cit.

70. "Behind the Mental Symptoms of AIDS," *Psychology Today*, December 1984, p. 12.

71. I. Grant, J.H. Atkinson "Neurogenic and Psychogenic Behavioral Correlates of HIV Infection," *Res Publ Assoc Res Nerv Ment Dis* 1990;68:291-304.

72. "Psycho Revisited," *International Healthwatch Report*, August 1990.

73. "Neuropsychiatric Manifestations of AIDS-Spectrum Disorders," op. cit.

74. See Appendix A, Part II.

75. D. Brody et al., "Olfactory Identification Deficits in HIV Infection," *American Journal of Psychiatry* February 1991 148(2)248-50.

76. B.J. Brewer, J. Miller, "HIV-Related Headache," VII International Conference on AIDS, Florence, 1991, Vol. 1, p. 206.

77. J. Goldstein, "Headache and Acquired Immunodeficiency Syndrome," *Neurol Clin* 1990 Nov;8(4):947-60.

78. C. Trenkwalder, E. Schielke et al., "Headache in HIV-Infected Patients," VII International Conference on AIDS, Florence, 1991, Vol. 1. p. 204.

79. A.F. Bell, J.S. Atkins et al., "HIV and Sensorineural Hearing Loss (SNHL)," IV International Conference on AIDS, Stockholm, 1988, Vol. 1, No. 7009.

80. R.G. Miller et al., "Peripheral Nervous System Dysfunction in AIDS," in M.L. Rosenblum et al., op. cit., p. 77.

81. Ibid., p. 68. The technical name for this condition is Distal Symmetric Peripheral Neuropathy.

82. G.J. Parry, "Peripheral Neuropathies Associated with Human Immunodeficiency Virus Infection," *Annals of Neurology* (Suppl. vol. 23) 1988 S49-53.

83. D.R. Cornblath et al., "Painful Sensory Neuropathy (PSN) in Patients with AIDS," III International Conference on AIDS, Wash. D.C., 1987, No. T.P.140; N.E. Rance et al., "Degeneration of the Fasciculus Gracilis in Patients with AIDS," *Annals of Neurology* 1986;20:142.

84. M.L. Rosenblum et al, op. cit., p. 39.

85. Ibid.

86. Ibid., p. 70.

87. Ibid., p. 65.

88. D.R. Cornblath, "Treatment of the Neuromuscular Complications of the Human Immunodeficiency Virus Infection," *Annals of Neurology* (Suppl. vol. 23) 1988 (S88-S91).

89. *Lancet*, 8 August 1987. pp. 343-344.

90. G. Hancock and E. Carim, op. cit., p. 13.

91. P. Richards, "AIDS and the Neurosurgeon," *Br J Neurosurg* 1987 1(2):163-71.

92. G. Hancock and E. Carim, op. cit., p. 28.

93. D. Wimberger et al., "AIDS im ZNS," [AIDS of the Central Nervous System] *Wien Klin Wochenschr* 1990 Jan 19;102(2):47-51 (Published in German).

94. "AIDS Update," *Nursing 88*, March 1988.

95. Ibid.

96. J.B. Clark, "Policy Considerations of Human Immunodeficiency Virus (HIV) Infection in U.S. Navy Aviation Personnel," *Aviation Space and Environmental Medicine* 1990 February 61(2):165-168.

97. Ibid.

98. *Preventive Law Reporter*, September 1988 University of Denver, National Center for Preventive Law, cited in "AIDS Side Effect Concern: Legal Expert Calls Dementia Work Hazard," by Julia Rubin, *Danville Commercial News*, (Illinois) 28 November 1988.

99. *International Healthwatch Report*, March/April 1989.

100. James S. Fulghum, III, "A Surgeon with AIDS" (letter) *JAMA* 1990:264(24)3147.

101. I. Grant et al., "Progressive Neuropsychological Deficit in HIV Infection," III International Conference on AIDS, Wash., D.C. 1987, No. M.P.145.

102. K. M. Einhaeupl, H. W. Pfister et al., "Frequent Early Inflammation in CSF in HIV-Positive Persons and Its Implications for the Diagnosis of HIV-encephalopathy," IV International Conference on AIDS, Stockholm, 1988, Vol. 1, No. 7008; S. Lunn et al., "A Preliminary Report on the Neuropsychologic Sequelae of HIV," *Arch Gen Psychiatry* 1991 Feb;48:139-142.

103. J.C. McArthur, "Neurologic Manifestations of AIDS," *Medicine* (Baltimore) November 1987;66(6):407-37. Dr. McArthur states: "The demonstration that HIV enters the central nervous system during *the earliest stages* of infection has major implications for antiviral agents which must penetrate brain parenchyma to clear the virus effectively. Other neurologic complications occur frequently, including myelopathies, peripheral neuropathies, opportunistic CNS infections, and CNS neoplasms. Many of these disorders are novel and incompletely characterized and their etiology is uncertain. *While treatment is available for several of these conditions, it is generally not curative, and is often poorly tolerated because of adverse effects. . . .*"

CHAPTER THREE
THE REALITY OF HETEROSEXUAL AIDS

1. "AIDS Epidemic Far From Abating," *Medical World News*, August 1991, p. 40.

2. Ibid.

3. *Medical Tribune*, 3 October 1991, p. 20; see also: K.K. Holmes et al., "The Increasing Frequency of Heterosexually Acquired AIDS in the United States (1983-88)," *American Journal of Public Health*, 1990;80:858. Dr. King Holmes and researchers from the University of Washington and the CDC reported the incidence of heterosexually acquired AIDS quadrupled from 0.9% in 1983 to 4.0% in 1988.

4. A.R. Moss et al., "Progression to AIDS in the San Francisco General Hospital Cohort Study," V International Conference on AIDS, Montreal, 1989, p. 60; A. Lifson et al., "The Natural History of HIV Infection in a Cohort of Homosexual and Bisexual Men: Clinical Manifestations, 1978-1989," V International Conference on AIDS, Montreal, 1989, p. 60.

5. M.G. Koch et al., "Particular Features of a Lentivirus Epidemic and Their Dynamic Consequences, Such as Transients, Crescents and a 10-Year's Moratorium on a Detection of Errors," V International Conference on AIDS, Montreal, 1989, p. 1052.

6. W. Greatbach and W. Holmes, "Additional Supporting Evidence from 3518 Cases of TA-AIDS that the Incubation Time of AIDS is Greater than 12 Years," VII International Conference on AIDS, Florence, 1991, Vol. 2, p. 1994. The researchers, from the State University College, Buffalo, NY state: "Our data continue to suggest that the incubation time of AIDS *is greater* than 12 years." HIV carriers remain infectious during this prolonged incubation period.

284 AIDS: RAGE AND REALITY

7. "AIDS Incidence Up 40% Among Heterosexuals," *Family Practice News*, 1 May 1992, p. 3. Dr. Thomas C. Quinn of the Johns Hopkins Medical Institutions noted the year 1991 saw a dramatic growth in the number of AIDS cases among heterosexuals, representing a 40% increase over 1990.

8. S.A. Colgate et al., "AIDS and A Risk-Based Model," *Los Alamos Science*, pp. 2-39; see particularly the section on "The Seeding Wave," pp. 36-39 by S.A. Colgate and J. H. Hyman.

9. B. De Rienzo et al., "Heterosexual Transmission of the Human Immunodeficiency Virus: A Seroepidemiological Study," *Arch Dermatol Res* 1989;281:369-72.

10. S.M. Blower et al., "Loglinear Models, Sexual Behavior and HIV: Epidemiological Implications of Heterosexual Transmission," *J Acquir Immune Defic Syndr* 1990;3(8):763-72; J.C. Barrett, "Monte Carlo Simulation of the Heterosexual Selective Spread of the Human Immunodeficiency Virus," *J Med Virol* 1988;26:99-109; F. Le Pont, S.M. Blower "The Supply and Demand Dynamics of Sexual Behavior: Implications for Heterosexual HIV Epidemics," *J Acquir Immune Defic Syndr* 1991;4:987-99.

11. B. Baccetti et al., "HIV Particles Detected in Spermatozoa in Patients with AIDS," VII International Conference on AIDS, Florence, 1991, Vol. 2, p. 284.

12. J. Krieger et al., "HIV Recovery from Semen: Minimal Impact of Clinical Stage of Infection and Minimal Effect on Semen Analysis Parameters," VI International Conference on AIDS, San Francisco, 1990, Vol. 1, p. 159; D. Anderson, "Prevalence and Temporal Variation of HIV-1 in Semen," VI International Conference on AIDS, San Francisco, 1990, Vol. 1., p. 263.

13. E. Axel et al., "HIV Targets Cells in Tests and Epididymides from AIDS Patients," V International Conference on AIDS, Montreal, 1990, p. 608; M.L. Rekart, "HIV Transmission by Artificial Insemination," IV International Conference on AIDS, Stockholm, 1989, Vol. 1, No. 4026.

14. Sheila Hutman, "AIDS: The Year in Review," *AIDS Patient Care*, December 1990:11-15.

15. V.E. Miller and V.L. Scofield, "Role of Spermatozoa in Sexual Transmission of AIDS," IV International Conference on AIDS, Stockholm, 1988, Vol. 2. No. 2550; E. Dussaix et al., "Potential Role of Spermatozoa in the Transmission of HIV," V International Conference on AIDS, Montreal, 1989, p. 114; O. Bagasra et al., "HIV-1 Replicates in Human Sperm Mitochondria of HIV-1-Seropositive Individuals," V International Conference on AIDS, Montreal, 1989, p. 583. In sperm, HIV replicates in the mitochondria, which appear like tiny rods inside the cell membrane. Some HIV-infected mitochondria resemble pods with HIV-like particles "bursting out" of these spores.

16. P. Van de Perre et al., "Detection of HIV p17 Antigen in Lymphocytes but Not Epithelial Cells from Cervicovaginal Secretions of Women Seropositive for HIV: Implications for Heterosexual Transmission of the Virus," *Genitourin Med* 1988;64:30-3.

17. Y. Hennin et al., "Prevalence of HIV in the Cervicovaginal Secretions of Women Seropositive for HIV: Correlation with the Clinical Status and Implications for Heterosexual Transmission," VI International Conference on AIDS, San Francisco, 1990, Vol. 1, p. 263.

18. J.A. Hill and D.J. Anderson, "Quantitation of Human Vaginal Leukocytes and Effects of Vaginal Secretions on Mechanisms of HIV Transmission," IV International Conference on AIDS, Stockholm, 1988, Vol. 2, No. 2551; These cells include CD4+ lymphocytes and macrophages. L. Belec et al., "Antibodies to HIV in Vaginal Secretions of Heterosexual Women," *J Infect Dis* 1989;160:385-91.

19. A. Lazzarin et al., "Man-to-Woman Sexual Transmission of the Human Immunodeficiency Virus. Risk Factors Related to Sexual Behavior, Man's Infectiousness, and Woman's Susceptibility, Italian Study Group on HIV Heterosexual Transmission," *Arch Intern Med* 1991;151:2411-16; N.S. Padian, "Sexual Histories of Heterosexual Couples with One HIV-Infected Partner," *Am J Public Health* 1990;80:990-1.

20. I. De Vincenzi et al., "Heterosexual Transmission of HIV: A European Study. II Female-to-Male Transmission," V International Conference on AIDS, Montreal, 1989, p. 74.

21. R.P. Brettle, et al., "Secretor Status and Susceptibility to Heterosexual Transmission of HIV," VII International Conference on AIDS, Florence, 1991, Vol. 1, p. 322.

22. L. Evans et al., "Infection of Colon Epithelial Cells by HIV-1," VI International Conference on AIDS, San Francisco, 1990, Vol. 2, p. 141.

23. M.P. Moyer et al., "HIV Infection of Gastrointestinal Cell Cultures," VI International Conference on AIDS, San Francisco, 1990, Vol. 2, p. 140.

24. D.P. Kotler et al., "HIV Infection of the Gastrointestinal Tract: Comparison of the Sensitivities of Hybridization and Immunoassay," V International Conference, Montreal, 1989, p. 669; M.P Moyer et al., "Expression of a Potential HIV Receptor on Human Gastrointestinal Epithelial Cells (GIECs)," V International Conference, Montreal, 1989, p. 606.

25. C.M. Mavligit et al., "Chronic Immune Stimulation by Sperm Alloantigens: Support for the Hypothesis that Spermatozoa Induce Immune Dysregulation in Homosexual Males," *JAMA* 1984;251:237-241; J.M. Richards et al., "Rectal Insemination Modifies Immune Responses in Rabbits," *Science* 1984;224:390-392. In a revealing study involving *monogamously* paired homosexual males, three-fourths of the passive partners manifested sperm induced immune dysregulation. Rectal insemination also alters immune responses in rabbits.

26. G.M. Mavligit et al., "Chronic Immune Stimulation by Sperm Alloantigens . . ." op. cit. The lining of the rectum is made up of a single layer of columnar epithelium which "is not only incapable of protecting against any abrasive effect, but also promotes the absorption of an array of sperm antigens, thus enhancing their exposure to the immune apparatus in the lymphatic and blood circulation." See also: P. Van de Perre et al., "Detection of HIV p17 Antigen in Lymphocytes but Not Epithelial Cells from Cervicovaginal Secretions of Women Seropositive for HIV: Implications for Heterosexual Transmission of the Virus," *Genitourin Med* 1988;64:30-3.

27. L.R. Braathen et al., "Langerhans Cells As Primary Target for HIV Infection," *Lancet*, 7 November 1987, p. 1094.

28. C. Miller et al., "Localization of SIV in the Reproductive Tract of Rhesus Macaques: Relationship to the Distribution of T Cells and Macrophages," VII International Conference on AIDS, Florence, 1991, Vol. 2, p. 121; B. Simon et al., "A Study of Langerhans Cells in the Cervical Epithelium of Women with HIV Infection," VI International Conference on AIDS, San Francisco, 1990, Vol. 2., p. 379; C. Miller et al., "Transmission of Simian Immunodeficiency Virus (SIV) Across the Genital Mucosas of Female and Male Rhesus Macaques," IV International Conference on AIDS, Stockholm, 1988, Vol. 2, No. 2581; C. Miller and M.B. Gardner "AIDS and Mucosal Immunity: Usefulness of the SIV Macaque Model of Genital Mucosal Transmission," *J AIDS* 1991;4:1169-1172.

29. A.M. Johnson et al., "Transmission of HIV to Heterosexual Partners of Infected Men and Women," *AIDS* 1989;3:367-72.

30. M.A. Chiasson et al. "Similar Risk of HIV Infection Through Heterosexual Transmission for Men and Women at a New York City STD Clinic," VII International Conference on AIDS, Florence, 1991, Vol. 1., p. 321.

31. R. Berkelman et al., "Women and AIDS: The Increasing Role of Heterosexual Transmission in the United States," VII International Conference on AIDS, Florence, 1991, Vol. 2, p. 49.

32. S. Chu et al., "Impact of the HIV Epidemic on Mortality Among Women 15 to 44 Years of Age, United States," VI International Conference on AIDS, San Francisco, 1990, Vol. 2, p. 267.

33. *JAMA* 1990;264:1807.

34. James Chin, "Current and Future Dimensions of the HIV/AIDS Pandemic in Women and Children," *Lancet* 1990;336:221-224.

35. "75% of HIV Cases Tied to Heterosexual Sex," *Ft. Worth Star Telegram*, (AP) 12 Nov. 1991.

36. James Chin, op. cit.

37. "World Health Organization Global Statistics," *AIDS* 1990;4:1305.

38. R.W. Goodgame, "AIDS In Uganda - Clinical and Social Features," *N Engl J Med* 1990;323:383-389.

39. Jane Perlez, "Toll of AIDS on Uganda's Women Puts Their Roles and Rights in Question," *NY Times*, 12 Oct. 1990, p. 11.

40. N. Hellmann et al., "HIV Infection among Patients in a Uganda STD Clinic," VI International Conference on AIDS, San Francisco, 1990, Vol. 1, p. 269; N. Hellmann et al., "Specific Heterosexual Risk Behaviors and HIV Seropositivity in an Uganda Health Clinic," VI International Conference on AIDS, San Francisco, 1990, Vol. 1, p. 269; M.J. Wawer, D. Serwadda et al., "Geographic and Community Distribution of HIV1 Infection in Rural Rakai District, Uganda," VI International Conference on AIDS, San Francisco, 1990, Vol. 2, p. 232.

41. E. M. Ankrah, et al., "The Environment, HIV Testing and Ugandan Women," VII International Conference on AIDS, Florence, 1991, Vol. 1, p. 451.

42. Kathleen Hunt, "Scenes from a Nightmare," *NY Times Magazine*, 12 August 1990.

43. *International Healthwatch Report*, November 1989, p. 2.

44. A.T. Manoka et al., "Non-Ulcerative Sexually Transmitted Diseases As Risk Factors for HIV Infection," VI International Conference on AIDS, San Francisco, 1990, Vol. 1, p. 158.

45. "Zimbabwe Depopulation," *International Healthwatch Report*, October 1990, pp. 6-7.

46. DPA News Service, 13 September 1991.

47. Xinjua News Service, 30 September 1991. In addition, researchers from the Ministry of Health in Tanzania and the University of Munich in Germany, have reported that in the Mbeya Region of Tanzania, 1 out of 10 blood donors are infected with HIV-1 [E. Naegele et al., "Transmission of HIV-1 through Blood Transfusions Despite Screening with HIVCHECK (TM)," VI International Conference on AIDS, San Francisco, 1990, Vol. 1, p. 274].

48. A. Chao, M. Bulterys et al., "Risk Factors for HIV-1 Seropositivity Among Pregnant Women in Rwanda," VII International Conference on AIDS, Florence, 1991, Vol. 1, p. 322; cf., Marc Bulterys et al., "Risk Factors for HIV-1 Seropositivity Among Rural and Urban Pregnant Women in Rwanda," VI International Conference on AIDS, San Francisco, 1990, Vol. 1, p. 269.

49. S. Allen et al., "HIV Infection in Urban Rwanda," *JAMA*;1991;266:1657-1663.

50. S. Benoit et al., "AIDS in Cote D'Ivoire: Progression of the Epidemic in West Africa," VI International Conference on AIDS, San Francisco, 1990, Vol. 1, p. 304; K.M. De Cock et al., "AIDS

the Leading Cause of Death in West Africa City (Abidjan)," VI International Conference on AIDS, San Francisco, 1990, Vol. 2, p. 115; J-M. N'Gbichi et al., "Comparison of Heterosexual Transmission of HIV-1 and HIV-2 Infections in Abidjan Cote D'Ivoire," VII International Conference on AIDS, Florence, 1991, Vol. 1, p. 304. Hospitalized patients and their spouses were examined for antibodies to HIV-1 and the emerging different strain of the AIDS virus HIV-2. Among 2270 hospitalized male patients the prevalence was 46.1% HIV-1, 4.7% HIV-2, 16.5% HIV-1 and HIV-2. Among 465 couples serologic concordance in the female spouse was 145/306 (47%) for HIV-1 and 19/49 (39%) for HIV-2.

51. M. Ntumbanzondo et al., "Large Increase in Health Care Utilization by HIV-Infected Employees At A Commercial Bank in Kinshasa, Zaire," VI International Conference on AIDS, San Francisco, 1990, Vol. 1, p. 172.

52. R.W. Ryder et al., "Heterosexual Transmission of HIV-1 Among Employees and Their Spouses at Two Large Businesses in Zaire," AIDS 1990;4:725-732. ". . . to asses the impact of HIV-1 infection on a large urban African workforce, we enrolled 7068 male employees, 416 female employees and 4548 female spouses of employees at two large Kinshasa businesses (a textile factory and a commercial bank) in a prospective study of HIV-1 infection. The HIV-1 seroprevalence rate was higher in male employees (5.8%) and their spouses (5.7%) at the bank than among male employees (2.8%) and their spouses (3.3%) at the textile factory. At both businesses HIV-1 seroprevalence was higher among employees in managerial positions (5.0%) than among workers in lower level positions (3.0%). . . . The HIV infection rate was higher among the female workers (7.7%) than among spouses of male workers (3.9%)."

53. International Healthwatch Report, October 1988, p. 5.

54. T. Prazuck et al., "Mother-to-Child Transmission of HIV Viruses: A Cohort Study in West Africa: Burkina Faso," VI International Conference on AIDS, San Francisco, 1990, Vol. 1, p. 277.

55. A. Bayley et al., "Surgical Pathology of HIV-Infected Patients in Zambia," VI International Conference on AIDS, San Francisco, 1990, Vol. 2, p. 212.

56. J.N. Simonsen et al., "HIV Infection Among Lower Socioeconomic Strata Prostitutes in Nairobi," AIDS 1990;4:139-144.

57. International Healthwatch Report, November, 1989; D. Clemetson et al., "Incidence of HIV Transmission within HIV-1 Discordant Heterosexual Partnerships in Nairobi, Kenya," VI International Conference on AIDS, San Francisco, 1990 Vol. 2, p. 448; D. Willerford, W. Emonyl et al., "Association Between Cervical Shedding of HIV and Cervicitis," VII International Conference on AIDS, Florence, 1991, Vol. 1, p. 321; Steve Rabin, "Kenya: AIDS as if it Mattered; Where Government Has a Will, Ways to Fight Can Be Found," Washington Post, 17 November 1991. Among HIV-infected women, cervical inflammation was associated with a 4.4-fold increased risk of cervical shedding (excreting the virus).

58. NY Times, International Edition, 18 November 1990, p. 15.

59. J.A. Dada, et al., "Prevalence Survey of HIV-1 and HIV-2 Infections in Female Prostitutes in Lagos State, Nigeria," VII International Conference on AIDS, Florence, 1991, Vol. 1, p. 371.

60. International Healthwatch Report, August 1990, p. 5.

61. R. Schall, "On the Population Size of the AIDS Epidemic Among the Heterosexual Black Population in South Africa," S Afr Med J 1990;78:507-510.

62. P.O. Way, and K. Stanecki, "How Bad Will It Be? Modelling the AIDS Epidemic in Eastern Africa," Paper prepared for the annual meeting of the American Association for the Advancement of Science, Wash., D.C., 14-19 February 1991.

63. Robert Massa, "Death in Florence," Village Voice, 9 July 1991.

64. C. Kunanusont et al., "Modes of Transmission for the High Rate of HIV Infection Among Male STD Patients and Male Blood Donors in Chiang Mai, Thailand," VII International Conference on AIDS, Florence, 1991, Vol. 2, p. 317; P. Sawanpanyalert et al., "Seroconversion Rate and Risk Factors for HIV-1 Infection Among Low-Class Female Sex Workers in Chiang Mai, Thailand: A Multi Cross-Sectional Study," VII International Conference on AIDS, Florence, 1991, Vol. 2, p. 320.

65. "Prostitutes Will Not Use Condoms," International Healthwatch Report, February 1992.

66. S.V. Apte et al., "Prevalence of Anti-HIV Antibodies Among Blood Donors in Bombay," VI International Conference on AIDS, San Francisco, 1990, Vol. 2, p. 233; Y.N. Singh et al., "HIV Infection in the Blood Donors of Delhi, India: 11/2 Years' Experience," J AIDS 1990;4:1008.

67. Omar Sattaur, "India Wakes Up to AIDS," New Scientist, 2 November 1991, pp. 25-29.

68. G. Bhave Geeta et al., "HIV Sero Surveillance in Promiscuous Females of Bombay India," VI International Conference on AIDS, San Francisco, 1990, Vol. 2, p. 234; K. Pavri et al., "HIV Antigen Positive Cultures and Retrovirus-Like Particles from an Asymptomatic Pregnant Prostitute from Tamil Nadu, India," IV International Conference on AIDS, Stockholm, 1988, Vol. 1, p. 1132; S.Y. Nath, et al., "HIV Prevention Interventions Among Prostitutes of India: Delhi Experience," VI International Conference on AIDS, San Francisco, 1990, Vol. 2, p. 104; R. Ramanathan et al., "Seroprevalence Among the Crime Related Population of Prisoners and Prostitutes," VI International Conference on AIDS, San Francisco, 1990, Vol. 1, p. 347.

69. M.A. Narayan et al., "HIV Serosurveillance in an AIDS Referral Centre in India," VI International Conference on AIDS, San Francisco, 1990, Vol. 2, p. 234.

70. *International Healthwatch Report*, February 1990.

71. M.A. Narayan et al., "HIV Serosurveillance in an AIDS Referral Centre in India," VI International Conference on AIDS, San Francisco, 1990, Vol. 2, p. 234, op. cit.

72. H. Rubsamen-Waigmann et al., "Spread of HIV-2 in India," VII International Conference on AIDS, Florence, 1991, Vol. 1, p. 370.

73. S.S. Sankari et al., "Trends of HIV Infections in Antenatal/Fertility Clinic - An Ominous Sign," VII International Conference on AIDS, Florence, 1991, Vol. 2, p. 355.

74. "Dark Tide of Aids in a Sea of Suffering," *Guardian Weekly*, 23 August 1992.

75. K. Jayapaul et al., "Sero-Epidemiological Study of HIV Infection In and Around Madras," VI International Conference on AIDS, San Francisco, 1990, Vol. 2, p. 234; John Pomfret, "AIDS Spreads While India Sleeps," *Daily Courier*, Grants Pass, Oregon, 20 April 1990.

76. R. Chan et al., "Epidemiology of HIV Infection in Singapore," VI International Conference on AIDS, San Francisco, 1990, Vol. 2, p. 234.

79. K. Soda et al., "Epidemiologic Status and Future Prediction of AIDS/HIV in Japan," VI International Conference on AIDS, San Francisco, 1990, Vol. 2, p. 234

78. Y. Dopngyou et al., "AIDS Surveillance in Sichuan, China," V International Conference on AIDS, Montreal, 1989, p. 1058.

79. S. Hameed et al., "AIDS Prevention and Its Countercurrents in Asia," V International Conference on AIDS. Montreal, 1989, p. 1058.

80. Rene Pastor, "AIDS Threatens Asia's Economic Boom, U.N. Says," Reuter, 23 January 1992.

81. N. Constantine et al., "HIV Seroprevalence in Egypt: A Two and Half Year Surveillance," V International Conference on AIDS, Montreal, 1989, p. 1001.

82. S. Yemen, G. Yayli et al., "HIV-1 Infection in Istanbul, Turkey," VII International Conference on AIDS, Florence, 1991, Vol. 1, p. 318.

83. James Chin, op. cit.

84. Ibid.

85. P. Muello, "AIDS in Brazil," (AP) 23 Nov. 1991, cf., E. Castilho, "Empirical Extrapolation Projection of AIDS Incidence in Brazil," V International Conference on AIDS, Montreal, 1989, p. 998; P. Giraldes et al., "HIV-1 Infection in Pregnant Women from Santos, Brazil," V International Conference on AIDS, Montreal, 1989, p. 999. As early as 1988, a significant rate (3.5%) of HIV disease was reported among pregnant women in the city of Santos, one of the major harbours in Brazil.

86. E. Cortes et al., "Seroprevalence of HIV-1, HIV-2 and HTLV-1 in Brazilian Bisexual Males," V International Conference on AIDS, Montreal, 1989, p. 1000; E. Cortes et al., "Seroprevalence of HIV-1, HIV-2, HTLV-1 in Male Prostitutes in Rio De Janeiro, Brazil," V International Conference on AIDS, Montreal, 1989, p. 1001.

87. R. Gonzalez et al., "Transition from Type 1 to Type 2 Transmission of HIV in the Americas: How Widespread the Trend?" VI International Conference on AIDS, San Francisco, 1990, Vol. 1, p. 302; cf., E. Castilho et al., "Patterns and Trends of Heterosexual Transmission of HIV Among Brazilian AIDS Cases," V International Conference on AIDS, Montreal, 1989, p. 998.

88. K. Sanches et al., "AIDS and Women in the State of Rio De Janeiro, Brazil," VII International Conference on AIDS, Florence, 1991, Vol. 1., p. 449; M. Guimaraes et al., "Heterosexual Transmission of HIV: A Multicenter Study in Rio De Janeiro, Brazil," VII International Conference on AIDS, Florence, 1991, Vol. 2, p. 320.

89. M. Boxaca et al., "HIV Infection in Heterosexuals from Buenos Aires City Consulting for Venereal Disease," V International Conference on AIDS, Montreal. 1989, p. 1012.

90. C. Wainstein et al., "Epidemiology of AIDS in Children in Buenos Aires, Argentina," VII International Conference ON AIDS, Florence, 1991, Vol. 1, p. 318.

91. G. Buchovsky et al., "HIV Epidemic at a Hemodialysis Center," IV International Conference on AIDS, Stockholm, 1988, Vol. 2, No. 7751; O. Fay et al., "HIV Infection in Voluntary Blood Donors in Argentina," V International Conference on AIDS, Montreal, 1989, p. 975.

92. G. Perez et al., "Retroviral Infections in Patients on Maintenance Hemodialysis," IV International Conference on AIDS, Stockholm, 1988, Vol. 2, No. 7752; cf., Z.F. Peixinho et al., "HIV-1 Antibodies in Hemodialysis Patients from São Paulo, Brazil," IV International Conference on AIDS, Stockholm, 1988, Vol. 2, No. 7753.

93. L. Mata et al., "Typology, Behavior, Bisexuality and HIV Infection of Homosexual Men of Costa Rica, 1985-1988," V International Conference on AIDS, Montreal, 1989, p. 1057.

94. F. Cleghorn et al., "Update on the Epidemiology of AIDS in Trinidad," VI International Conference on AIDS, San Francisco, 1990, Vol. 1, p. 304.

95. Ibid.

96. I. Garris et al., "The Wave-Like Progression of AIDS in the Dominican Republic," V International Conference on AIDS, Montreal, 1989, p. 975.

97. J.L. Mora et al., "Development of HIV/AIDS Epidemic in the Country Ranking 4th in Number of Cases in the Americas," VI International Conference on AIDS, San Francisco, 1990, Vol. 1, p. 304.

98. B. Enrique et al., "Distribution and Trends of AIDS Cases By Socioeconomic Strata in Mexico," VI International Conference on AIDS, San Francisco, 1990, Vol. 1, p. 303.

99. H. Flor, "Nationwide HIV-1 Seroprevalence in Blood Donors in Mexico," VII International Conference on AIDS, Florence, 1991, Vol. 1, p. 370.

100. C. Avila et al., "HIV Transmission in Paid Plasma Donors in Mexico City, Mexico," IV International Conference on AIDS, Stockholm, 1988, Vol. 2, No. 7681.

101. M. De Lourdes Garcia et al., "HIV-1 Tendencies and Risk Factors in 5040 Homo and Bisexual Men in Mexico (1985-1989)," VI International Conference on AIDS, San Francisco, 1990, Vol. 2, p. 259.

102. Stanley Monteith, M.D., AIDS: The Unnecessary Epidemic, (Sevierville, TN: Covenant House Books, 1991), p. 61. This outstanding book may be ordered from: AIDS Book, 618 Frederick St., Santa Cruz, CA 95062.

103. V.V. Pokrovsky et al., "Epidemiological Investigation of the First Case of AIDS Detected in the USSR," IV International Conference on AIDS, Stockholm, 1988, Vol. 1, No. 4184.

104. A. Koslov et al., "First Cases of HIV-1 Infection in Leningrad, USSR," VI International Conference on AIDS, 1990, San Francisco, Vol. 2., p. 243.

105. I. Eramova et al., "Transmission of HIV Infection in the Male Homosexual Population in the USSR," VI International Conference on AIDS, San Francisco, 1990, Vol. 2, p. 214. James Chin, "Current and Future Dimensions of the HIV/AIDS Pandemic in Women and Children," Lancet 1990;336:221-224. These areas are classified by the WHO as areas manifesting Pattern III type of HIV transmission, indicating that no predominant mode of AIDS transmission has emerged .

106. S.E. Clarke et al., "Increasing HIV-1 Infection in Women - England, Wales, and Northern Ireland," VII International Conference on AIDS, Florence, 1991, Vol. 2, p. 326.

107. H.W. Jaffe et al., "National Case-Control Study of Kaposi's Sarcoma and Pneumocystis Carinii Pneumonia in Homosexual Men: Part 1, Epidemiological Results," Ann Int Med 1983;99:145-151.

108. Ibid.

109. R.A. Coates et al., "Transmission of HIV in Male Sexual Contacts of Men with ARC or AIDS," IV International Conference on AIDS, Stockholm, 1988, Vol. 1, No. 4113.

110. H.W. Jaffe et al., op. cit.

111. D.G. Ostrow et al., Sexually Transmitted Diseases in Homosexual Men (New York: Yorke Medical Books, 1984), p. 204.

112. Darrow et al., "Gay Report on STDs," Am J Pub Health 1981;71:1005-1011.

113. H.L. Kazal et al., "The Gay Bowel Syndrome. Clinico-pathologic Correlation in 260 Cases," Ann Clin Lab Sci 1976;6:184.

114. D. Abrams and R. Pierce, "AIDS and Parasitism," Lancet, 23 June 1984, p. 1411.

115. W. Winkelstein et al., "Sexual Practices and Risk of Infection by the Human Immunodeficiency Virus," JAMA 1987;257:321-325.

116. E.V. Morse et al., "The Male Street Prostitute: A Vector for Transmission of HIV Infection into the Heterosexual World," Soc Sci Med 1991;32:535-539.

117. P.M. Davies et al., "Heterosexual Behavior in a Cohort of Homosexually Active Men in England and Wales," VI International Conference on AIDS, San Francisco, 1990, Vol. 2, p. 259.

118. G. Bennet at al., "A Potential Source for the Transmission of HIV into the Heterosexual Population: Bisexual Men Who Frequent "Beats," Med J Aust 1989:151:314-318.

119. R.B. Hays et al., "Why Are Young Gay Men Engaging in High Rates of Unsafe Sex?" VI International Conference on AIDS, San Francisco, 1990, Vol. 2, No. 261.

120. T.A. Kellog et al., "Prevalence of HIV-1 Among Homosexual and Bisexual Men in the S.F. Bay Area: Evidence of Infection among Young Gay Men," VII International Conference on AIDS, Florence, 1991, Vol. 2, No. 298.

121. R. Fulton and R.E. Kennedy, Jr., "Are Bisexuals Under-Recognized Among White Men with AIDS in the U.S.?" VII International Conference on AIDS, Florence, 1991, Vol 1., p. 85.

122. D.K. Lewis et al., "Sexual Behavior and Self Identity in Male Bisexual and Heterosexual IV Drug Users," VI International Conference on AIDS, San Francisco, 1990, Vol. 2, p. 272.

123. P.M. Davies et al., "Heterosexual Behavior in a Cohort of Homosexually Active Men in England and Wales," VI International Conference on AIDS," San Francisco, 1990, Vol. 2, p. 259.

124. Personal letter sent to Congressman William Dannemeyer in 1987. A copy of the letter was sent to every member of Congress.

125. R. Beach et al., "Patterns of HIV Infection in Central America," VI International Conference on AIDS, San Francisco, 1990, Vol. 2, p. 228.

126. D.L. Murphy "Heterosexual Contacts of Intravenous Drug Abusers: Implications for the Next Spread of the AIDS Epidemic," *Adv Alcohol Subst Abuse* 1987;7:89-97.

127. J.B. Glaser et al., "Heterosexual HIV Transmission Among the Middle Class," *Arch Int Med* 1989;149:645-649.

128. S. De Wit and N. Clumeck, "Heterosexual Transmission of AIDS," [published in French] *Rev Med Brux* 1989:10:336-339.

129. J.A. van den Hoek et al., "HIV Infection and STD in Drug Addicted Prostitutes in Amsterdam: Potential for Heterosexual Transmission," *Genitourin Med* 1989;65:146-150.

130. D.E. Kanouse et al., "Prostitute Use by Heterosexual Males in the U.S., 1982," VI International Conference on AIDS, San Francisco, 1990, Vol. 2, p. 266.

131. "STDs - AIDS," (UPI) 20 December 1990.

132. *Annual Report*, United States Department of Health and Human Services, Division of STD/HIV Prevention, 1989, p. 3.

133. Ibid., p. 4.

134. Ibid.

135. Ibid., cf., S. Saffrin et al., "Prevalence and Risk Factors for HIV-1 Infection in Patients with Acute Pelvic Inflammatory Disease (PID)," V International Conference on AIDS, Montreal, 1989, p. 230.

136. N.J. Alexander, "Sexual Transmission of HIV: Virus Entry into the Male and Female Genital Tract," *Fertility and Sterility*, 1990;54:1-18.

137. P. Wambugu et al., "Are Sexually Transmitted Diseases (STD) Opportunistic Infections in Infected Women?" VII International Conference on AIDS, Florence, 1991, Vol. 1, p. 313.

138. N.J. Alexander, op. cit.

139. D. Anderson et al., "Prevalence and Temporal Variation of HIV-1 in Semen," VI International Conference on AIDS, San Francisco, 1990, Vol. 1, p. 263; J.J. Goedert et al., "Heterosexual Transmission of HIV: Association with Severe T4-Cell Depletion in Male Hemophiliacs," III International Conference on AIDS, Wash., D.C., 1987, No. W.2.6.; D.S. Burke et al., "Increased 'Viral Burden' in Late Stages of HIV Infection," V International Conference on AIDS, Montreal, 1989, p. 156.

140. *International Healthwatch Report*, October 1988.

141. J.J. Gonzalez et al., "HIV Carriers: Increasing Infectivity with Progression to AIDS Has Important Implications for the AIDS Epidemic among Heterosexuals," V International Conference on AIDS, Montreal, 1989, p. 149.

142. M. Laga et al., "Risk Factors for HIV Infection in Heterosexual Partners of HIV-Infected Africans and Europeans," IV International Conference on AIDS, Stockholm, 1988, Vol. 1, No. 4004.

143. *Ft. Worth Star Telegram*, 30 July 1985.

144. Jay A. Levy, "The Host Range of HIV and Its Relationship to Tissue Tropism and Pathogenesis," IV International Conference on AIDS, Stockholm, 1988, Vol. 2, No. 2586. Dr. Levy states: "HIV replicates to high titer in human T cells and infects macrophages. . . . Moreover, human monolayer cells lacking CD4 expression can be infected with some HIV isolates and HIV can be recovered from bowel epithelial cells. These observations underscore the wide tropism of HIV [the virus' affinity for infecting a broad spectrum of cells] and suggest other receptors or mechanisms for its infection of human cells." See also: C. Cheng-Mayer, D. Seto et al., "Biologic Features of HIV that Correlate with Virulence in the Host," IV International Conference on AIDS, Stockholm, 1988, Vol. 2, No. 2590. Dr. Levy and his colleagues at the Cancer Research Institute at the University of California School of Medicine state: "Progression of disease in those infected correlated with the emergence of an HIV strain that in, in comparison to the initial virus identified, *is more cytopathic [cell-killing] and has higher replicating capabilities in a wide variety of different human cells.* . . . These observations indicate that *a more cytopathic HIV with a high replicative ability emerges concomitant with progression of disease in the host.*"

145. S. Colgate et al., *Los Alamos Science*, op. cit., p. 20.

146. G.F. Bolz et al., "Simulating the Epidemic Dynamics of HIV-Infection Using Stochastic Processes over Random Graphs," V International Conference on AIDS, Montreal, 1989, p. 151.

147. S. Colgate et al., op. cit., *Los Alamos Science*, p. 21.

148. S.A. Colgate et al., "A Risk Based Model of the Early Growth of AIDS in the United States," IV International Conference on AIDS, Stockholm, 1988, Vol. 2, No. 4697.

149. J.J. Gonzalez et al., "HIV Carriers: Increasing Infectivity with Progression to AIDS Has Important Implications for the AIDS Epidemic Among Heterosexuals," V International Conference on AIDS, Montreal, 1989, p. 149.

150. F. Chiodi et al., "Human Immunodeficiency Virus Isolates Differ in Replication Potential in Vitro," III International Conference on AIDS, Wash., D.C. 1987, No. MP. 11; V.M. Zhdanov et al., "Comparative Study of HIV Strains," III International Conference on AIDS, Wash., D.C., 1987, No. MP. 7.

151. S. Colgate et al., op. cit., Los Alamos Science, p. 19.

152. M.M. Goodenow, T. Juet et al., "HIVs Are Highly Polymorphic," IV International Conference on AIDS, Stockholm, 1988, Vol. 2, No. 1575.

153. Mark Ellis, "Super AIDS Worry for Doctors," Daily Mirror, England, Dec. 16, 1991.

154. N H. Rubsamen-Waigman et al., "Two West-African Isolates of HIV-2 with Marked Tropism for Macrophages, One of Which Is Highly Divergent and Genetically Equidistant between HIV-2(ROD) and SIV(MAC)," V International Conference on AIDS, Montreal, 1989, p. 537.

155. I. Onorato et al., "Warning of the Next Epidemic: Surveillance for HIV-2 Infection in High-Risk Populations, United States 1988-90," VII International Conference on AIDS, Florence, 1991, Vol. 1, p. 315; S.A. Quattara et al., "Evolution of HIV-1, HIV-2 and AIDS Epidemics in Ivory Coast Between 1985 and 1987," IV International Conference on AIDS, Stockholm, 1988, Vol. 1, No. 5015.

156. F.E. McCutchan et al., "Genetic Relationships Among International HIV-1 Isolates," VII International Conference on AIDS, 1991, Florence, Vol. 2, p. 63. "Isolates from North America are relatively homogeneous and similar to known prototypes. In Asia and South America, disparate patterns were observed in different locales. One Asian country exhibited isolates principally of the North American/European region type while another exhibited broad genetic diversity of isolates. In South America, both homogeneous and heterogeneous locales were also identified in terms of HIV-1 diversity.... The genetic diversity of HIV-1 in Africa and specific regions of Asia and South America may be more extensive than previously appreciated."

157. G.L. Myers, C.R. Linder, and K.A. MacInnes, "Genealogy and Diversification of the AIDS Virus," Los Alamos Science, Fall, 1989, pp. 47-53.

158. H. Von Briesen, W. Enzensberger et al., "Biological and Genetic Characterization of HIV-Isolates from Blood and Cerebrospinal Fluid of AIDS Patients with Neurological Symptoms," IV International Conference on AIDS, Stockholm, 1988, Vol. 2, No. 1580.

159. M. Tersmette et al., "Differences in Risk of AIDS and AIDS Mortality in 49 Individuals Infected with Low- and High-Virulent HIV Variants," V International Conference on AIDS, Montreal, 1989, p. 599.

160. S. Colgate et al., op. cit., Los Alamos Science, p. 20.

161. R.A. Feinstein et al., "Chlamydia Trachomatis Cervical Infection and Oral Contraceptive Use Among Adolescent Girls," J Adolesc Health Care 1989 Sep;10(5):376-81; D. Avonts et al., "Incidence of Uncomplicated Genital Infections in Women Using Oral Contraception or an Intrauterine Device: A Prospective Study," Sex Transm Dis 1990 Jan-Mar;17:23-9; J.R. Daling et al., "Risk factors For Condyloma Acuminatum in Women," Sex Transm Dis ;1986;13:16-8; F.E. Willmott, H.J. Mair, "Genital Herpesvirus Infection in Women Attending a Venereal Diseases Clinic," Br J Vener Dis 1978;54:341-3.

162. M.K. Oh et al., "Sexually Transmitted Diseases and Sexual Behavior in Urban Adolescent Females Attending a Family Planning Clinic," J Adolesc Health Care 1988 January;9(1):67-71

163. G. Bousfield, "The Pill and Venereal Disease," Br Med J 1973;1(851):491; W.W. Darrow, "Changes in Sexual Behavior and Venereal Diseases," Clin Obstet Gynecol 1975;18:255-67; L.H. Pereira et al., "Cytomegalovirus Infection Among Women Attending a Sexually Transmitted Disease Clinic: Association with Clinical Symptoms and Other Sexually Transmitted Diseases," Am J Epidemiol 1990;131:683-92; F. Plummer et al., "Co-Factors in Male-Female Transmission of HIV," IV International Conference on AIDS, Stockholm, 1988, Vol. 2, No. 4554; P. Piot et al., "AIDS: An International Perspective," Science 1988; 239:573-9; J. Mati et al., "Contraceptive Use and HIV Infection Among Women Attending Family Planning Clinics in Nairobi, Kenya," VI International Conference on AIDS, San Francisco, 1990, Vol. 1, p. 158; cf., F.E. Riphagen, "Contraception and AIDS prevention," Contraception 1989;39:577-8.

164. Cecil Textbook of Medicine, op. cit., p. 1705.

165. J.N. Simonsen et al., "HIV Infection Among Lower Socioeconomic Strata Prostitutes in Nairobi," AIDS 1990;4:139-144 citing I.A. Trait et al., "Chlamydia Infection of the Cervix in Contacts of Men with Non-gonococcal Cervicitis," Br J Vener Dis 1980;56:257-261; J.D.Oriel, "Genital Yeast Infections," Br Med J 1972;4:761-764; C.J. Grossman, "Interactions Between Gonadal Steroids and the Immune System," Science 1985;227:257-261.

166. R.P. Dickey, M.D., Ph.D. Managing Contraceptive Pill Patients, (Durant, OK: Creative Infomatics, Inc., 1987), p. 172.

167. "The Pill and Ovarian Cysts," International Healthwatch Report, July 1988.

168. K.E. Brock et al., "Sexual, Reproductive and Contraceptive Risk Factors for Carcinoma-In-Situ of the Uterine Cervix in Sydney," *Med J Aust* 1989;150:125-30.

169. R.P. Dickey, op. cit., pp. 110-111;112-113;114-117;171-172;194-196; see also: C.R. Kay et al., "Oral Contraception and Genital Tract Malignancy," *Lancet* 1989;1:783-4.

170. N. Hasley et al., "Smoking as a Risk Factor for Heterosexual Transmission of HIV-1 in Haitian Women," V International Conference on AIDS, Montreal, 1989, p. 57.

171. *Cecil Textbook of Medicine*, op. cit., p. 1443.

172. *The Pill and the IUD: Some Facts for an Informed Choice*, Couple to Couple League, 3621 Glenmore Ave, Cincinnati, Ohio 45211.

173. J. Urquhart, "Effect of the Venereal Diseases Epidemic on the Incidence of Ectopic Pregnancy–Implications for the Evaluation of Contraceptives," *Contraception* 1979;19:455-80.

174. S. Hafez et al., "Contraceptives, HIV Infections and Heterosexual Transmission," V International Conference on AIDS, Montreal, 1989, p. 481; see also: G.E. Bignardi, "Candidiasis in Women Fitted with an Intrauterine Contraceptive Device," *Br J Obstet Gynaecol* 1988;95:1083-4; B. Foxman R.R. Frerichs, "Epidemiology of Urinary Tract Infection: I. Diaphragm Use and Sexual Intercourse," *Am J Public Health* 1985;75:1308-13.

175. A. Ravinathan et al., "Oral Contraception, IUD, Condom Use & Man to Woman Heterosexual Transmission of STD/HIV Infection," VII International Conference on AIDS, Florence, 1991, Vol. 1, p. 448.

176. T.M. Hooton et al., "Escherichia Coli Bacteriuria and Contraceptive Method," *JAMA* 1991;265:64-69.

177. T.M. Hooton et al., "Association Between Bacterial Vaginosis and Acute Cystitis in Women Using Diaphragms," *Arch Intern Med* 1989;149:1932.

178. "Life-Threatening Hypersensitivity to Latex Called a Growing Problem, *Family Practice News*, 15 May 1992, pp. 1, 30.

179. C.D. Lytle et al., "Virus Leakage Through Natural Membrane Condoms," V International Conference on AIDS, Montreal, 1989, p. 597.

180. N.E. MacDonald et al., "High-Risk STD/HIV Behavior Among College Students," *JAMA* 1990;263:3155-9; M. Levine et al., "Condom Usage Decisions Among Gay Men," V International Conference on AIDS, Montreal, 1989, p. 808; G. Farr et al., "Acceptability of Condom Use Among Patients at a Sexually Transmitted Disease Clinic," VI International Conference on AIDS, San Francisco, 1990, Vol. 2, p. 266. "Even though the majority of these patients were convinced that condoms help reduce the likelihood of HIV transmission, they chose not to use them."

181. *Dallas Times Herald*, 18 February 1989, p. A9; see also: D.L. Cohn et al., "Condom Usage for Anal Intercourse in a Longitudinal Study of Homosexual and Bisexual Men," IV International Conference on AIDS, Stockholm, 1988, Vol. 2, No. 6540.

182. W. Rozenblum et al., "HIV Transmission by Oral Sex," IV International Conference on AIDS, Stockholm, 1988, Vol. 2, No. 4562.

183. "Oral Sex Transmits AIDS," *International Healthwatch Report*, October 1990.

184. *British Medical Journal*, 14 March 1987, p. 706.

185. M. Piazza et al., "Passionate Kissing and Microlesions of the Oral Mucosa: Possible Role in AIDS Transmission," *JAMA* 1989;262:244-245.

186. D. Ajdukovic et al., "Susceptibility to HIV of Blood Lymphocytes Transformed by Antigens/Mitogens of Oral Flora," IV International Conference on AIDS, Stockholm, 1988, Vol. 2, No. 2613.

187. R.P. Dickey, op. cit., p. 172.

188. D. Perlman, "New Test Finds High Incidence of Wart Virus," *San Francisco Chronicle*, 28 January 1991. The researchers studied 467 coeds at the University of California at Berkeley using a newly developed PCR test. The conventional test method had only been able to detect the presence of HPV in 11% of the women.

CHAPTER FOUR
TRANSMISSION THROUGH OTHER BODY FLUIDS

1. *MMWR*, 1 April 1988, Vol. 37, No. S-4.

2. *New York Times*, 18 January 1991.

3. J.R. Winkler et al., "Periodontal Disease in HIV-Infected Male Homosexuals," III International Conference on AIDS, Wash., D.C., 1987, No. WP.144.

4. P.C. Fox et al., "Salivary Alterations in HIV-Infected Persons," IV International Conference on AIDS, Stockholm, 1988, Vol. 2, No. 2614.

5. C-K. Yeh et al., "Oral Mucosa Alterations in HIV-1 Infected Individuals," IV International Conference on AIDS, Stockholm, 1988, Vol. 2, No. 7577; S. Engelbert et al., "Oral Findings in Patients with Asymptomatic HIV Disease," V International Conference on AIDS, Montreal, 1989, p. 469; M. Grassi, J.R. Winkler, P.A. Murray, D. Greenspan, J.S. Greenspan. "Oral Manifestations of HIV Infections: Current Status and Perspectives," *Schweizerische Monatsschrift Fur Zahnmedizin* 1987;97:1537-44 (Published in German).

6. P. Romagnoli et al., "Dendritic Cells of the Oral Mucosa in HIV Infection," VII International Conference on AIDS, Florence, 1991, Vol. 1, p. 243. According to researchers from the University of Florence and the National Health Service, "The expression of molecules involved in antigen presentation is impaired in DCs or oral tissues *even in the absence of lesions*." See also: S.C. Knight et al., "Effect of HIV on Antigen Presentation by Dendritic Cells and Monocytes," VII International Conference on AIDS, Florence, 1991, Vol. 1, p. 63; E. Langhoff et al., "Prolific HIV-1 Growth in Human Dendritic Cells," VII International Conference on AIDS, Florence, 1991, Vol. 2, p. 40. Dr. William Haseltine and other scientists from the Dana-Farber Cancer Institute in Boston, have found a "prolific growth" of HIV-1 in human dendritic cells. "The prolific viral replication in dendritic cells is unexpected . . . and can serve as a significant source of viral spread."

7. D. Ajdukovic et al., "Oral Bacteria Stimulation of Production of HIV," III International Conference on AIDS, Wash., D.C. 1987, No. MP.102; see also: M. Gornitsky, D. Pekovic, "Involvement of Human Immunodeficiency Virus (HIV) in Gingiva of Patients with AIDS," *Advances in Experimental Medicine and Biology* 1987;216A:553-62.

8. D. Ajdukovic et al., "Susceptibility to HIV of Blood Lymphocytes Transformed by Antigens/Mitogens of Oral Flora. IV International Conference on AIDS, Stockholm, 1988, Vol. 2, No. 2613.

9. D.D. Chitwood et al., "HIV Seropositivity of Needles from Shooting Galleries in South Florida," *American Journal of Public Health* 1990;150-152; D.C. Des Jarlais et al., "Shooting Galleries and AIDS: Infection Probabilities and 'Tough' Policies," *AJPH* 1990;142-143.

10. D. Ajdukovic et al., "Oral Bacteria Flora: Role in the Infectivity of HIV," V International Conference on AIDS, Montreal, 1989, p. 475. See also: D. Pekovic et al., "Detection of Human Immunosuppressive Virus in Salivary Lymphocytes from Dental Patients with AIDS," *Am J Med* 1987;82:188-9; L.I. Zon et al., "IgA Deficiency and Salivary Transmission of Human Immunodeficiency Virus," *Lancet* 1986;2:1039-1040.

11. J.S. Greenspan et al., "Oral Lesions of HIV Disease: Implications in Pathogenesis, Diagnosis and Care," IV International Conference on AIDS, Stockholm, 1988, Vol. 2, No. 7574; A. Sinicco et al., "Oral Lesions in 327 Anti-HIV Positive Subjects," IV International Conference on AIDS, Stockholm, 1988, Vol. 2, No. 7568; F. Lazada-Nur et al., "Recurrent Oral Aphthae in HIV-Infected Homosexual Males," V International Conference on AIDS, Montreal, 1989, p. 471.

12. E.A.J.M. Schulten et al., "Oral Manifestations of HIV-Infection in a Dutch Population," IV International Conference on AIDS, Stockholm, 1988, Vol. 2, No. 7565.

13. D. Ajdukovic et al., "Oral Bacteria Stimulation of Production of HIV," III International Conference on AIDS, Wash., D.C. 1987, No. MP. 102; see also: B.D. Johnson, D. Engel, "Acute Necrotizing Ulcerative Gingivitis. A review of Diagnosis, Etiology and Treatment," *Journal of Periodontology* 1986;57:141-50; J.J.Pindborg, J.J. Thorn et al., [Acute Necrotizing Gingivitis in an AIDS Patient] *Tandlaegebladet* 1986;90:450-3 (Published in Danish).

14. A.M. Quart et al., "Periodontal Disease in Heterosexual Patients with AIDS," V International Conference on AIDS, Montreal, 1989, p. 474; J. Engelman et al., "Oral Manifestations of HIV Infection in a Cohort of Homosexual and Bisexual Men," IV International Conference on AIDS, Stockholm, 1988, Vol. 2, No. 7580.

15. J.R. Winkler et al., "Periodontal Disease in HIV-Infected Male Homosexuals," III International Conference on AIDS, Wash., D.C., 1987, No. WP. 144; see also: J.R. Winkler et al., "Clinical Documentation of HIV-Associated Periodontitis and Gingivitis," IV International Conference on AIDS, Stockholm, 1988, Vol. 2, No. 7571; J.R. Winkler et al., "The Microbiology of HIV-Associated Periodontal Lesions," IV International Conference on AIDS, Stockholm, 1988, Vol. 2, No. 7570; A. Zakarian et al., "HIV-Related Ulcerative Gingivitis and Periodontitis," IV International Conference on AIDS, Stockholm, 1988, Vol. 2, No. 7573; D.D. Pekovic et al., "AIDS-Associated Periodontal Disease," IV International Conference on AIDS, Stockholm, 1988, Vol. 2, No. 7569; J.A. Phelan et al., Major (Giant) Aphthous-Like Ulcers in Patients with AIDS," IV International Conference on AIDS, Stockholm, 1988, Vol. 2, No. 7586; C.A. Williams et al., "Necrotizing Stomatitis Associated with AIDS," IV International Conference on AIDS, Stockholm, 1988, Vol. 2, No. 7572; D. Croser et al., "The Oral Manifestations of HIV Disease, Can They Predict Disease Progression?" A Study of 143 Patients with Reference to Disease Status, CD4 Lymphocyte Count, and HIV p24 Antigen Presence," VII International Conference on AIDS, Florence, 1991, Vol. 1, p. 241; A. Quart et al., "Dental and Oral Complaints Among Intravenous Drug Users in a Methadone Maintenance Treatment Program," VII International Conference on AIDS, Florence, 1991, Vol. 2, p. 373.

16. A.M. Quart et al., "Periodontal Disease in Heterosexual Patients with AIDS," V International Conference on AIDS, Montreal, 1989, p. 474.

17. D. Greenspan et al., "Human Papillomavirus Types in Oral Warts in Association with HIV Infection," IV International Conference on AIDS, Stockholm, 1988, Vol. 2, No. 7587.

18. G. Ficarra et al., "Epstein-Barr Virus and Human Papilloma Virus Detection in Oral Hairy Leukoplakia and Normal Oral Mucosa of HIV-Infected Patients," VII International Conference on AIDS, Florence, 1991, Vol. 1, p. 254.

19. D.D. Pekovic et al., "Origin, Role and Infectivity of Salivary HIV," IV International Conference on AIDS, Stockholm, 1988, Vol. 2, No. 1602.

20. G. Lecatsas et al., "Retrovirus-Like Particles in Salivary Glands, Prostate and Testes of AIDS Patients," Proc Soc Exp Biol Med 1985;178:653-655.

21. M. Gravell et al., "Transmission of Simian Acquired Immunodeficiency Syndrome (SAIDS) with Type D Retrovirus Isolated from Saliva or Urine," Proc Soc Exp Biol Med 1984;177:491-4.

22. M. Jennings et al., "Infection with Simian Immunodeficiency Virus (SIV) Via Conjunctival and Oral Mucosae in a Newborn Rhesus Macaque," V International Conference on AIDS, Montreal, 1989, p. 594.

23. C. Hammerle et al., "Langerhans Cells in Rhesus Monkey Oral Mucosa Before and After Infection with Simian Retrovirus Serotype 1," V International Conference on AIDS, Montreal, 1989, p. 597.

24. D.W. Archibald et al., "Salivary Antibodies as a Means of Detecting HTVL-III/LAV Infection," J Clin Microbiol 1986;24:873-875.

25. A.S. Goldstein et al., "Analysis of HIV Antibodies in Serum Versus Whole Saliva," IV International Conference on AIDS, Stockholm, 1988, Vol. 2, No. 1601.

26. C. Major et al., "Evaluation of Saliva as an Alternative to Blood for HIV Seroprevalence Testing," VI International Conference on AIDS, San Francisco, 1990, Vol. 3, p. 241.

27. J.R. Winkler et al., "Correlation of HIV in Gingival Crevicular Fluid," V International AIDS Conference, Montreal, 1989, p. 472.

28. "Saliva Is Better in Tests for AIDS, Say Thai Doctors," The Straits Times, Singapore, 26 January 1988, p. 10.

29. Ibid.

30. W. Panmoung, et al., "Salivary Anti-HIV Assay by ELISA Test," VI International Conference on AIDS, San Francisco, 1990, Vol. 3, p. 242.

31. "Saliva Test for AIDS Developed," The Tampa Tribune, 21 Sept. 1991; "Quick AIDS Test in Sight," Gainesville Sun, 21 Sept. 1991.

32. T. Ze'ev et al., "Mucosal Immune Symptoms in HIV1 Infection; Activity of Specific Antibodies in Parotid Saliva," V International AIDS Conference, Montreal, 1989, p. 645.

33. Slaff and Brubaker, The AIDS Epidemic (New York: Warner Books, 1985), p. 42.

34. F. Barre-Sinoussi et al., "Resistance of AIDS Virus at Room Temperature," Lancet, 28 September 1985, pp. 721-722.

35. JAMA Medical News, 22/29 November 1985, p. 2866.

36. L. Resnick et al., "Stability and Inactivation of HTLV-III/LAV under Clinical and Laboratory Experiments," JAMA 1985;225:1887-1891.

37. S.L. Loskoski et al., "Survival of the Human Immunodeficiency Virus [HIV] Under Controlled Drying Conditions," III International Conference on AIDS, Wash., D.C. 1987, No. MP.229; see also: P. Gilligan and L. Smiley, "HIV Survival in Blood Cultures," IV International Conference on AIDS, Stockholm, 1988, Vol. 1, No. 9008 [Researchers from the University of North Carolina School of Medicine].

38. L. Rabeneck et al., "Acute HIV Infection Presenting with Painful Swallowing and Esophageal Ulcers," JAMA 1990;263:2318-2322.

39. C. Graziosi et al., "Lymphoid Tissues Function as 'Reservoirs' for HIV Infection," VII International Conference on AIDS, Florence, 1991, Vol. 1, p. 63.

40. K. Hisashi et al., "Virologic and Serologic Characteristics of HIV-1 Infection in Children," VI International Conference on AIDS, San Francisco, 1990, Vol. 2, p. 166.

41. MMWR, 1 April 1988, Vol. 37, No. S-4.

42. MMWR, 1 Aug. 1987, Vol. 36, No. 2S.

43. Cf., MMWR, 1 April 1988, Vol. 37, No. S-4, op. cit..

44. "AIDS Viruses Multiply Rapidly in Mouth," International Healthwatch Report, January, 1989.

45. V. Wahn et al., "Horizontal Transmission of HIV Infection between Two Siblings," Lancet, 20 September 1986.

46. Theodore M. Hammett, Ph.D., "Precautionary Measures and Protective Equipment: Developing a Reasonable Response," U.S. Department of Justice, National Institute of Justice, AIDS Bulletin, February, 1988.

47. A.L. Belman et al., "Pediatric AIDS: Neurologic Syndromes," III International Conference on AIDS, Wash., D.C. 1987, No. W.5.3; J. Vincent et al., "Neurologic Symptoms as the Initial

Presentation of HIV Infection in Pediatric Patients," V International Conference on AIDS, Montreal, 1989, p. 316.

48. G. Shearer et al., "Behavioral Changes in Children with HIV Infection," V International Conference, Montreal, 1989, p. 316.

49. T.P. Swales et al., "Neurocognitive Functioning among Infants Exposed Perinatally to HIV," V International Conference on AIDS, Montreal, 1989, p. 317; T. Calvelli et al., "Divergence of Onset of Neurologic and Immunologic Impairment in Infants Born to HIV Seropositive Mothers," V International Conference, Montreal, 1989, p. 317.

50. J. Hittelman et al., "Neurodevelopmental Assessment of Children with Symptomatic HIV Infection," V International Conference on AIDS, Montreal, 1989, p. 316.

51. H. Mendez et al., "Response to Childhood Immunizations in Children with HIV Infection," IV International Conference on AIDS, Stockholm, 1988, Vol. 1, No. 5109.

52. M. Mvula et al., "Measles and Measles Immunization in African Children with HIV," IV International Conference on AIDS, Stockholm, 1988, Vol. 1, No. 5110.

53. P.A. Brunell, "Varicella," Cecil Textbook of Medicine, op. cit., pp. 1788-1790.

54. Y.D. Park et al., "Stroke in Pediatric AIDS," IV International Conference on AIDS, Stockholm, 1988, Vol. 1, No. 7061.

55. Reed Bell, M.D., "Health Care Risks from Daycare Diseases," cited in Who Will Rock the Cradle? Phyllis Schlafly, ed., (Washington, D.C.: Eagle Forum Education & Legal Defense Fund, 1989), pp. 115-122. This is the premier work on the social, economic, medical and psychological effects of daycare. It is available through: Eagle Forum, Box 618, Alton, Illinois 62002.

56. Li Jian Jun et al., "Detection of HIV-1 Proviral DNA and Viral RNA in Urine Pellets from HIV-1 Seropositive Individuals," VI International Conference on AIDS, San Francisco, 1990, Vol. 2, p. 164. Using a reverse transcriptase/polymerase chain reaction (RT/PCR) technique, the researchers found HIV-1 proviral DNA in 69% of fresh urine centrifuged pellets from seropositive individuals. ". . . The HIV-1 infected lymphocytes found in urine may possibly be due to secondary contamination from the genito-urinary tract (e.g., prostate, bladder, urethra, vagina)." See also: Y Cao et al., "Predominant IgG Antibodies to HIV-1 in the Urine of HIV-1 Seropositive Individuals," IV International Conference on AIDS, Stockholm, 1988, Vol. 2, No. 1603.

57. T. Gottfried et al., "Detection of HIV-1 Antibodies in Urines of Asymptomatic and ARC/AIDS Patients," V International Conference on AIDS, Montreal, 1989, p. 375.

58. J.V. Parry et al., "Sensitive and Specific Methods for Detecting Anti-HIV in Urine," VI International Conference on AIDS, San Francisco, 1990, Vol. 3, p. 241.

59. A. Francis et al., "Evaluation of Urine as an Alternative to Blood for HIV Prevalence Testing," VII International Conference on AIDS, Florence, 1991, Vol. 2, p. 342.

60. C. Miller et al., "Detection of HIV Antibodies in Urine; Blinded Prospective Comparison with Serum Testing in Low and High Prevalence Cohorts," VI International Conference on AIDS, San Francisco, 1990, Vol. 2, p. 317. The sensitivity of the test was 100%; specificity 98.9%.

61. Family Practice News, 1 February 1992, p. 2.

62. William H. Wickett, Jr., M.D., Herpes: Cause & Control (New York: Pinnacle Books, 1982), pp. 33-34.

63. H.M. Balfour, Jr., M.D., and R.C. Heussner, Herpes Diseases and Your Health (Minneapolis: University of Minnesota Press, 1985), pp. 56-57.

64. E.A. Velongia et al., "An Outbreak of Herpes Gladiatorum at a High School Wrestling Camp," N Eng J Med 1991;325:906-910.

65. D. Torre et al., "Transmission of HIV-1 Infection Via Sports Injury," Lancet, 23 June 1990, pp. 1105, 1532.

66. Grants Pass Courier, (AP) 5 May 1990.

67. L.R. Braathen et al., "Langerhans Cells as a Primary Target for HIV Infection," Lancet, 7 November 1987, p. 1094.

68. E. Tschachler et al., "The Skin Represents a Site of Virus Replication During the Course of Infection with Human Immunodeficiency Virus (HIV)," III International Conference on AIDS, Wash., D.C., 1987, No. TP.107. The researchers state: "Epidermal Langerhans cells (LC) represent a persistent, distinct population of antigen presenting leukocytes within the skin. . . .
Extensive electromicroscopic analysis of skin and mucosal biopsies from an AIDS patient . . . revealed mature HIV-like virions in the extracellular space surrounding Langerhans cells (LC) as well as developmental forms of HIV-like particles budding from LC surface membranes.
Moreover, cocultivation of a punch biopsie from normal appearing skin of this AIDS patient with mononuclear phagocytes from a non-infected donor, resulted in the detection of high levels of reverse-transcriptase activity in the culture supernatant. This latter finding implies that ACTIVE VIRUS CAN BE RESCUED FROM THE SKIN OF HIV-INFECTED INDIVIDUALS."

69. G. Ramirez et al., "Latent Infection of Epidermal Langerhans Cells in HIV Positives?" IV International Conference on AIDS, Stockholm, 1988, Vol. 1, No. 2089.

70. J. Ramsauer et al., "Langerhans Cells (LC) in the Pathogenesis of HIV Infection," IV International Conference on AIDS, Stockholm, 1988, Vol. 1, No. 2089.

71. D.M. Phillips & A.S. Bourinbaiar, "Infection of CD4 Negative Epithelia in Vitro," VI International Conference on AIDS, San Francisco, 1990, Vol. 2, p. 337. Researchers from the Population Council in New York City state: "HIV can be transmitted either by direct exposure to infected blood or through indirect exposure across [intact] epithelial barrier as it occurs in milk-borne transmission. . . . Although the exact mechanism responsible for multiple types of HIV entry is not well known, the possibility of simultaneous viral uptake via three different mechanisms by the same CD4-negative epithelial cell indicates the complexity of modes of HIV infection and may have important consequences on the preventive strategies against HIV."

72. P. Weinbreck et al., "Breast-Feeding and HIV-1 Transmission," IV International Conference on AIDS, Stockholm, 1988, Vol. 1, No. 5102. "CASE REPORT: A previously healthy white woman with no HIV risk factors delivered her second child vaginally. Because of blood loss, she received 2 blood units after delivery. . . . Breast-feeding was established on the first day and continued for 4 weeks with no nipple difficulties. Twenty-seven months later, the mother was admitted for AIDS with p. carinii pneumonitis. The mother and the child were HIV-1 seropositive, the father and older siblings were negative, one of the two blood donors was tested retrospectively and was a a male homosexual who was HIV-1 seropositive. The mother's frozen blood sample taken during the fourth month of pregnancy was retrospectively tested and was negative for HIV."

73. M. Pezzella et al., "The Presence of HIV-1 Genome in Human Colostrum from Asymptomatic Seropositive Mothers," VI International Conference on AIDS, San Francisco, 1990, Vol. 2, p. 165

74. S. Solomon et al., "Transmission of HIV Infection Through Breast Milk," V International Conference on AIDS, Montreal, 1989, p. 1025.

75. R.L. Colebunders et al., "Breastfeeding and Transmission of HIV," IV International Conference on AIDS, Stockholm, 1988, Vol. 1, No. 5103; S. Hira, "Breast Milk as a Risk Factor for HIV-1 Transmission," V International Conference on AIDS, Montreal, 1989, p. 374.

76. B.K. Rao et al., "Histopathologic Features of Inflammatory Skin Disorders in HIV-Infected Patients," VII International Conference on AIDS, Florence, 1991, Vol. 1, p. 256.

77. A.P. Lozar, M.D., M.P.H. and H.H. Roenigk, MD, "AIDS and Psoriasis," *Cutis* 1987;39:347-351.

78. M. Cuisini et al., "Muco-cutaneous Manifestations in HIV Positive Subjects," III International Conference on AIDS, Wash., D.C., 1987, No. TP.164; L. Morfeldt-Manson et al., "Dermatitis of the Face and Yellow Toe Nail Changes Indicate Progression to AIDS/OI in Patients with HIV Infection," V International Conference on AIDS, Montreal, 1989, p. 349; B.K. Rao & C.J. Cockrell, "Histopathologic Features of Inflammatory Skin Disorders in HIV Infected Patients," VII International Conference on AIDS, Florence, 1991, Vol. 1, p. 256.

79. M. Froschl et al., "HIV Infection in Women," IV International Conference on AIDS, Stockholm, 1988, No. 7275.

80. L. Morfeldt-Manson et al., "Dermatitis of the Face and Yellow Toe Nail Changes Indicate Progression to AIDS/OI in Patients with HIV Infection," V International Conference on AIDS, Montreal, 1989, p. 349.

81. L.R. Braathen et al., "Langerhans Cells as a Primary Target for HIV Infection," *Lancet*, 7 November 1987, p. 1094.

82. "AIDS Virus May Pass Through Intact Skin," *International Healthwatch Report*, September 1988.

CHAPTER FIVE
SECONDARY DISEASES

1. Rick Weiss, "Viruses: the Next Plague?" *Washington Post*, 8 October 1989.

2. In precise medical terminology, the word "casual" pertains to accidental injuries or to accidents. Cases involving medical workers, patients and others who contract AIDS through a needlestick injury or accidental exposure to blood or other body fluids should be defined as "casual" transmission [*Dorland's Illustrated Medical Dictionary*, op. cit., p. 281].

3. B.E. Laughon et al., "Prevalence of Enteric Pathogens in Homosexual Men with and without AIDS," *Gastroenterology* 1988;94:984-993; D.W. Cameron et al., "Altered Serologic Response to Natural Human Infection with Haemophilus Ducreyi, Due to HIV Infection," VI International Conference on AIDS, San Francisco, 1990, Vol. 1, p. 255.

4. R. Veronesi, "AIDS in Developing Countries," III International Conference on AIDS, Wash., D.C., 1987, No. MP.48; O. Kashala et al., "HIV-1, HTLV-1, and HTLV-2 Infection Among Leprosy Patients and Their Contacts in Zaire," VII International Conference on AIDS, 1991, Florence, Vol. 1, p. 375.

5. C. Pean et al., "Natural History of M. Leprae and HIV Co-Infection," V International Conference on AIDS, Montreal, 1989, p. 427.

6. L.A. Lettau, "Nosocomial Transmission and Infection Control Aspects of Parasitic and Ectoparasitic Diseases, Part II: Blood and Tissue Parasites," *Infect Control Hosp Epidemiol* 1991;12:111-121.

7. *Cecil Textbook of Medicine*, op. cit., pp. 1879-1881.

8. Ibid.

9. K.M. Cahill, *The AIDS Epidemic* (New York: St. Martin's Press, 1983) pp. 126, 135.

10. W.H. Gerlich, R. Thomssen, "Outbreak of Hepatitis B in a Butcher Shop," *Dtsch Wochenschr* 1982;107:1627-1630.

11. K.M. De Cock et al., "Fulminant Delta Hepatitis in Chronic Hepatitis B Infection," *JAMA* 1984;252:2746-2748.

12. A.M. Mutch et al., "An Outbreak of Hepatitis B and D in Butchers," *Scand J Infect Dis* 1987;19:179-184.

13. R.S. Remis et al., "Case Control of a Cluster of HIV Seroconversions Among Hemophilia Patients Implicating Heat-Treated Donor-Screened Factor Concentrates," IV International Conference on AIDS, 1988, Stockholm, 1988, Vol. 2, No. 7740; P. Gilligan and L. Smiley, "HIV Survival in Blood Cultures," IV International Conference on AIDS, Stockholm, 1988, Vol. 1, No. 9008. Researchers from the University of North Carolina state: "The collection and processing of blood cultures presents a potential risk for HIV exposure to individuals handling these specimens." They examined the survival of HIV in several blood culture systems. They incubated HIV-infected cells in broth bottles at 37 degrees Celsius (98.6 degrees Fahrenheit) and examined the supernatant fluids for virus-associated reverse transcriptase (RT) activity every 3 or 4 days for 42 days. Infectious virus was "readily recovered" from all specimens incubated in the broth bottles after 2 and 7 days. "These data indicate the need to follow strict infection control guidelines when performing blood cultures."

14. F.N. Judson, "Sexually Transmitted Viral Hepatitis and Enteric Pathogens," *Urologic Clinics of North America* 1984;11:177-185.

15. C. Hankansson et al., "Intestinal Parasitic Infection and Other Sexually Transmitted Diseases in Asymptomatic Homosexual Men," *Scandinavia Journal of Infectious Diseases* 1984; Vol. 16, No. 2.

16. H.L. Kazal et al., "The Gay Bowel Syndrome. Clinico-pathologic Correlation in 260 Cases," *Ann Clin Lab Sci* 1976;6:184.

17. *Cecil Textbook of Medicine*, op. cit., pp. 1590-1591.

18. J.D.H. Porter et al., "Food-Borne Outbreak of Giardia Lamblia," *AJPH* 1990;80:1259-1260.

19. J.E. Brody, "Test Unmasks a Parasitic Disease," *New York Times*, 26 October 1989.

20. *Cecil Textbook of Medicine*, op. cit., pp. 1802-1803.

21. Ibid., pp. 1886-1888.

22. Ibid., pp. 1648-1651.

23. Ibid., pp. 1646-1648.

24. Ibid., pp. 1881-1883.

25. M.R. Skeels et al., "*Cryptosporidium* Infection in Oregon Public Health Clinic Patients 1985-88: The Value of Statewide Laboratory Surveillance," *AJPH* 1990;80:305-308.

26. H. Albrecht et al., "Rotavirus Associated Diarrhea in HIV-Infected Patients, VII International Conference on AIDS, Florence, 1991, Vol. 1, p. 252.

27. L. Corey and K.K. Holmes, "Sexual Transmission of Hepatitis A in Homosexual Men," *N Eng J Med* 1980;302:435-438.

28. Jeanne Kassler, *Gay Men's Health: A Guide to the AID Syndrome and Other Sexually Transmitted Diseases* (New York: Harper and Row, 1983), p. 52.

29. D. Williams, "Parasitic Infectious Diseases as Sexually Transmitted Infections," in Pearl Ma and Donald Armstrong, *The Acquired Immunodeficiency Syndrome and Infections of Homosexual Men*, (New York: Yorke Medical Books, 1984), p. 78.

30. A. Rompalo and H. Hunter Handsfield, "Overview of Sexually Transmitted Diseases in Homosexual Men," in Ma and Armstrong, op. cit., p. 8.

31. C.B. Panosian and S.L. Gorbach, "Bacterial Diarrhea in Homosexual Men," in Ma and Armstrong, op. cit., pp. 63-76.

32. D.G. Ostrow et al., *Sexually Transmitted Diseases in Homosexual Men* (New York: Plenum Medical Book Co., 1983), p. 117.

33. P.J. Buchanan and J. Gordon Muir, M.D., "Gay Times and Diseases," *The American Spectator*, August 1984.

34. H.L. Kazal et al., "The Gay Bowel Syndrome. Clinico-pathologic Correlation in 260 Cases," *Ann Clin Lab Sci* 1976;6:184; L. McKusick et al., "AIDS and Sexual Behavior Reported by Gay Men in San Francisco," *Amer J Pub Health* 1985;75:493-496.

35. B.E. Laughon et al., "Prevalence of Enteric Pathogens in Homosexual Men with and without AIDS," *Gastroenterology* 1988;94:984.

36. Ibid.

37. *Cecil Textbook of Medicine*, op. cit., pp. 821-822.

38. B.S. Levy et al., "Intensive Hepatitis Surveillance in Minnesota: Methods and Results," *Am J Epidemiol* 1977 February;105(2):127-34.

39. C.P. Schade and D. Komorwska, "Continuing Outbreak of Hepatitis A Linked with Intravenous Drug Abuse in Multnomah County," *Public Health Rep* 1988 Sep-Oct;103(5):452-4599.

40. T. Kosatsky and J.P. Middaugh, "Linked Outbreaks of Hepatitis A in Homosexual Men in Food Service Patrons and Employees," *Western Journal of Medicine* 1986;144:307-310.

41. E.B. Keeffe, "Clinical Approach to Viral Hepatitis in Homosexual Men," *Med Clin North Am* 1986;70:567-586.

42. M. Navarro, "Federal Officials See Sharp Rise of Hepatitis Among Gay Men," *New York Times*, 6 March 1992; "Hepatitis A Among Homosexual Men – United States, Canada and Australia," *JAMA* 1992;267:1587-1588.

43. C.R. Boughton et al., "Viral Hepatitis: A Four-Year Hospital and General-Practice Study in Sydney. 2. Transmission of Viral Hepatitis Among Residential Contacts in Sydney," *Med J Aust* 1982;20;1:174-176.

44. R.M. Frace, J.A. Jahre, "Policy for Managing a Community Infectious Disease Outbreak," *Infect Control Hosp Epidemiol.* 1991;12:364-367.

45. C. Poirot, "Worthington Hotel Billed for Hepatitis Shots," *Ft. Worth Star-Telegram*, 4 May 1989.

46. J.V. Parry et al., "Diagnosis of Hepatitis A and B by Testing Saliva," *J Med Virol* 1989 Aug;28(4):255-60.

47. P.J. Grob, H.J. Joller-Jemelka, "Hepatitis-C-Virus (HCV), Anti-HCV and Non-A-, Non-B-Hepatitis," *Schweiz Med Wochenschr* 1990 Feb 3;120(5):117-24 [Published in German]; E. Tabor, "The Three Viruses of Non-A, Non-B Hepatitis." *Lancet*, 1985 March 30;1(8431):743-745; A.M. Lever, "Non A/Non B Hepatitis," *J Hosp Infect* 1988;11 Suppl. A:150-160.

48. *Cecil Textbook of Medicine*, op. cit., 823; C.H. Thorne et al., "A Histologic Comparison of Hepatitis B with Non-A, Non-B Chronic Active Hepatitis," *Arch Pathol Lab Med* 1982 Sep;106(9):433-6; B. Berris, "Chronic viral diseases," *Can Med Assoc J* 1986 Dec 1;135(11):1260-8; R. Wejstal et al., "Chronic Non-A, Non-B Hepatitis. A Long-Term Follow-Up Study in 49 Patients," *Scand J Gastroenterol* 1987;22:1115-1122.

49. M.S. Khuroo et al., "Incidence and Severity of Viral Hepatitis in Pregnancy," *Am J Med* 1981 Feb;70:252-255.

50. P.J. Grob, H.J. Joller-Jemelka, op. cit.; J.M. Barrera et al., "Incidence of Non-A, Non-B Hepatitis After Screening Blood Donors for Antibodies to Hepatitis C Virus and Surrogate Markers," *Ann Intern Med* 1991;115:596-600; J.I. Esteban et al., "High Rate of Infectivity and Liver Disease in Blood Donors with Antibodies to Hepatitis C Virus," *Ann Intern Med*;1991;115:443-449; D. Marchesi et al., "Outbreak of Non-A, Non-B Hepatitis in Centre Haemodialysis Patients: A Retrospective Analysis," *Nephrol Dial Transplant* 1988;3:795-799; See also N. Muss, "Epidemic Outbreak of Non-A, Non-B Hepatitis in a Plasmapheresis Center. I: Epidemiological Observations," *Infection* 1985 Mar-Apr;13(2):57-60.

51. J. Feldschuh, op. cit., pp. 73-81.

52. G.P. Wormser et al., "Seroprevalence of Hepatitis C (HCV) in HIV-1 Infected IVDUs in the New York City Vicinity: 1987-1990," VII International Conference on AIDS, Florence, 1991, Vol. 1, p. 235.

53. D.G. Kelen et al., "Seroprevalence of HIV, HTLV, HCV and HBV among Emergency Department Patients and Potential Risk to Health Care Workers," VII International Conference on AIDS, Florence, 1991, Vol. 2, p. 433.

54. N P. Kuhnl et al., "[Hepatitis C antibodies in non-A, non-B hepatitis patients and members of HIV risk groups (pilot study)] HCV-Antikorper bei NANBH-Patienten and HIV-Risikogruppen-Angehorigen (Pilotstudie)," *Beitr Infusionther* 1990;26:30-2 (Published in German).

55. G.P. Wormser et al., "Hepatitis C in HIV-Infected Intravenous Drug Users and Homosexual Men in Suburban New York City," *JAMA* 1991;12;265:2958; M. Kiese et al., "Epidemiology of Hepatitis C in Homosexual Men," *Klinische Wochenschrift* 1990; 68:1082; S. Watanabe et al., "Electron Microscopic Evidence of Non-A, Non-B Hepatitis Markers and Virus-like Particles in Immunocompromised Humans," *Hepatology* 1984;4:628-632; J.G. McHutchison et al., "Assessment of Hepatitis C Antibody Tests in Homosexual Men with Hyperglobulinemia," *J Infect Dis* 1991 ;164:217-218; J.A. van den Hoek et al., "Prevalence, Incidence, and Risk Factors of Hepatitis C Virus Infection Among Drug Users in Amsterdam," *J Infect Dis* 1990;162:823-826; G. Hess et al.,

"[Diagnosis of hepatitis C virus (HCV) infection: diagnostic value of the anti-HCV test] Diagnose der Hepatitis-C-Virus(HCV)-Infektion: Diagnostische Wertigkeit des Anti-HCV-Tests," Z Gastroenterol 1990 May;28(5):251-252 (Published in German).

56. C.K. Fairley et al., "Epidemiology and Hepatitis C Virus in Victoria," Med J Aust 1990;153:271-273.

57. R.S. Tedder et al., "Hepatitis C Virus: Evidence for Sexual Transmission," British Med J 1991;302:1299-1302; A. Sanchez-Quijano et al., "Hepatitis C Virus Infection in Sexually Promiscuous Groups," Eur J Clin Microbiol Infect Dis 1990;9:610-612; A. Sonnerborg et al., "Hepatitis C Virus Infection in Individuals with or without Human Immunodeficiency Virus Type 1 Infection," Infection 1990 Nov-Dec;18(6):347-351; A. Sanchez-Quijano et al., "Hepatitis C Virus Infection in Sexually Promiscuous Groups," Eur J Clin Microbiol Infect Dis 1990;9:610-612.

58. M.E. Eyster et al., "Heterosexual Co-Transmission of Hepatitis C Virus (HCV) and Human Immunodeficiency Virus (HIV)," Ann Intern Med 1991;115:764-768.

59. G. Shi, "[An Epidemiological Investigation on an Outbreak of Non-A, Non-B Hepatitis Occurring after a Dinner Party]," Chung Hua Liu Hsing Ping Hsueh Tsa Chih 1990 Oct;11(5):263-6 [Abstract in English]; K. Hino "A Small Epidemic of Enterically Transmitted Non-A, Non-B Acute Hepatitis," Gastroenterol Jpn 1991 Jul;26 Suppl 3:139-141; S. Chakraborty et al., "Non-A Non-B Viral Hepatitis: A Common-Source Outbreak Traced to Sewage Contamination of Drinking Water," J Commun Dis 1982;14:41-46; D.C. Wong et al., Epidemic and Endemic Hepatitis in India: Evidence for a Non-A, Non-B Hepatitis Virus Aetiology," Lancet 1980;2(8200):876-9; M. Iqbal "An Outbreak of Enterically Transmitted Non-A, Non-B Hepatitis in Pakistan," Am J Trop Med Hyg 1989 ;40:438-443; K. Abe, "Experimental Transmission of Non-A, Non-B Hepatitis by Saliva," J Infect Dis 1987 May;155(5):1078-9; B. Nouasria et al., "Direct Evidence that Non-A, Non-B Hepatitis is a Waterborne Disease," Lancet 1984;14;2:94.

60. D.P. Francis et al., "Occurrence of Hepatitis A, B, and Non-A/Non-B in the United States. CDC Sentinel County Hepatitis Study I," Am J Med 1984 Jan;76(1):69-74; H. Myint et al., "A Clinical and Epidemiological Study of an Epidemic of Non-A Non-B Hepatitis in Rangoon," Am J Trop Med Hyg 1985 Nov;34(6):1183-9.

61. M.J. Alter, "Hepatitis C: A Sleeping Giant?" Am J Med;1991;91:112S-115S.

62. E. Tabor, "The Three Viruses of Non-A, Non-B Hepatitis," Lancet, 30 March 1985, pp. 743-745; M.J. Alter et al., "Sporadic Non-A, Non-B Hepatitis: Frequency and Epidemiology in an Urban U.S. Population," J Infect Dis 1982;145:886-893.

63. M.E. Eyster et al., "Heterosexual Co-transmission of HIV and HCV," VI International Conference on AIDS, San Francisco, 1990, Vol. 1, p. 266.

64. R.S. Klein et al., "Occupational Risk for Hepatitis C Virus Infection Among New York City Dentists," Lancet 1991;338:1539-1542.

65. G. Antonio, op. cit., p. 18.

66. V. Beral et al., "Kaposi's Sarcoma Among Persons with AIDS: A Sexually Transmitted Disease?" Lancet 1991;335:123-128; A.E. Friedman-Kien et al., "Kaposi's Sarcoma in HIV-Negative Homosexual Men," Lancet 1991;335:168-169.

67. V. Beral et al., "Risk of Kaposi's Sarcoma and Sexual Practices Associated with Faecal Contact in Homosexual or Bisexual Men with AIDS," Lancet 1992;339:632-635.

68. C.P. Archibald et al., "Risk Factors for Kaposi's Sarcoma in the Vancouver Lymphadenopathy-AIDS Study," J Acquir Immune Defic Syndr 1990; 3 (suppl. 1):S18-S23.

69. W.K. Darrow et al., "Kaposi's Sarcoma and Exposure to Faeces," Lancet 1992;339:685.

70. Ibid.

71. E.B. Keeffe, "Clinical Approach to Viral Hepatitis in Homosexual Men," Med Clin North Am 1986;70:567-586. "The annual incidence for HBV infection in homosexual men is 16% to 28% higher than that for hepatitis A. Transmission of HBV infection in homosexual men is facilitated by a large number of sexual partners, high HBsAg carrier rate, high infectivity of carriers (positive HBeAg), and the specific sexual practices of oral-anal and anal-genital contact with exposure to HBV on open mucosal surfaces."

72. J. Kassler, op. cit., p. 39.

73. D.G. Ostrow, op. cit., p. 204.

74. M.J. Alter and D. P. Francis, "Hepatitis B Virus Transmission between Homosexual Men: A Model for AIDS," in Ma and Armstrong, op. cit., pp. 97-106.

75. MMWR, 7 June 1985, p. 523.

76. "Update on Hepatitis B Prevention," MMWR 1987;36:353-365.

77. Ibid.

78. A.C. Street et al., "Persistence of Antibody in Healthcare Workers Vaccinated Against Hepatitis B," Infect Control Hosp Epidemiol 1990;11:525-530.

79. Ibid.

80. Ibid.

81. Ibid.

82. M.T. Pasko et al., "Persistence of Anti-HBs Among Health Care Personnel Immunized with Hepatitis B Vaccine," *Am J Public Health* 1990;80:590-593.

83. D. Nyanjom et al., "Unusual Hepatitis B Markers in HIV Seropositive Patients," IV International Conference on AIDS, Stockholm, 1988, Vol. 1, No. 7204; F. Mazzotta et al., "Hepatitis Viruses in HIV-Infected. Clinical and Epidemiological Correlations," VII International Conference on AIDS, Florence, 1991, Vol. 1, p. 234.

84. J.F. Colin et al., "Influence of HIV and Hepatitis C Virus in Infections on Chronic Hepatitis B in French Homosexual Men," VII International Conference on AIDS, 1991, Vol. 1, p. 251.

85. A. Cargnel et al., "Chronic HBsAg Positive Hepatitis in HIV Infection," V International AIDS Conference, Montreal, 1989, p. 257.

86. R.J.C. Gilson et al., "Interaction Between Hepatitis B Virus (HBV) and HIV in Homosexual Men," IV International Conference on AIDS, Stockholm, 1988, Vol. 2, No. 3671.

87. Y. Lazizi et al., "Reappearance of Hepatitis B Virus (HBV) in Immune Patients Infected with HIV-1," IV International Conference on AIDS, Stockholm, 1988, Vol. 1, No. 7205.

88. C.A. Lee et al., "Plasma-Derived Hepatitis B Vaccination in Anti-HIV Positive Patients with Hemophilia," IV International Conference on AIDS, Stockholm, 1988, Vol. 1, No. 5110; S.P. Buchbinder et al., "The Interaction of HIV and Hepatitis B Vaccination in a Cohort of Homosexual and Bisexual Men," V International Conference on AIDS, Montreal, 1989, p. 259; M. Gesemann et al., "Antibody Response to a Recombinant Hepatitis B Vaccine in Anti-HIV Positive Vs. Anti-HIV Negative Persons," III International Conference on AIDS, Wash., D.C., 1987, No. THP.131; B.N. Odake et al., "Randomized Clinical Trial of Plasma and Recombinant Hepatitis B Virus Vaccines in Gay Men," III International. Conference on AIDS, Wash., D.C., 1987, THP.119.

89. N. Bodsworth. B. Donovan, "The Effect of HIV on Chronic Hepatitis B: A Study of 150 Homosexual Men." V International Conference on AIDS, Montreal, 1989, p. 259.

90. W.W. Bond et al., "Survival of Hepatitis B Virus after Drying and Storage for One Week," *Lancet* 1981;1:550-551.

91. J.L. Lauer et al., "Transmission of Hepatitis B Virus in Clinical Laboratory Areas," *J Infect Dis* 1979;140:513-516.

92. W.W. Bond et al., "Inactivation of Hepatitis B Virus by Intermediate-to-High-Level Disinfectant Chemicals," *J Clin Microbiol* 1983;18:535-538.

93. C.P. Pattison et al., "Epidemic Hepatitis in a Clinical Laboratory: Possible Association with Computer Card Handling," *JAMA* 1974;230:854-857.

94. T.P. Bello et al. "An Institutional Outbreak of Hepatitis B Related to a Human Biting Carrier," *J Infect Dis* 1982;146:642-656.

95. M.J. Alter et al., "The Changing Epidemiology of Hepatitis B in the United States," *JAMA* 1990;263:1218-1222.

96. Ibid.

97. P.R.J. Gangadharam, V.K. Perumal et al., "Association of Plasmids and Virulence of *Mycobacterium avium intracellulare* Complex," III International Conference on AIDS, Wash., D.C., 1987, No. WP.69.

98. *Cecil's Textbook of Medicine*, op. cit., pp. 1694-1696.

99. M. Kaplan et al., "HTLV-I and HTLV-II Infection in HIV-Infected Patients: Report of 45 Co-infected Patients," VI International Conference on AIDS, San Francisco, 1990, Vol. 2, p. 248; D. Metzger et al., "HIV and HTLV-I/II Infection Among Opiate Addicts In and Out of Methadone Treatment in Philadelphia," VI International Conference on AIDS, San Francisco, 1990, Vol. 2, p. 248; P. W. Tuke et al., "The Use of Novel Methodology for the Determination of the Prevalence of HTLV-I/II Infection in an HIV-1 Positive Intravenous Drug User Cohort in Dublin," VII International Conference on AIDS, Florence, 1991, Vol. 1, p. 162.

100. P.S. Dixon, A.J. Bodner et al., "Tropical Spastic Paraperesis (TSP) and HTLV-I Infection in the U.S." IV International AIDS Conference, Stockholm, 1988, Vol. 2, No. 4663.

101. S.C. Lo, R.Y.-H. Wang et al., "Fatal Infection of Non-Human Primates with the Virus-Like Infectious Agent (VLIA-sb51) Derived from a Human Patient with AIDS," IV International Conference on AIDS, Stockholm, 1988, Vol. 2, No. 2662.

102. R.Y. Wang et al., "Direct Detection of a Newly Identified Virus-Like Infectious Agent by PCR in Blood (PBL) from Patients with AIDS," V International Conference on AIDS, Montreal, 1989, p. 681.

103. Katie Leishman, "Insects and AIDS," *Atlantic Monthly*, September, 1987, pp. 56-72.

104. V.L. Ng et al., "Characterization of Proteins Associated with Two Novel Retroviruses Isolated from AIDS-Associated Lymphoma Tissue," V International Conference on AIDS, Montreal, 1989, p. 625.

105. K.M. Cahill, op. cit., pp. 126, 135.

106. E. Gonczol et al., "Cytomegalovirus Replicates in Differentiated But Not in Undifferentiated Human Embryonal Carcinoma Cells," *Science* 1984;224:159-161.

107. *Sexually Transmitted Diseases: 1980 Status Report*, NIAID Study Group, U.S. Department of Health and Human Services, Public Health Service, National Institutes of Health, NIH Publication No. 81-2213, p. 316.

108. W.L. Drew et al., "Prevalence of Cytomegalovirus in Homosexual Men," *J Infect Dis* 1981;143:188.

109. *Ann Intern Med* 1986;104:38-41.

110. G.H. Murata et al., "Community-Acquired Bacterial Pneumonias in Homosexual Men: Presumptive Evidence for a Defect in Host Resistance," *AIDS Res* (1984-85)1(6):379-93. ". . . in the absence of apparent risk factors, when compared to heterosexual controls, the homosexual group had a much higher frequency of bacteremia [bacteria in the blood], complicated primary infections, multilobar involvement, required longer antibiotic therapy, and took longer to defervesce [lose their fever]."

111. P.A. Selwyn et al., "Increased Risk of Bacterial Pneumonia in HIV-Infected Intravenous Drug Users Without AIDS," *AIDS* 1988 August 2(4):267-72; R. Stoneburner et al., "Increasing Pneumonia Mortality in NYC, 1980-1986: Evidence for a Larger Spectrum of HIV-Related Disease in Intravenous Drug Users," IV International Conference on AIDS, Stockholm, 1988, Vol. 1, No. 7133.

112. E.W. Hook et al., "Failure of Intensive Care Unit Support to Influence Mortality from Pneumococcal Pneumonia," *JAMA* 1983;249:1055; *Cecil Textbook of Medicine*, op. cit., pp. 1554-1560.

113. J. Ward, "Antibiotic-Resistant Strains of *S. pneumoniae*: Clinical and Epidemiologic Aspects," *Rev Infect Dis* 1981;3:254.

114. *Cecil Textbook of Medicine*, op. cit., p. 1560.

115. "Agent Summary Statement Agent: HIVs Including HTLV-III, LAV, HIV-1, and HIV-2," CDC, *MMWR*, 1 April 1988, Vol. 34/No S-4, p. 3.

CHAPTER SIX
AIDS AND INSECTS

1. As cited in Katie Leishman, "AIDS and Insects," *Atlantic Monthly*, September 1987, pp. 56-72. Leishman's report is an in-depth comprehensive examination of the subject. It is well worth obtaining and reading.

2. G.L. Myers, C.R. Linder, and K.A. MacInnes, "Genealogy and Diversification of the AIDS Virus," *Los Alamos Science*, Fall, 1989, pp. 47-53.

3. C.A. Stein et al., "Molecular Characterization of AZT Resistant Viruses from the HIV Cohort at the Royal London Hospital," VII International Conference on AIDS, Florence, 1991, Vol. 2, p. 75; D.D. Richman et al., "Resistance to HIV Drugs," V International Conference on AIDS, Montreal, 1989, p. 198; H. Mohri et al., "Quantitation of AZT-Resistant HIV-1 in the Blood of Treated and Untreated Patients," VI International Conference on AIDS, San Francisco, 1990, Vol. 3, p. 116.

4. G. Crowley, "Is a New Virus Emerging?" *Newsweek*, 27 July 1992, p. 41.

5. C.S. Pannuti et al., "Relationship Between the Prevalence of Antibodies to Arbovirus and Hepatitis B Virus in the Vale do Ribiera Region, Brazil," *Rev Inst Med Trop Sao Paolo* 1989;31:103-109; S.S.A. Karim et al., "The Prevalence and Transmission of Hepatitis B Virus Infection in Urban, Rural and Institutionalized Black Children of Natal/KwaZulu, South Africa," *Intl J Epidemiol* 1988;17:168-173; N. Nagaratum et al., "Some Aspects of HB Ag in Hepatitis in Sri Lanka," *Trop Geogr Med* 1975;27:177-180.

6. S.J. Dick et al., "Hepatitis B Antigen in Urban-Caught Mosquitoes," *JAMA* 1974;229:1627-1629.

7. M.M. Newkirk et al., "Fate of Ingested Hepatitis B Antigen in Blood-Sucking Insects," *Gastroenterology* 1975;69:982-987. See also: "Bed Bugs, Insects and Hepatitis B," *Br Med J* 1979;2:752;.

8. S.F. Lyons et al., "Survival of HIV in the Common Bedbug," *Lancet*, 5 July 1985.

9. J.C. Chermann et al., HIV-Related Sequences in Insects from Central Africa," III International Conference on AIDS, Wash., D.C., 1987, No. MP.37.

10. L.J. Moncany et al., "Sequencing of PCR-Amplified HIV-1 Related Sequences Found in the DNA of Insects from Central Africa," V International Conference on AIDS, Montreal, 1989, p. 630.

11. A.C. Bayley et al., "HTLV-III Serology Distinguishes Atypical and Endemic Kaposi's Sarcoma in Africa," *Lancet* 16 February 1985, pp. 359-361.

12. K. Leishman, op. cit., p. 60.

13. M. Klinghoffer, M.D., "AIDS – The Unanswered Questions," *Journal of Civil Defense,* December, 1990, P.O. Box 310, Starke, Florida, 32061

14. For further information on their findings contact: Institute of Tropical Medicine, 1780 Northeast 168th St., Miami, Florida 33462.

15. D. Serwadda et al., "Slim Disease: A New Disease in Uganda and Its Association with HTLV-III Infection," *Lancet,* 19 October 1985, pp. 849-852.

16. R.B. Hornick, "The Typhus Group," in *Cecil Textbook of Medicine,* op cit., pp. 1739-1742.

17. For more information on the prevention and control of lice write: The National Pediculosis Association, P.O. Box 149, Newton, MA 02161

18. K. Leishmann, op. cit., p. 65.

19. W.T. O'Connor, M.D. "AIDS Survival Guide," *American Survival Guide,* June, 1990, pp. 28-67 citing R.J. Brenner et al., "Health Implications of Cockroach Infestations," *Infections in Medicine,* October 1987, p. 349. Copies of Dr. O'Connor's article are available from the HIVE Foundation, P.O. Box 808, Vacaville, CA 95696.

20. *Cecil Textbook of Medicine,* op. cit., p. 1925.

21. A. Kelly, C. Fry, "Outbreak of Norwegian Scabies Among Health Care Workers," V International AIDS Conference, Montreal, 1989, p. 273.

22. M. Arico et al., "Localized Norwegian Scabies as an Opportunistic Infestation in AIDS," VII International Conference on AIDS, Florence, 1991, Vol. I, p. 256.

23. Robert E. Shope, "Arthropod-Borne Viral Diseases," in *Cecil,* op cit., pp. 1814-1815. See also: R.E. Shope, G.E Gather, "Arboviruses," in E.H. Lennette, N.J. Schimdt, *Diagnostic Procedures for Viral Rickettsial and Chlamydial Procedures,* 5th edition, Wash., D.C., American Public Health Association, 1979, pp. 767-814.

24. K. Leishman, op. cit., p. 59; see also G. Antonio, op. cit., pp. 71-74; 105-107.

CHAPTER SEVEN
AIDS AND TB: A LETHAL CONNECTION

1. M. Shaffer, "Resistant TB Threat Widens," *Medical Tribune,* 12 December 1991, p. 1.

2. *MMWR* 1989;38:313-325.

3. *Medical Tribune,* 20 August 1992, p. 3.

4. *The Blade,* Toledo, Ohio, 18 February 1990, cited in *The Cutting Edge,* August 1990.

5. Kristin White, "HIV and Tuberculosis – An Old Plague Returns with Added Fury," *AIDS Patient Care,* December 1990:16-19.

6. Adapted from the *New York Times,* "TB Cases Strike in 13 States," *Ft. Worth Star Telegram,* 24 January 1992, p. 1. There frequently is a lengthy lag time between when certain aspects of AIDS are announced by medical officials and their being reported by the popular press. The outbreaks described in the article just cited had been reported by the CDC almost two years previously. See also: "Outbreak of Multidrug Resistant Tuberculosis – Texas, California, and Pennsylvania, *MMWR* 1990;30:369-372.

7. A.E. Pitchenik, "Tuberculosis Control and the AIDS Epidemic in Developing Countries," *Ann Intern Med* 1990;113:89-91; "From the Centers for Disease Control: Tuberculosis Outbreak Among HIV-Infected Persons," *JAMA* 1991;266:2058,2061; "Resolutions Taken at the World Conference on Lung Health, Boston, 1990," *Bulletin of the International Union Against Tuberculosis and Lung Disease* 1990 (Jun-Sep);65:7-9.

8. A.L. Kritski et al., "Association Between Active Pulmonary Tuberculosis (APT) and HIV in Rio de Janeiro, Brazil," IV International Conference on AIDS, Stockholm, 1988, Vol. 2, No. 5561; A.L. Kritski et al. "Tuberculosis and AIDS-Rio De Janeiro, Brazil:1983-1988," V International Conference on AIDS, Montreal, 1989, p. 428.

9. M.L. Garcia et al., "Increasing Trends of Tuberculosis and HIV/AIDS in Mexico," VII International Conference on AIDS, Florence, 1991, Vol. 1, p. 292.

10. A.V. Bollinger, "Homeless Contaminate Public Areas in the City," *NY Post,* 16 October 1990.

11. "Tuberculosis Cases Tied to Hospitals," *Dallas Morning News,* 1 August 1992, p. 10A.

12. "Concurrent with the AIDS epidemic, New York City TB incidence rates have increased 60% between 1980 and 1986." R.L. Stoneburner et al., "Evidence for a Causal Association between HIV Infection and Increasing Tuberculosis Incidence in New York City," III International Conference on AIDS. Wash., D.C., 1987, No. THP.67.

13. S. Handwerger, D. Mildvan et al., "Tuberculosis and the Acquired Immunodeficiency Syndrome at a New York City Hospital: 1978-1985," *Chest* 1987 Feb;91:176-180; see also: F.P. Duncanson et al., "Mycobacterium Tuberculosis Infection in the Acquired Immunodeficiency Syndrome. A Review of 14 Patients." *Tubercle* 1986 (Dec);67:295-302; C. Pedersen et al., "Tuberculosis in Homosexual Men with HIV Disease," *Scand J Infect Dis* 1987; 19:289-290.

14. "Do Worldwide Outbreaks Mean Tuberculosis Again Becomes Captain of All These Men of Death," *JAMA* 1992;267:369-373;1174-1175.

15. N.H. Graham et al., "Prevalence of Tuberculin Positivity and Skin Test Anergy in HIV-1 Seropositive and Seronegative Intravenous Drug Abusers," *JAMA* 1992;267:369-373.

16. "Do Worldwide Outbreaks Mean Tuberculosis Again Becomes Captain of All These Men of Death," *JAMA* 1992;267:1174-1175.

17. *Cecil Textbook of Medicine,* op. cit., p. 1686.

18. P. Arnow, S. Offutt et al., "HIV Infected Patients with Pulmonary Tuberculosis: Risk of Exposure for Health Care Workers," III International Conference on AIDS, Wash., D.C. 1987, No. TP.212.

19. N. Daramola et al., "Association of HIV Serostatus with Confidential and Unlinked Antibody Testing in an STD Clinic," VI International Conference on AIDS, San Francisco, 1990, Vol. 2, p. 252. The researchers note: "Between September, 1988 and March, 1989, 1008 specimens were collected for evidence of antibody to HIV; *81% of the specimens were from patients who declined confidential HIV testing.*" Medical authorities were not allowed to know the identities of the patients found to be HIV positive.

20. L. Monno et al., "Emergence of Drug-Resistant Tuberculosis Among AIDS Patients," VII International Conference on AIDS, Florence, 1991, Vol. 2, p. 257.

21. E. Laroche et al., "Survival Experience After TB Diagnosis in 1452 AIDS Cases: Implications for Expansion of the AIDS Definition," VI International Conference on AIDS, San Francisco, 1990, Vol. 1, p. 298.

22. K. Brudney et al., "Poor Compliance is the Major Obstacle in Controlling the HIV-Associated Tuberculosis (TB) Outbreak," V International Conference on AIDS, Montreal, 1989, p. 427.

23. Ibid.

24. I. Errante et al., "Tuberculosis (TB) and HIV Infection," IV International Conference on AIDS, Stockholm, 1988, Vol. 2, No. 7552. Infectious disease specialists from Italy have reported: ". . . the poor compliance by [HIV-infected] drug addicts for long term TB prophylaxis or therapy raises concern about diffusion of TB in the general population." See also: L. Monno et al., "Emergence of Drug-Resistant Tuberculosis Among AIDS Patients," VII International Conference on AIDS, Florence, 1991, Vol. 2, p. 257. "Standard treatments for tuberculosis were frequently ineffective. . . . Our data are alarming since HIV infected patients can become a worrisome reservoir of unresponsive TB in the general population."

25. Dennis Fiely, "Drug-Resistant Strains of TB Pose New Threat," *The Columbus Dispatch,* 5 September 1989, p. 3c.

26. "Use of BCG Vaccines in the Control of Tuberculosis," *MMWR,* 4 November 1988, p. 663.

27. *Cecil Textbook of Medicine,* op. cit., p. 1685.

28. Ibid., p. 1686.

29. Ibid, p. 1688.

30. *JAMA* 1992;267:1174-1175.

31. *Cecil Textbook of Medicine,* op. cit., p. 1683.

32. W.W. Stead, "Pathogenesis of Tuberculosis: Clinical and Epidemiologic Perspective," *Rev Infect Dis* 1989 Mar-Apr;11 Suppl 2:S366-368.

33. "Use of BCG Vaccines in the Control of Tuberculosis," *MMWR,* 4 November 1988, p. 663.

34. Rebecca Voelker, "New Push to Control Drug-Resistant TB," *Medical World News,* 20 January 1992.

35. *Cecil Textbook of Medicine,* op. cit., p. 1687.

36. CDC pamphlet, *Tuberculosis, The Connection Between TB and HIV.*

37. Cedric A. Mims, *The Pathogenesis of Infectious Diseases* (New York: Academic Press, 1977), pp. 27-28.

38. *MMWR* 1989;38:313-325.

39. M.D. Hutton, W.W. Stead et al., "Nosocomial Transmission of Tuberculosis Associated with a Draining Abscess," *J Infect Dis* 1990;161:286-95. This article provides a graphic description of how easily TB can spread in a medical facility.

40. *International Healthwatch Report,* May 1990; see also: A.J. Frew, R.T. Mayon-White et al., "An Outbreak of Tuberculosis in an Oxfordshire School," *Br J Med Chest* 1987 (July);81:293-5.

41. J.J. Sacks, E.R. Brenner et al., "Epidemiology of a Tuberculosis Outbreak in a South Carolina Junior High School," *Am J Public Health* 1985 Apr;75(4):361-5.

42. P. Schuch, A. Schicht and A. Windorfer, "Zur Ausbreitung der Tuberkulose," [Spreading of tuberculosis] *Deutsche Medizinische Wochenschrift* 1982 Sep 24;107(38):1429-31 (Published in German).

43. V.R. Rao, R.F. Joanes et al., "Outbreak of Tuberculosis after Minimal Exposure to Infection," *British Medical Journal*, 1980 (July 19):281:187-9.

44. A.R. Bosley, G. George, M. George, "Outbreaks of Pulmonary Tuberculosis in Children," *Lancet* 1986 May 17;1 (8490):1141-3.

45. "Interstate Outbreak of Drug-Resistant Tuberculosis Involving Children - California, Montana, Nevada, Utah," *MMWR*, 7 October 1983, pp. 516-518.

46. W.W. Stead, "Tuberculosis Among Elderly Persons: An Outbreak in a Nursing Home," *Ann Intern Med* 1981;94(5):606-10.

47. W.W. Stead, A.K. Dutt, "Tuberculosis in Elderly Persons," *Annu Rev Med* 1991;42:267-76.

48. W.W. Stead, J.P. Lofgren et al, "Tuberculosis as an Endemic and Nosocomial Infection Among the Elderly in Nursing Homes," *N Engl J Med* 1985;;312:1483-7.

49. "Tuberculosis on the Rise in Nursing Homes and Prisons," *International Healthwatch Report*, August, 1988.

50. *New York Times*, 16 November 1991.

51. D. Morse et al., "Increasing Tuberculosis in Association with AIDS/HIV Among New York State Prison Inmates," V International Conference on AIDS, Montreal, 1989, p. 82.

52. "Prevention and Control of Tuberculosis in Correctional Institutions," *MMWR* 1989;38:313-325 cited in *JAMA* 1989;262:3259-3262.

53. Ibid.

54. D. Morse et al., op. cit., p. 82.

55. T. Gottfried et al., "Detection of HIV-1 Antibodies in Urines of Asymptomatic and ARC/AIDS Patients," V International Conference on AIDS, Montreal, 1989, p. 375.

56. M.D. Hutton, W.W. Stead et al., "Nosocomial Transmission of Tuberculosis Associated with a Draining Abscess," *J Infect Dis* 1990 Feb;161(2):286-95.

57. R.H. George, P.R. Gully et al., "An Outbreak of Tuberculosis in a Children's Hospital," *J Hosp Infect* 1986 Sep;8(2):129-42.

58. C.E. Haley, R. C. McDonald et al., *Infect Control Hosp Epidemiol* 1989 May;10(5):204-210.

59. "Nosocomial Transmission of Multidrug-Resistant Tuberculosis to Health Care Workers and HIV-Infected Patients in an Urban Hospital – Florida," *MMWR* 12 October 1990, pp. 718-722.

60. "Nosocomial Transmission of Multidrug-Resistant Tuberculosis Among HIV-Infected Persons – Florida and New York, 1988-1991," *MMWR*, 30 October 1991, p. 588.

61. "*Mycobacterium Tuberculosis* Transmission in a Health Clinic - Florida, 1988." *MMWR*, 14 April, 1989, pp. 236-243.

62. S.W. Dooley et al., "Tuberculosis Infection Among Health Care Workers in an AIDS Unit in Puerto Rico: Evidence for Nosocomial Transmission," VII International Conference on AIDS, Florence, 1991, Vol. 3, p. 310; see also: S.W. Dooley Jr. et al., "Guidelines for Preventing the Transmission of Tuberculosis in Health-Care Settings, with Special Focus on HIV-Related Issues," *MMWR* 1990 December 7;39 RR 17:1-29; G. Di Perri et al., "Nosocomial Epidemic of Active Tuberculosis Among HIV-Infected Patients," *Lancet*, 1989 December 23-30;2(8678-8679):1502-1504; CDC, "Tuberculosis Outbreak Among Persons in a Residential Facility for HIV-Infected Persons – San Francisco," *MMWR* 1991 September 27;40(38):649-652; "AIDS Linked to Explosion of TB Cases," *Traverse City-Record Eagle* (Michigan) 24 June 1990.

63. G. Leoung et al., "Risk of TB Transmission in HIV Infected Patients Receiving Aerosolized Pentamadine Treatment," VI International Conference on AIDS, San Francisco, 1990, Vol. 1, p. 226. "Because cough and bronchospasm are frequent side effects of aerosolized pentamadine treatments, airborne transmission of infectious diseases is a growing concern."

64. "Tuberculosis Cases Tied to Hospitals," *Dallas Morning News*, 1 August 1992.

65. A. Pablos-Mendez et al., "Drug-Resistant Tuberculosis in AIDS and ARC," V International Conference on AIDS, Montreal, 1989, p. 422.

66. C. Ciesielski et al., "Surveillance for HIV/AIDS-Related Tuberculosis (TB) in the United States," V International Conference on AIDS, Montreal, 1989, p. 423.

67. M. Ciacco et al., "Evidence of Another Epidemic: Tuberculosis and HIV in NYC," V International Conference on AIDS, Montreal, 1989, p. 423.

68. Ibid.

69. A.V. Bollinger, "Homeless Contaminate Public Areas in the City," *NY Post*, 16 October 1990.

70. A.V. Bollinger, "TB Alert: Epidemic Has Put the Entire City at Risk," *NY Post*, 15 October 1990.

71. Ibid.

72. Ibid.

73. Ibid.

74. Ibid.

75. Ibid.

76. B.M. Anita et al., "High Rates of HIV Among Municipal Tuberculosis (TB) Clinic Patients with Inactive As Well As Active TB," VI International Conference on AIDS, San Francisco, 1990, Vol. 1, p. 307.

77. K.G. Castro et al., "Reported AIDS Patients with Tuberculosis in the United States," VI International Conference on AIDS, San Francisco, 1990, Vol. 1, p. 307.

78. *MMWR* 1991;40:129-131.

79. G.R. Fitzgerald, H. Grimes et al., "Hepatitis-Associated Antigen-Positive Hepatitis in a Tuberculosis Unit," *Gut* 1975 Jun;16(6):421-8.

80. Dr. John R. Seale, Royal Society of Medicine, "Problems Associated with Aids," Vol. III, Minutes of Evidence (8 April - 13 May 1987) and Memoranda.

81. W. Travis et al., "Lymphoid Pneumonitis in 50 Adult HIV-Infected Patients: Lymphocytic Interstitial Pneumonitis Versus Nonspecific Interstitial Pneumonitis," VII International Conference on AIDS, Florence, 1991, Vol. 2, p. 65.

82. G. Ramaswamy et al., "Diffuse Alveolar Damage and Interstitial Fibrosis in Acquired Immunodeficiency Syndrome Patients Without Concurrent Pulmonary Infection," *Arch Pathol Lab Med* 1985 May; 109:408-412.

83. D. Druckman et al., "Lymphoid Interstitial Pneumonitis in the Clinical Setting of HIV Disease," IV International Conference on AIDS, Stockholm, 1988, Vol. 1, No. 7244.

84. C.C. Linnemann, Jr., et al., "Human Immunodeficiency Virus and Antigen in Bronchoalveolar Lavage Fluid from Adult Patient with AIDS," IV International Conference on AIDS, Stockholm, 1988, Vol. 1, No. 7136.

85. C.C. Linnemann, Jr., et al., "Presence of Human Immunodeficiency Virus (HIV) in the Alveolar Macrophages (AM) from Bronchoalveolar Lavage (BAL) Fluid of Patients with AIDS," V International Conference on AIDS, Montreal, 1989, p. 677.

86. J.M. Wallace et al., "Cellular and T-Lymphocyte Subpopulation Profiles in Bronchoalveolar Lavage Fluid from Patients with Acquired Immunodeficiency Syndrome and Pneumonitis," *Am Rev Respir Dis* 1984 Nov;130:786-790.

87. M. Evans et al., "HIV Detected within Alveolar Macrophages in Vivo by Immunocytochemistry from Induced Sputum Samples," VII International Conference on AIDS, Florence, 1991, Vol. 1, p. 144.

88. J.M. Ziza et al., "[Lymphocytic Interstitial Pneumopathy in AIDS-Related Complex. Presence of the LAV Virus in the Bronchoalveolar Lavage Fluid]," *Presse Med* 1986 Jul 5-12;15:1267-1269 (Published in French).

89. J.M. Brechot et al., "Alveolar Hemorrhage Among HIV Individuals," VII International Conference on AIDS, Florence, 1991, Vol. 1, p. 219.

90. S.Z. Salahuddin et al., "Human T Lymphotropic Virus Type III Infection of Human Alveolar Macrophages," *Blood* 1986 (July) 68:281-284.

91. Ibid.

92. G. Zambruno et al., "HIV-1 Proviral DNA Is Present in Epidermal Langerhans Cells of HIV-Infected Patients: Detection Using the Polymerase Chain Reaction," VII International Conference on AIDS, Florence, 1991, Vol. 2, p. 60.

93. Dr. John R. Seale, Royal Society of Medicine, "Problems Associated with Aids," Vol. III, Minutes of Evidence (8 April - 13 May 1987) and Memoranda, op. cit.

94. K.J. Chayt et al., "Detection of HTLV-III in Lungs of Patients with AIDS and Pulmonary Involvement," *JAMA* 1986;256:2356-2359; J.D. Morris et al., "Lymphocytic Interstitial Pneumonia in Patients at Risk for the Acquired Immune Deficiency Syndrome," *Chest* 1987;91:63-67.

95. W. Travis et al., "Lymphoid Pneumonitis in 50 Adult HIV-Infected Patients: Lymphocytic Interstitial Pneumonitis Versus Nonspecific Interstitial Pneumonitis," VII International Conference on AIDS, Florence, 1991, Vol. 2, p. 65.

96. Dr. John R. Seale, Royal Society of Medicine, "Problems Associated with Aids," Vol. III, Minutes of Evidence (8 April - 13 May 1987) and Memoranda, op. cit.

97. P.A. Palsson, *Slow Virus Diseases of Animals and Man,* edited by R.H. Kimberlin (Amsterdam: North Holland Publishing Co., 1976), p. 37.

98. D. Narayan et al., "Lentiviral Diseases of Sheep and Goats: Chronic Pneumonia of Leukoencephalomyelitis and Arthiritis," *Rev Infect Dis* 1985;7:89-98; D. Narayan et al., "Slow Virus Replication: The Role of Macrophages in the Persistence and Expression of Visna Viruses of Sheep and Goats," *J Gen Virol* 1982;59:345-356.

99. E. Baenda et al., "Characterization of Transmitters of M. Tuberculosis (M. Tb) in Zaire by HIV-1 Serostatus Level of Immunosuppression and Clinical Status," VII International Conference on AIDS, Florence, 1991, Vol. 1, p. 307.

100. Joshua Lederberg, "Pandemic as a Natural Evolutionary Phenomenon," *Social Research* 1988;55 (3):343-359.

101. "Prevention and Control of Tuberculosis in Correctional Institutions," *MMWR* 1989;38:313-325 cited in *JAMA*;1989;262:3258-3262

102. "Nurses Infected with TB," *Peoria Journal Star,* 16 July 1987. Dr. Schrepfer noted that health authorities had claimed that other secondary infections associated with AIDS, including various types of pneumonia, were not a threat to healthy people. "But they said that about TB as well," he said.

103. T.C. Eickhoff, M.D., "Tuberculosis–The Plague of the '90s?" *Infectious Disease News,* July 1992, p. 6.

104. Thomas Butler, Yersinia Infections, *Cecil Textbook of Medicine,* op. cit., pp. 1661-1663.

105. "Tough TB Strain Immune to Drugs," *Washington Times,* 22 November 1991, p. B4.

CHAPTER EIGHT
WHY PATIENTS ARE AT RISK

1. "The Dentist and the Patient," *People Magazine,* 22 October 1990.

2. "Florida Officials Firm on Law: Statute Said to Prohibit AIDS Warnings to Dentist's Patients," *Dallas Morning News,* 29 July 1990.

3. *International Healthwatch Report,* September 1990.

4. *Surgeon General's Report on AIDS,* 1986, pp. 22-23 cited in G. Antonio, *A Critical Evaluation of the Surgeon General's Report on AIDS* (Ft. Worth: Dominion Press, 1987), p. 5.

5. E. Moran, "Facing Up to AIDS in the Health Care Setting," *RT Image* 30 April 1990, p. 43. Moran states: "[CDC] guidelines have not prevented the AIDS contamination of some 69 health care workers to date."

6. James S. Fulghum, III, "A Surgeon with AIDS" (letter) *JAMA* 1990;264(24)3147.

7. J. Tokars et al., "Percutaneous Injuries During Surgical Procedures," VII International Conference on AIDS, Florence, 1991, Vol. 2, p. 83.

8. J.R. Smith, J.M. Grant, "The Incidence of Glove Puncture During Caesarian Section and Various Potential Solutions," V International Conference on AIDS, Montreal, 1989, p. 167.

9. *International Healthwatch Report,* March, 1991.

10. "Oral Surgeon Who Died of AIDS Treated Many Children," Detroit (UPI), 14 July 1991.

11. E. Walsh, "Dentist's Death Shakes Tiny Town," *Washington Post,* 20 July 1991.

12. *Washington Post,* 19 April 1991, p. A3.

13. *International Healthwatch Report,* February 1988 citing *The Globe and Mail* [Canada], 18 February 1988.

14. *Dallas Morning News,* 3 December 1990.

15. Alicia Mundy, "The Death of a Doctor," *Trouble,* June/July 1991.

16. J.R. Smith, J.M. Grant, op. cit.

17. "Infected Doctor Tells 328 Patients of Risk," *Washington Times,* 17 June 1991.

18. "Transmission of HIV Infection During an Invasive Dental Procedure – Florida," CDC Update, *JAMA* 1991;265:563-568.

19. C. Y. Ou et al., (CDC) "Strain Specific DNA Probes to Study the Epidemiology of HIV Infection," V International Conference on AIDS, Montreal, 1989, p. 159.

20. Editorial, *The Washington Times,* 28 May 1991, p. C2.

21. *Time,* 11 February 1991, p. 10.

22. N. Bodsworth et al., "The Effect of HIV on Chronic Hepatitis B: A Study of 150 Homosexual Men," V International Conference on AIDS, Montreal, 1989, p. 258.

23. R.J.C. Gilson et al., "Interaction Between Hepatitis B Virus and HIV in Homosexual Men," IV International Conference on AIDS, Stockholm, 1988, Vol. 2, No. 3671.

24. D.J. Weber, W.A. Rutala, "Hepatitis B Immunization Update," *Infect Control Hosp Epidemiol* 1989;10:541-546.

25. D. Rimland et al., "Hepatitis B Outbreak Traced to an Oral Surgeon," *N Engl J Med* 1977;296:953-958.

26. M.A. Kane, L.A. Lettau, "Transmission of HBV from Dental Personnel to Patients," *J Am Dental Assoc* 1985;110:634-636.

27. F.E. Shaw et al., "Lethal Outbreak of Hepatitis B in a Dental Practice," *JAMA* 1986;255:3260-3264.

28. L.A. Lettau et al., *JAMA*, 21 February 1986, pp. 934-937.

29. "Mass Hepatitis B Outbreak in Doctor's Office," *International Healthwatch Report*, December 1991.

30. *Wall St. Journal*, 18 January 1989.

31. F. Bellis et al., "Neuropsychological Tests in HIV-patients: Which Tests?" VI International Conference on AIDS, San Francisco, 1990, Vol. 2, p. 390.

32. M. Dalakas et al., "AIDS and the Nervous System," *JAMA* 1989;261:2396-2399 citing M.C. Dalakas, G.H. Pezeshkpour, "Neuromuscular Diseases Associated with HIV Infection," *Ann Neurol* 1988;23(suppl):38S-48S.

33. *USA Today*, 15 May 1992, p. 1D.

34. C. Gorman, "Should You Worry about Getting AIDS from Your Dentist?" *Time*, 20 July 1991.

35. *Medical Economics*, 2 December 1991, pp. 43-45.

36. F. S. Rhame, "The HIV Infected Surgeon," *JAMA*, 25 July 1990, Vol. 264, p. 507.

37. *News-Democrat*, Belleville, IL, 1 January 1989.

38. P. Kelly, "Counseling Patients with HIV," *RN Magazine*, February 1992, pp. 54-58.

39. Editorial, *Washington Times*, 28 May 1991, p. C2.

40. *American Medical News*, 18 March 1991, p. 25.

41. Ibid.

42. *Physicians Financial News*, 30 September 1991, pp. 3-4.

43. *Physicians Financial News*, 15 June 1991, p. 3.

44. J. Cobb, "After Safe Sex, Safe Surgery?" *Br Med J*, 27 June 1987;294:1667-1668.

45. D.D. Smith, "Physicians and Acquired Immunodeficiency Syndrome," (letter) *JAMA* 1990;264:452.

CHAPTER NINE
HEALTH CARE WORKERS UNDER SIEGE

1. T.C. Eickhoff, "Tuberculosis–The Plague of the '90s?" *Infectious Disease News*, July 1992, p. 6.

2. *Daily Mirror*, 8 May 1992.

3. W. Robbins, "Nurse Infected by AIDS Embraced by Town," *New York Times*, 8 October 1990, p. A8.

4. *Medical Economics*, 2 December 1991, pp. 43-45.

5. K. Hsia et al., "HIV DNA Is Present in a High Percentage of Peripheral Blood Mononuclear Cells in Infected Individuals," V International Conference on AIDS, Montreal, 1989, p. 614.

6. R. Marcus et al., "CDC's Healthcare Workers Surveillance Project: An Update," IV International Conference on AIDS, Stockholm, 1988, Vol. 1, No. 9015.

7. G.P. Wormer et al., "Estimated Risk of HIV Infection Among Surgeons Practicing in the New York City Area," V International Conference on AIDS, Montreal, 1989, p. 796.

8. *RT Image*, 30 April 1990, p. 46.

9. J. Seale, "Aids Virus Infection: Prognosis and Transmission," *J Roy Soc Med* 1985;78:613-615.

10. "AZT First-Aid Treatment Fails," *Medical Tribune*, 14 June 1990.

11. I. Hewlett et al., "Viral Gene Expression Assessed by PCR in HIV-1 Infected H9 Cells," V International Conference on AIDS, Montreal, 1989, p. 635.

12. M.E. Chamberland et al., "Health Care Workers with AIDS," *JAMA* 1991;266:3459-3462.

13. S. Okie, "HIV-Infected Workers Undercounted; CDC's Low Tally of Accidental Contacts Seen Leading to Complacency," *Washington Post*, 16 January 1990.

14. J. Feldschuh, op. cit., p. 100.

15. D. Tandberg et al., "Under-Reporting of Contaminated Needlestick Injuries in Emergency Health Care Workers," *Ann Emerg Med* 1991;20:66-70.

16. N. D. Korniewicz et al., "The Use of Latex and Vinyl Gloves for Protection Against HIV Infection," IV International Conference on AIDS, Stockholm, 1988, Vol. 1, No. 9007.

17. "Medical Gloves Fail Leak Tests Badly," *The Vancouver Sun*, 20 October 1990.

18. J. McCann, "Test Finds 60% of Surgical Gloves Leak," *Medical Tribune*, 8 March 1990.

19. *New York Times*, 18 October 1990.

20. A.L. Reingold et al., "Failure of Gloves and Other Protective Devices to Prevent Transmission of Hepatitis B Virus to Oral Surgeons," *JAMA* 1988;259:2558-2560.

21. A. Ehrnst et al., "Efficient Isolation of HIV from Plasma During Different Stages of HIV Infection," *J Med Virology* 1988;26:23-32.

22. J. Feldschuh, op. cit., p. 76.

23. *Cecil Textbook of Medicine*, op. cit., p. 825.

24. "What is Leaky Can Be Risky: A Study of Integrity of Hospital Gloves," *Infect Control Hosp Epidemiol* 1989;10:553-556.

25. J.G. Wright et al., "Mechanisms of Glove Tears and Sharp Injuries Among Surgical Personnel," *JAMA* 1991:266:1668-1671.

26. L.R. Braathen et al., "Langerhans Cells as a Primary Target for HIV Infection," *Lancet*, 7 November 1987, p. 1094.

27. K. Lafferty, A.P. Wyatt, (letter) *Brit Med J*, 8 August 1987, p. 392.

28. CDC, "Recommendations for Prevention of HIV Transmission in Health-Care Settings," Supplement, *MMWR*, 21 August 1987, p. 15S.

29. J.M. Garden et al., "Papillomavirus in the Vapor of Carbon Dioxide Laser-Treated Verrucae [warts]," *JAMA* 1988;259:1199-1202.

30. G.K. Johnson, W.S. Robinson, "HIV-1 in the Vapors of Surgical Power Instruments," *J Med Virol* 1991;33:47-50.

31. C. Ortiz, "Masks May Not Shield Surgeons from AIDS, UCSF Researcher Says," *Contra Costa Times*, 1 October 1990.

32. D.L. Lewis, R.K. Boe, "Cross Infection Risks Associated with Current Procedures for Using High-Speed Dental Handpieces," *J Clin Microbiol*, February 1992, pp. 401-406.

33. L.A. Lettau et al., "Nosocomial Transmission and Infection Control Aspects of Parasitic and Ectoparasitic Diseases, Part II. Blood and Tissue Parasites," *Infect Control Hosp Epidemiol* 1991;12:111-121.

34. W.D. Williamson et al., "Asymptomatic Congenital CMV Infection," *AJDC* 1990;144:1365-1368.

35. S. Stagno et al., "Congenital CMV Infection," *N Engl J Med* 1977;296:1254-8..

36. I. Gurevich. P. Tafuro, "Caring for the Infectious Patient: Risk Factors During Pregnancy," *Infection Control*, 1984:5:482-485.

37. E.L. Pantelick et al., "Hepatitis B Infection in Hospital Personnel During an Eight-Year Period: Policies for Screening and Pregnancy in High Risk Areas," *Am J Med* 1981;70:924-927.

38. A. Cargnel et al., "Chronic HBsAg Positive Hepatitis in HIV Infection, V International AIDS Conference, Montreal, 1989, p. 257.

39. S.J. Naides, "Infection Control Measures for Human Parvovirus B19 in the Hospital Setting," Infect Control Hosp Epidemiol 1989;10:326-329; F. Leoncini et al., "Parvovirus B19 as an Associated Cause of Anemia in AIDS Patients Treated with Zidovudine [AZT]," VII International Conference on AIDS, Florence, 1991, Vol. 1, p. 258.

40. I. Gurevich, P. Tafuro, op. cit.

41. E.R. Annis, "No Disease Should Be Placed on a Pedestal," *Private Practice*, January 1989.

42. "High Rate of TB Infection Found Among Hospital Doctors," *Medical World News*, June 1992, p. 31.

43. L. Vikhanski, "Resistant TB Spreading in Hospitals; Said to Result in 89% Mortality Rate," *Medical Tribune*, 20 August 1992.

44. "Hospital Staffs' Risks of TB May Be High," *Medical Tribune*, 11 June 1992, p. 6.

45. Ibid. This issue of the *Medical Tribune* presented a "Special Report on Tuberculosis" detailing the dramatic rise in TB among medical workers treating AIDS patients and mentioning the

need for wearing air-tight face masks when treating TB patients. Yet, on the same page they show an emaciated TB patient sitting on an examining bench with two doctors in the room neither of whom are wearing masks. One is standing with his hands in his pockets casually looking at the TB patient's chest x-rays, the other is talking on the phone.

46. J. Slaff, *The AIDS Epidemic* (New York: Warner Books) pp. 201, 251-252.

47. L.A. Chambers et al., "Long-Incubation HIV-Infection in a Donor, Recipient and Children, III International AIDS Conference, Wash., D.C., 1987, No. MP.242.

48. H.J. Alter et al., "Prevalence of HIV Type 1 p24 Antigen in U.S. Blood Donors – An Assessment of the Efficacy of Testing in Donor Screening," *N Engl J Med* 1990;323:1312-7.

49. *International Healthwatch Report*, June 1991.

50. "Test Directly Measures HIV," *Medical Tribune*, 21 May 1992, p. 40.

51. N. Daramola et al., "Association of HIV Serostatus with Confidential and Unlinked Antibody Testing in an STD Clinic," VI International Conference on AIDS, San Francisco, 1990, Vol. 2, p. 252.

52. M. Specter, "New Technique Helps in Detecting the AIDS Virus; Method Multiplies DNA in Blood Sample," *Washington Post* 26 May 1988. The PCR "DNA Fingerprinting" test for HIV is available through Cetus Corp., Emoryville, California. NOTE: They will *not* give out information about performing the test to anyone except physicians and will only officially perform the test "for research purposes."

53. S. Salvi et al., "Unambiguous Detection of HIV-1 Proviral DNA in Newborns from Infected Mothers by Polymerase Chain Reaction," VII International Conference on AIDS, Florence, 1991, Vol. 1, p. 123; see also: *New Engl J Med* 1989;320:1649-1654.

54. M. Pezella et al., "HIV Genome in Anti-HIV Seronegative Partners of HIV Infected Subjects by In Situ." IV International Conference on AIDS, Stockholm, 1988, Vol. 2, No. 1611. "Our preliminary data show that the SERONEGATIVE REGULAR SEX PARTNERS OF HIV INFECTED SUBJECTS MAY BE HIV INFECTED." See also: C. Papetti et al., "High Prevalence of HIV Heterosexual Transmission in One Hundred Stable Couples," VI International Conference on AIDS, San Francisco, 1990, Vol. 2, p. 101. "Seronegative at risk partners should *all* be tested for HIV genome."

55. *Federal Register*, Vol. 56, No. 144, 26 July 1991, Part V: Equal Employment Opportunity Commission, 29 CFR Part 1630, p. 35745, citing ADA section 1630.2(r) Direct Threat. However, see M. Barnes et al., "Neuropsychological Impairment of HIV-Infected Persons: Legal Implications for the Workplace," V International Conference on AIDS, Montreal, 1989, p. 828.

56. *The FACT Report*, citing the *New York Times*, 5 June 1987.

57. N. Kass et al., "Perceived Discrimination in Health Care and Employment Among Homosexual Men," VI International Conference on AIDS, San Francisco, 1990, Vol. 1, p. 329.

58. B. O'Bryen et al., "The Army HIV Five Year Testing Experience: 1985-1990," VI International Conference on AIDS, San Francisco, 1990, Vol. 3, p. 250.

59. *Medical Tribune*, 1 April 1987.

60. J.L. Gerberding et al., "Longterm Follow-up of Health Care Workers with PCR and Antibody Testing to Detect Delayed Seroconversion," VI International Conference on AIDS, San Francisco, June 1990, Vol. 1, p. 275; A.A. Imrie et al., "Negative Western Blots Do Not Exclude HIV-1 Infection. Experience in a Public Health Laboratory," VII International Conference on AIDS, Florence, 1991, Vol. 2, p. 335.

61. "Having AIDS," *Br Med J* 1987;295:320-321.

62. *Physician's Financial News*, 15 June 1991, p. 3.

63. *American Medical News*, 18 March 1991, p. 21.

CHAPTER 10
THE THREAT OF "SAFE SEX"

1. Laud Humphreys, *Out of the Closet: The Sociology of Homosexual Liberation* (Englewood Cliffs, NJ: Premiere Hall, 1972), pp. 165-167.

2. *Surgeon General's Report on AIDS*, 1986, C. Everett Koop, U.S. Public Health Service.

3. *Understanding Family Structures to Meet Children's Needs*, a curriculum received by all public schools in New York City, cited in *Education Newsline* (April, 1992), P.O. Box 3200, Costa Mesa, CA 92628. The last part of the quote states: ". . . and should avoid exclusionary practices by presuming a person's sexual orientation, reinforcing stereotypes, or speaking of lesbians/gays as 'they' or 'them.'"

4. D. Noebel et al, citing Dr. Olav H. Alvig, *American Medical News*, 20 December 1985.

5. H.W. Jaffe et al., "National Case-Control Study of Kaposi's Sarcoma and *P. carinii* Pneumonia in Homosexual Men," *Ann Int Med* 1983;99:145-151.

6. Enrique T. Rueda, *The Homosexual Network*, (Old Greenwich, Conn.: Devin Adair, 1982), p. 239.

7. D. Johnson et al., "Perceived Changes in Sexual Practices Among Homosexual Men," III International Conference on AIDS, Wash., D.C. 1987, No. TP. 188. Among homosexuals interviewed in this study, 25% *admitted* they were continuing to engage in anal sodomy without a condom, 39% *admitted* having two or more partners in the previous month (24+ partners annually), 24% *admitted* recently having anonymous sodomy partners. F. Hickson et al., "Unsafe Sexual Behavior Among Gay Men: A critique of the Relapse Model," VII International Conference on AIDS, Florence, 1991, Vol. 2, p. 36. W. Winkelstein et al., "Sexual Practices and Risk of Infection by the Human Immunodeficiency Virus – The San Francisco Men's Health Study," *JAMA* 1987;257:321-325; L.A. Kingsley et al., "Sexual Transmission Efficiency of Hepatitis B Virus and HIV Among Homosexual Men," *JAMA* 1990;264:23-234. See also: Paul Cameron, Ph.D., et al., "Effect of Homosexuality Upon Public Health and Social Order," *Psychological Reports*, 1989;64:1167-1179.

8. M. Enochs et al., "HIV Seroprevalence of STD Clinics in Houston, Texas," V International Conference on AIDS, Montreal, 1989, p. 90.

9. M.T. Osterholm, "The Surveillance of Clinical Viral Hepatitis B and Primary, Secondary, and Early Latent Syphilis in Homosexual and Bisexual Men in MN: Implications for HIV Transmission," III International Conference on AIDS, Wash., D.C. 1987, No. T.7.5. "Among homosexual men declining rates of syphilis and other bacterial STDs among homosexual and bisexual men MAY NOT REFLECT a concurrent reduction in the transmission of selected viral STDs, such as viral hepatitis type B [AND HIV]. We believe these results may have significant implications when interpreting the impact of risk reduction programs on HIV transmission nationally."

10. "Reported Cases of Gonorrhea on the Upswing Among Homosexuals," *International Healthwatch Report*, November 1989.

11. A. Parachini, "AIDS-Condom Study Grant Cut Off by U.S.," *Los Angeles Times*, 10 August 1988.

12. M. Adib et al., "Relapse in Safer Sexual Practices Among Homosexual Men," VI International Conference on AIDS, San Francisco, 1990, Vol. 2, p. 262.

13. Phyllis Schlafly, Editor, *Child Abuse in the Classroom*, (Alton, IL: Pere Marquette Press, 1984).

14. J. Reissman, E. Eichel, J.G. Muir, *Kinsey, Sex and Fraud*, (1990) available through Huntington House Publishers, P.O. Box 53788, Lafayette, LA 70505. This book is an invaluable resource for combatting the myth that "one in ten people are homosexual."

15. *One Teenager in Ten*, Edited by Ann Heron, (Boston: Alyson Books, 1983).

16. *Focus on the Family Citizen*, 15 April 1992.

17. Deborah Anne Dawson, "The Effects of Sex Education on Adolescent Behavior," *Family Planning Perspectives* 18 No. 4 (1986):164.

18. For more information on abstinence-based materials for public schools write: Project Respect, P.O. Box 97, Golf, IL 60029. See also: Randy Engel, *Sex Education – The Final Plague*, Published by Human Life International, 7845-E Airpark Road, Gaithersburg, MD 20879.

19. Melvin Anchell, M.D., *What's Wrong with Sex Education?* (Selma, AL: Hoffman Center for the Family, 1991), 5266 Citizens Parkway, Selma, AL 36701.

20. P. Schlafly, op. cit. p. 163-164.

21. Ray Ballmann, *The How and Why of Homeschooling* (Wheaton, IL: Crossway Books, 1987). This book provides a comprehensive overview of the subject.

CHAPTER ELEVEN
THE AMERICANS WITH DISABILITES ACT

1. C. Muggeridge, "Gay Rights Advancing Under the Banner of AIDS," *Wall Street Journal*, 21 September 1989.

2. *The Advocate*, May 28, 1985.

3. William Dannemeyer, *Homosexuality: Shadow in the Land*, (San Francisco: Ignatius Press, 1990). Gives a riveting account of how the American Psychiatric and Psychological Associations were strong-armed into abruptly changing the classification of homosexuality from a mental illness and disorder to a "preference."
During his tenure in the U.S. House of Representatives Congressman Dannemeyer fought a courageous uphill battle for sound health measures to combat AIDS and has been an intrepid advocate of the Judeo-Christian ethic. His book provides a compelling, comprehensive analysis of the homosexual movement and its impact on American society.

4. Ibid.

5. C. Muggeridge, op. cit.

6. John Sloan, "Dangerously Vague Act Will Enrich Many Lawyers," *Dallas Morning News*, 8 October 1989. Mr. Sloan was commenting on the ADA prior to its final passage. The final version of the bill contains some amending language but remains onerous for private businesses. Sloan has since joined the Executive Committee of the President's Committee on Employment of People with Disabilities.

7. *Kansas Statutes Annotated*, Vol. 3A, p. 802, No. 44-1002.

8. *Kentucky Revised Statutes*, Official Edition, p. 269, No. 207.140.

9. George Orwell, *1984* (New American Library: New York, 1961), pp. 246-247. In describing "Newspeak," Orwell wrote: "The word *free* still existed in Newspeak, but it could only be used in such statements as "This dog is free from lice" or "This field is free from weeds." It could not be used in its old sense of "politically free" or "intellectually free," since political and intellectual freedom no longer existed even as concepts, and were therefore of necessity nameless. Quite apart from the suppression of definitely heretical words, *reduction of vocabulary was regarded as an end in itself*, and no word that could be dispensed with was allowed to survive. Orwell's description of the diminution of language is worth pondering. Daniel Siegal, professor of history at Hobart and William Smith Colleges states: "Our brightest students are getting a "dumbed down" education. Half the country's students, the group referred to as 'college bound,' are entering college so badly prepared that they perform far below potential – a fact with grave implications for our ability to compete with other nations in the future." ["The Other Crisis in Our Schools," *Reader's Digest*, April 1992.]

10. *The American Heritage Dictionary*, op. cit., p. 374.

11. ADA 42 USC 12188, Sec. 308. ENFORCEMENT.

12. ADA Sec. 2(a).

13. *Federal Register*, Vol. 56, No. 144, 26 July 1991, Part V: Equal Employment Opportunity Commission, 29 CFR Part 1630, Equal Employment Opportunities for Individuals with Disabilities; Final Rule, pp. 35740-35741.

14. Ibid.

15. Ibid., p. 35735.

16. *American Psychiatric Association: Diagnostic and Statistical Manual of Mental Disorders*, Third Edition, Revised, [*DSM-III-R*] op. cit., (Wash., D.C.: American Psychiatric Association, 1987).

17. *Federal Register*, op. cit., pp. 35741.

18. Ibid.

19. Ibid.

20. For a further understanding of Multiple Personality Disorder see: James G. Friesen, Ph.D., *Uncovering the Mystery of MPD* (San Bernardino, CA: Here's Life Publishers, 1991).

21. *Ft. Worth Star-Telegram*, November 30, 1989.

22. R. Smothers, "Disturbed Past of Killer of 7 Is Unraveled," *NY Times*, 16 September 1989.

23. C. Suplee, "Berserk! Violent Employees Obsessed with Revenge Are Turning the Workplace into a Killing Zone," *Washington Post*, 1989, (d.n.a.). "The problem of psychotic employees in the workplace "has fostered a brisk market in litigation against businesses for failing to anticipate violent behavior on the part of employees."

24. L.H. Rockwell, Jr., "Disabling the Economy," *The Free Market*, September 1992.

25. *DSM-III-R*, op. cit.

26. Ibid.

27. Ibid.

28. Ibid.

29. Ibid.

30. Ibid., V65.20 Malingering.

31. ADA SEC. 101. Definitions.

32. ADA SEC. 103. Defenses.

33. "Witches Rights," *Reader's Digest*, September 1989. See also: "The Coming [Legal] Nuclear Attack Against Christianity," by Attorney Shelby Sharpe, Esq., of the Rutherford Institute. Available from FACT, Box 90140 Arlington, TX 76004 ($3).

34. ADA SEC. 301. Definitions (Public Accommodations).

35. ADA SEC. 302.

36. ADA SEC. 102. Discrimination.

37. *Federal Register*, op. cit., p. 35744.

38. Ibid.

39. See: *Kansas Statutes Annotated*, Vol. 3A, p. 802, No. 44-1002. "The term "physical handicap" means the physical condition of a person, whether congenital or acquired by accident, injury or disease which constitutes a substantial disability, but *is unrelated to such person's ability to engage in a particular job or occupation.*"

40. *The American Heritage Dictionary*, op. cit., p. 1086.

41. *Federal Register*, op. cit., p. 35748.

42. Ibid., p. 35730.

43. Ibid., p. 35747.

44. Ibid., p. 35729.

45. Ibid., p. 35750.

46. Ibid., p. 35728, Section 1630.2(m).

47. L.H. Rockwell, Jr., op. cit.

48. *Federal Register*, op. cit., p. 35752.

49. ADA, 42 USC 12117, Sec. 107 ENFORCEMENT.

50. Civil Rights Act of 1991, Public Law 102-166, 21 November 1991, SEC. 1977A. Damages in Cases of Intentional Discrimination in Employment.

51. ADA, SEC. 308. ENFORCEMENT.

52. "See You in Court," *Nation's Business*, July 1989.

53. ADA, SEC. 511. DEFINITIONS.

54. *Federal Register*, op. cit., p. 35742.

55. Ibid., p. 35731.

56. Ibid., p. 35742.

57. Ibid., p. 35747.

58. Ibid., pp. 35743, 35745.

59. *The Advocate*, May 28, 1985.

60. *Federal Register*, op. cit., p. 35741.

61. *Federal Register*, op. cit., p. 35740 citing the Federal Rehabilitation of 1973 in *School Board of Nassau County v. Arline*, 480 U.S. 273 [1987].

62. L.H. Rockwell, Jr., op. cit.

63. Ibid.

CHAPTER TWELVE
ENDING THE DELUSION

1. J. Feldschuh, op. cit., pp. 107-108.

2. *Today*, 2 June 1992 (published in England).

3. B.R. Edlin et al., "A Nosocomial Outbreak of Isoniazid and Streptomycin-Resistant Tuberculosis among AIDS Patients at a New York City Hospital," VII International Conference on AIDS, Florence, 1990, Vol. 1, p. 225.

4. T. Butler, "Yersinia Infections," *Cecil Textbook of Medicine*, op. cit., pp. 1661-1664.

5. *Wisconsin Light*, 8 January 1992.

6. N.D. Rosenberg, "HIV Spreading to Teenage Girls," *Milwaukee-Journal*, 20 January 1992.

7. AIDS Conference held in Washington, D.C., 8 May 1992, as reported on the "Talk Back With Bob Larson," radio show, Denver, CO.

8. K.L. McDonald et al., "Results of Blood Donor Screening for HIV in Minnesota: Implications for Sequential EIA and Western Blot Test Specificity," IV International Conference on AIDS, Stockholm, 1988, Vol. 2, No. 7699.

9. N. Daramola et al., "Association of HIV Serostatus with Confidential and Unlinked Antibody Testing in an STD Clinic," VI International Conference on AIDS, San Francisco, 1990, Vol. 2, p. 252.

10. A. Francis et al., "Evaluation of Urine as an Alternative to Blood for HIV Prevalence Testing." VII International Conference on AIDS, Florence, 1991, Vol. 2, p. 342; A.S. Goldstein et al., "Analysis of HIV Antibodies in Serum Versus Whole Saliva," VI International Conference on AIDS, San Francisco, 1990, Vol. 3, p. 242.

11. O. Recchia et al., "Seroepidemiological Study on Association Between HIV and Chlamydia Trachomatis Infection," VII International Conference on AIDS, Florence, 1990, Vol. 2, p. 320; M.

Laga et al., "Non-Ulcerative STDs as Risk Factors for HIV Infection," VI International Conference on AIDS, San Francisco, 1990, Vol. 1, p. 258.

12. N. Gregory, "Relapse of Secondary Syphilis Following Influenza Vaccination in an HIV-Infected Patient," IV International Conference on AIDS, Stockholm, 1988, Vol. 2, No. 7632.

13. N.J. Alexander, "Sexual Transmission of HIV: Virus Entry into the Male and Female Genital Tract," *Fertility and Sterility*, 1990:54:1-18.

14. "Recommendations for Diagnosing and Treating Syphilis in HIV-Infected Patients," *MMWR*, 7 October 1988;37:600-602. Both nontreponemal and treponemal tests for syphilis can be negative in HIV patients with secondary syphilis. See also: J.S. Haas et al., "Seroreversion of Treponemal Tests During HIV Infection," V International Conference on AIDS, Montreal, 1989, p. 360.

15. P. Hay et al., "Failure of Benzathine Penicillin to Eradicate Syphilis in HIV Positive Patients," V International Conference on AIDS, Montreal, 1989, p. 361. Researchers state: "Benzathine penicillin is unreliable for the treatment of syphilis in HIV positive patients."

16. R. Malessa et al., "Neurosyphilis in HIV-Infected Patients: Evidence of Unreliable Serologic Response," V International Conference on AIDS, Montreal, 1989, p. 360; J.R. Berger et al., "Syphilitic Myelopathy with HIV: A Treatable Cause of Spinal Cord Disease, V International Conference on AIDS, Montreal, 1989, p. 360.

17. D. Morse et al., "Increasing Tuberculosis in Association with AIDS/HIV among New York State Prison Inmates," V International Conference on AIDS, Montreal, 1989, p. 82.

18. K. Castro et al., "HIV Transmission in Correctional Facilities," VII International Conference on AIDS, Florence, 1991, Vol. 1, p. 364.

19. *International Healthwatch Report*, September 1990.

20. R.P. Wenzel, "Prevention and Treatment of Hospital-Acquired Infections," in *Cecil Textbook of Medicine*, op. cit., p. 1541.

21. "Pap Smears May Fail to Spot Cancer in HIV Patients," *Family Practice News*, 1 June 1992.

22. W. Panmoung et al., "Salivary Anti-HIV Assay by Elisa Test," VI International Conference on AIDS, San Francisco, 1990, Vol. 3, p. 242.

23. B. Greenberg et al., "HIV Seroprevalence in Patients Attending New York City Department of Health TB Clinics," VI International Conference on AIDS, San Francisco, 1990, Vol. 1, p. 307; C. Ciesielski et al., "Surveillance for HIV/AIDS-Related Tuberculosis in the United States," V International Conference on AIDS, Montreal, 1989, p. 423.

24. "Two-Day Assay for Tuberculosis Proves Accurate," *Medical Tribune*, 12 December 1991.

25. G. Antonio, op. cit., p. 105.

26. *Dallas Morning News*, January, 1991 (d.n.a).

27. *Medical Tribune*, 11 June 1992, p. 15.

28. R. Restak, "Worry About Survival of Society First; Then AIDS Victims' Rights," *Washington Post*, 8 September 1985.

29. *N Engl J Med* 1989;320:1458-1462. "A prolonged period of latency may be more common than previously realized."

30. *N Engl J Med* 1989;320:1487-1489. Dr. William Haseltine cautions: these findings raise the "the sobering possibility that HIV-1 infections may be transmitted by blood and organ donors who are silently infected . . . Reliable cost-effective methods for detecting silent infections are urgently needed."

31. *Br Med J* 1989;298:713-716.

32. "Test Directly Measures HIV," *Medical Tribune*, 21 May 1992, p. 40.

33. *Dallas Morning News*, 6 September 1987, p. 3A.

34. Joshua Lederberg, "Pandemic as a Natural Evolutionary Phenonmenon," *Social Research* 1988;55 (3):343-359.

35. Jacqueline Kasun, *The War Against Population* (San Francisco: Ignatius Press, 1988), pp. 115-155.

36. For more information write: Project Respect, Box 97, Golf, IL 60029.

37. E. Rueda, op. cit., p. 37.

38. UTA *Shorthorn* 1990 (d.n.a.).

EPILOGUE
BREAKING THE DEADLY SILENCE

1. Roy Masters, "Media Hysteria and the Remolding of the American Mind," *New Dimensions Magazine*, April 1990, p. 58.

2. *DSM-III-R*, op. cit., pp. 157-159

3. E. Annis, op. cit.

4. J. Seale, Royal Society of Medicine, "Problems Associated with Aids," Vol. III, Minutes of Evidence (8 April - 13 May 1987) and Memoranda, op. cit.

5. *Dallas Gay News*, 20 May 1983.

6. J. Feldschuh, op. cit., pp. 114, 197 citing T. Imagawa et al., "HIV Type 1 Infection in Homosexual Men Who Remain Seronegative for Prolonged Periods," *New Engl J Med* 1989;320:1458-1462.

7. J. Feldschuh, op. cit., p. 111. citing Allen White, "Leaders Urge Donors: 'Write Protest Letters to Irwin Blood Bank,'" *Bay Area Reporter*, 1 August 1988; Karen Everett, "Community Blood Drives Reinstated in Castro," *San Francisco Sentinel*, 19 August 1988.

8. Lorraine Day, M.D., *AIDS What the Government Isn't Telling You*, (Palm Desert, CA: Rockford Press, 1991), 44-489 Town Center Way, Suite D-412, Palm Desert, CA 92260.

9. J. Feldschuh, op cit., p. 67.

10. Ibid., p. 118.

11. E. Annis, op. cit.

12. *Titus* 1:15 (KJV).

13. S. Handwerger et al., "Tuberculosis and the Acquired Immunodeficiency Syndrome at a New York City Hospital," *Chest*, 1987;91:176-180.

14. G. Antonio, op. cit., p. 142.

15. *Federal Register*, op. cit., p. 35747.

16. *New York Times*, 23 April 1992, pages B1-B2.

17. Compare this view with *Genesis* 19:1-29 *and Romans* 1:18-32 (KJV). See also: Greg L. Bahnsen, *Homosexuality: A Biblical View* (Grand Rapids: Baker Book House, 1978). Dr. Bahnsen's trenchant work is the most comprehensive book published on the subject.

18. For a riveting account of how the American Psychiatric and Psychological Associations were strong-armed into changing the classification of homosexuality from a mental disease to a "preference" see: William Dannemeyer, *Homosexuality: Shadow in the Land*, (San Francisco: Ignatius Press, 1990). Congressman Dannemeyer's book provides a clear, compelling examination of the homosexual movement and its impact on American society.

19. In his eye-opening work, *Are Gay Rights Right?*, attorney Roger Magnuson gives several graphic illustrations of how the homosexual lobby is implementing its agenda. One particularly chilling case occurred in Madison, Wisconsin. Two young women, Ann Hacklander and Maureen Rowe were renting an apartment and looking for a roommate to share the expense. When a female who expressed an interest in living with them disclosed she was a lesbian, they told her politely they would prefer someone else. The lesbian took the matter immediately to the Madison Equal Opportunities Commission (MEOC), an agency charged with enforcement of the Madison homosexual privileges law. MEOC summoned Hacklander and Rowe to a meeting that proved to be a four-and-a-half hour self-criticism session. Reduced to tears at the meeting, Hacklander sad she felt like she was in Red China, not the United States. The result of the meeting was an agreement exacted by the MEOC. The two women would each be required to pay the lesbian $1500, would be forced to attend a sensitivity training class taught by homosexuals, would have their housing situation monitored by MEOC for two years, and would apologize to the aggrieved lesbian in a formal letter. When Rowe, a recent college graduate, claimed the settlement would bankrupt her, she was told her bankruptcy was of no consequence to the MEOC [Roger Magnuson, *Are Gay Rights Right?* (Portland: Multnomah Press, 1990), p. 71]. Mr. Magnuson is an honors graduate of Harvard Law School. His work provides a powerful analysis of the impact of homosexual privileges laws and their effects on society.

20. Ibid., pp. 90-91; 139-144.

21. Paul deParrie and Mary Pride, *Unholy Sacrifices of the New Age*, (Wheaton, IL: Crossway Books, 1988), p. 132 citing Ellen Goodman, "'Harvesting for Organs Goes Too Far," *Oregonian*, 11 December 1987. See also *Weeping in Ramah* by J.R. Lucas (Wheaton, IL: Crossway Books, 1985). Both books are essential reading in order to comprehend the dire ramifications of the utilitarian ethic.

22. Eugen Kogon, *The Theory and Practice of Hell* (New York: Berkley Books, 1980), "Scientific Experiments," pp. 153-175.

23. "U.S. Scientists Succeed in Transplanting Human Cells," Associated Press, Los Angeles, 14 September 1988,

24. Philip J. Hilts, "Mice Implants Created Model of Human Immune System; Potential 'Extraordinary' for AIDS Research," *Washington Post*, 15 September 1988.

25. J.M. McCune et al., "The Evaluation of Antiviral Compounds in the SCID-hu Mouse," VI International Conference on AIDS, San Francisco, 1990, Vol. 2, p. 107.

26. *Romans* 3:8, 13-18 (KJV).

27. W.E. Bullock, "Leprosy," in *Cecil Textbook of Medicine*, op. cit., pp. 1696-1701.

28. R. Jacobson, M.D., "The Face of Leprosy in the United States Today," *Arch Dermatol*, December 1990, pp. 1627-1630 citing the WHO Expert Committee on Leprosy, *Sixth Report*, Geneva Switzerland: World Health Organization, 1988, Technical Report Series No. 768.

29. G.A. Filice, D.W. Fraser, "Management of Household Contacts of Leprosy Patients," *Ann Intern Med* 1978;88:538.

30. C. Kennedy et al., "Leprosy and HIV Infection: A Closer Look at the Lesions," *Int J Dermatol* 1990;29:139-140.

31. C. Pean et al., "Natural History of M. Leprae and HIV Co-Infection," V International AIDS Conference, Montreal, 1989, p. 427.

32. O. Kashala et al., "HIV-1, HTLV-1 and HTLV-II Infection Among Leprosy Patients and their Contacts in Zaire," VII International Conference on AIDS, Florence, 1991, Vol. 1, p. 375.

33. *Leviticus* chapters 13 and 14 (KJV).

34. *Luke* 5:12-14; *Matthew* 8:2-4; *Mark* 1:40-44 (KJV).

35. *Deuteronomy* 23:12-13 (KJV). If this basic Mosaic injunction regarding disposal of human waste (i.e., excrement goes in the ground and is not for contact or consumption) the pandemics of AIDS, hepatitis, Kaposi's sarcoma, "gay bowel" syndrome, etc., which plague male homosexuals would have been avoided. Dr. Selma Dritz, a spokeswoman for the San Francisco Department Health, admitted that at least 1 out of 10 patients reported because of positive fecal samples or cultures for ameba, giardia and shigella infections were employed as food handlers. Sixty to 70% of these carriers were homosexual males, most of whom became infected through deviant acts involving the direct handling ("mudrolling"), manipulation ("fisting") and ingestion ("rimming" and "eating scat," etc., *ad nauseam*) of others' feces. Dr. Dritz comments: "We need vaccines that will create sufficient widespread immunity . . . to interrupt transmission of the pathogens by all routes" [S. Dritz, "Medical Aspects of Homosexuality," *N Engl J Med* 1980;302:463-464]. The notion of developing a vaccine for diseases spread by intentional fecal-oral contact is medically ludicrous. There is no such thing as "safe excrement ingestion." Willful voluntary ingestion of human excrement is a biological and psychological perversion. Individuals who engage in such conduct desperately need intensive reparative therapy to overcome their unhealthy compulsions.

36. Cf, *Romans* 1:27-32 (KJV).

37. *Matthew* 27:44 (KJV).

38. *Luke* 23:40-43 (KJV).

39. *John* 11:25 (KJV).

40. *I Peter* 1:18-19 (KJV).

41. *Zechariah* 9:11 (KJV).

42. J. Seale, "Problems Associated with Aids," op. cit.

43. Ibid.

44. L. Kramer, "Who Says AIDS Is Hard to Get?" *Newsweek*, 13 April 1992.

45. Judith Reisman, Ph.D., *A Content Analysis of The Advocate (1972-1991) and The 1991 Gay Yellow Pages*, The Institute for Media Education, P.O. Box 7404, Arlington, VA 22207, pp. 57-58. Dr. Reisman is also the author of *Soft Porn Plays Hardball*, a book which convincingly demonstrates the harmful effects of so-called "soft-core" pornography.

46. Edmund Bergler, M.D., "Homosexuality: Disease or Way of Life?" (New York: Collier Books, 1971), p. 281.

47. *Focus on the Family Citizen*, 18 May 1992 citing Eric M. Pollard, *The Washington Blade*, 31 January 1992.

48. Stanley Monteith, M.D., *AIDS The Unnecessary Epidemic* (Sevierville, TN: Covenant House Books, 1991). Available through: AIDS Book, 618 Frederick St., Santa Cruz, CA 95062. Dr. Monteith's work provides an extraordinary firsthand account of the political machinations which have blocked effective disease control measures from being enacted.

49. E. Annis, op. cit.

APPENDIX A
HIV BRAIN DETERIORATION

1. M.R. Lee, D.D. Ho, M.E. Gurney, "Functional Interaction and Partial Homology Between Human Immunodeficiency Virus and Neuroleukin," *Science*, 1987 August 28; 237(4818):1047-51.

2. D. Wimberger, J. Kramer, H. Kollegger, G. Mayrhofer and H. Imhof, "AIDS im ZNS," [AIDS of the Central Nervous System] *Wien Klin Wochenschr* 1990 Jan 19;102(2):47-51 (Published in German). Institutional address: Zentrales Institut fur Radiodiagnostik Universitat Wien.

3. G. Hancock and E. Carim, op. cit., p. 144.

4. M. Teresa, M. Ocana et al., "Neuropsychological Study of the AIDS Dementia Complex: A Preliminary Report," VII International Conference on AIDS, Florence, 1991, Vol. 1, p. 204.

5. R.M. Levy, D.E. Bredesen, M.L. Rosenblum, "Neurologic Complications of HIV Infection," *American Family Physician* 1990 Feb;41(2):517-36 Institutional address: Northwestern University Medical School, Chicago, Illinois.

6. R.H. McAllister, M.J. Harrison and M. Johnson, "HIV and the Nervous System," *British Journal of Hospital Medicine*, Jul;1988;40(1):21-6.

7. L.M. Grimaldi, R.P. Roos et al., "Restricted Heterogeneity of Antibody to gp120 and p24 in AIDS," *Journal of Immunology* 1988 Jul 1; 141(1):114-7.

8. Y. Koyanagi, S. Miles "Dual Infection of the Central Nervous System by AIDS Viruses with Distinct Cellular Tropisms," *Science*, 1987 May 15; 236(4803):819-22.

9. P. Gallo. A. De Rossi, A. Amadori, B. Tavolato, L. Chieco-Bianchi, "Central Nervous System Involvement in HIV Infection," *AIDS Research and Human Retroviruses*, 1988 Jun; 4(3):211-21.

10. A. Srinivasan, D. Dorsett, D. York, C. Bohan, R. Anand, "Human Immunodeficiency Virus Replication in Human Brain Cells. Brief Report," *Archives of Virology* 1988; 99(1-2):135-41.

11. D. Dormont, F. Boussin, Y. Merrouche, "Interactions Between HIV Virus and the Nervous System: Recent Pathogenic Data and Hypotheses," *Nouvelle Revue Francaise D Hematologie* 1988; 30(1-2):21-9 (Published in French).

12. C.L. Achim, M.K. Morey, C.A. Wiley, "Expression of Major Histocompatibility Complex and HIV Antigens within the Brains of AIDS Patients," *AIDS* 1991 May;5(5):535-41.

13. M.M. Derix, J. de Gans, J. Stam, P. Portegies, Dept. of Neurology, Academisch Medisch Centrum, Amsterdam," Mental Changes in Patients with AIDS," *Clin Neurol Neurosurg* 1990;92(3):215-22.

14. S. Snyder, J.J. Strain, G. Fulop, "Evaluation and Treatment of Mental Disorders in Patients with AIDS," *Compr Ther* 1990 Aug;16(8):34-41.

15. M.M. Beckham, "Neurologic Manifestations of AIDS," *Crit Care Nurs Clin North Am* 1990 Mar;2(1):29-32.

16. I. Grant, R.K. Heaton, "Human Immunodeficiency Virus-Type 1 (HIV-1) and the Brain," *J Consult Clin Psychol* 1990 Feb;58(1):22-30.

17. H. Hollander "Neurologic and Psychiatric Manifestations of HIV Disease," *J Gen Intern Med* 1991 Jan-Feb;6(1 Suppl):S24-31.

18. M.H. Stoler, T.A. Eskin, S. Benn, R.C. Angerer, L.M. Angerer, "Human T-cell Lymphotropic Virus Type III Infection of the Central Nervous System. A Preliminary in situ Analysis," *JAMA* 1986 November 7;256(17):2360-4.

19. J.M. Orenstein, F. Jannotta, "Human Immunodeficiency Virus and Papovavirus Infections in Acquired Immunodeficiency Syndrome: An Ultrastructural Study of Three Cases," *Human Pathology* 1988 Mar; 19(3):350-61.

20. K.T. Lin et al., "An Autopsy-Proved Case of AIDS in Taiwan," *Asian Pacific Journal of Allergy and Immunology* 1987;5:25-31.

21. T.E. Schlapfer, H.U. Fisch, "HIV Infection of the Central Nervous System: psychiatric consequences," *Schweiz Med Wochenschr* 1988;118:571-6 (Published in German). Institutional address: Psychiatrische Poliklinik der Universitat Bern.

22. N. Diederich, A. Karenberg and U.H. Peters "Psychopathologic Pictures in HIV Infection: AIDS Lethargy and AIDS Dementia," *Fortschritte Der Neurologie, Psychiatrie Und Iherr Grenzbebietefortschr Neurol Psychiatr* 1988 Jun; 56(6):173-85 (Published in German). Institutional address: Universitats-Nervenklinik Koln.

23. L.G. Epstein, L.R. Sharer and D.C. Gajdusek, "Hypothesis: AIDS Encephalopathy is Due to Primary and Persistent Infection of the Brain with a Human Retrovirus of the Lentivirus Subfamily," *Med Hypotheses* 1986 Sep;21(1):87-96. Epstein and Sharer are from UMD-NJ Medical School, Newark, NJ and Gajdusek is from National Institutes of Health, Bethesda, MD.

24. B.A. Navia, R.W. Price, "The Acquired Immunodeficiency Dementia Complex as the Presenting or Sole Manifestation of Human Immunodeficiency Virus Infection," *Archives of Neurology* 1987 January 44(1):65-69.

25. D.H. Gabuzda, M.S. Hirsch, "Neurologic Manifestation of Infection with Human Immunodeficiency Virus. Clinical Features and Pathogenesis," *Annals of Internal Medicine* 1987 September 107(3):383-91.

26. I.J. Koralnik, P. Burkhard et al., "Effect of Zidovudine on Early Neurological Manifestations of HIV Infection," VII International Conference on AIDS, Florence, 1991, Vol. 1, p. 187.

27. G. Villa, D. Monteleone et al., "Cognitive Impairment in AIDS and Asymptomatic HIV-Seropositive Subjects," VII International Conference on AIDS, Florence, 1991, Vol. 1, p. 191.

28. M. Schroder, S. Spieles et al. "Event-related Potentials (P3) in the Course of HIV-Infection," VII International Conference on AIDS, Florence, 1991, Vol. 1, p. 192.

29. D. Naber, C. Perro et al., "Psychiatric Symptoms and Neuropsychological Deficits in HIV-Infected Patients," VII International Conference on AIDS, Florence, 1991, Vol. 1, p. 193.

30. S.E. McManis, G.R. Brown et al., "Neuropsychiatric Impairment in HIV+ Persons," VII International Conference on AIDS, Florence, 1991, Vol. 1, p. 198.

31. N.R. Karlsen, I. Reinvang, "Slowed Reaction Time in Asymptomatic HIV-Positive Patients," VII International Conference on AIDS, Florence, 1991, Vol. 1, p. 201.

32. E.L. Kramer, J.J. Sanger, "Brain Imaging in Acquired Immunodeficiency Syndrome Dementia Complex," *Seminars in Nuclear Medicine* 1990 Oct;20(4):353-63.

33. T.P. Bridge, L.J. Ingraham, "Central Nervous System Effects of Human Immunodeficiency Virus Type 1," *Annu Rev Med* 1990;41:159-68.

34. S. Lunn, M. Skydsbjerg et al., "A Preliminary Report on the Neuropsychologic Sequelae of Human Immunodeficiency Virus," *Archives of General Psychiatry* 1991 Feb;48(2):139-42.

35. G. Bono, C. Zandrini, "Neuropsychological and Neurophysiological Abnormalities in HIV-Infection. Their Relevance and Predictive Value," *Acta Neurol* (Napoli) 1990;12:4-8, Neuro-Aids Unit, IRCCS C. Mondino, Universita di Pavia, Italy.

APPENDIX B
NOW FOR A LITTLE CONDOM SENSE

1. Dr. Theresa Crenshaw, Congressional Testimony for Children and Teenagers to the Select Committee of Children, Youth and Families, 18 June 1987, p. 3.

2. M.A. Fischl et al., "Heterosexual Transmission of Human Immunodeficiency Virus (HIV), Relationship of Sexual Practices to Sero Conversion," III International Conference on AIDS, Wash., D.C., 1987.

3. A. Parachini, "AIDS-Condom Study Grant Cut Off by U.S.," *Los Angeles Times*, 10 August 1988.

4. A. Parachini, "Condoms and AIDS: How Safe is 'Safe'?" *Los Angeles Times*, 18 August 1987.

5. Nancy E. Dirubbo, "Condom Barrier," *American Journal of Nursing*, 87 No. 10 (1987):1306.

6. Richard Smith, "The Condom," unpublished paper, October 1990, p. 6.

7. Ibid., p. 13 and Dirubbo, p. 1306.

8. Based on a failure rate of 18+ percent. William R. Grady et al, "Contraceptive Failure in the United States: Estimates from the 1982 National Survey of Family Growth," *Family Planning Perspectives*, 18 No. 5(1988):207.

9. U.S. Department of Education, "Will 'Safe Sex' Education Effectively Combat AIDS?" 22 January 1988, p. 16.

10. Deborah Anne Dawson, "The Effects of Sex Education on Adolescent Behavior," *Family Planning Perspectives* 18 No. 4 (1986):164. Critical discussion of this article is found in Jacqueline Kasun, "Sex Education: A New Philosophy for America?" published by The Rockford Institute Center on The Family in America, p. 4.

11. Douglas Kirby, "Sexuality Education: A More Realistic View of its Effects," *Journal of School Health* 55 No. 10(1985):422.

12. James W. Stout and Frederick P. Rivara, "Schools and Sex Education: Does It Work?" *Pediatrics*, 83 No. 3(1989):378.

13. Douglas Kirby, speaking at the Sixteenth Annual Meeting of the National Family Planing and Reproductive Health Association, 2 March 1988, Washington, D.C. as cited in Kasun, op. cit.

14. Douglas Kirby et al., "Six School-Based Clinics: Their Reproductive Health Services and Impact on Sexual Behavior," *Family Planning Perspectives*, 23 No. 1 (1991):6-16.

ABOUT THE AUTHOR

GENE ANTONIO is a leading human rights activist and investigative journalist who has extensively researched the AIDS epidemic since 1984. He is the author of the highly acclaimed national best-seller, *The AIDS Cover-Up?* Antonio has testified before federal, state and municipal legislators regarding AIDS and human rights issues.

For the past several years he has been the Executive Editor of the *International Healthwatch Report*, a newsletter providing critical information which is frequently ignored or misrepresented in the media. He has been a guest on numerous local and national radio and television shows. An effective public speaker, Antonio conducts seminars for civic and medical organizations and other concerned groups.

To receive the *International Healthwatch Report*, simply send a contribution of twenty-five dollars ($25.00 US funds) or more to FACT, Box 90140, Arlington, TX 76004.

Videotapes and other educational materials are also available:

THE REAL FACTS ABOUT AIDS (video)
by Gene Antonio
Contribution of $19.00 (+$3 p/h)
Suitable for adults and young people.

AIDS AND DENTISTRY (audio cassette)
by Gene Antonio
Contribution of $9.00 (+$2.00 p/h)
Suitable for dental professionals and patients.

Additional copies of *AIDS: RAGE AND REALITY*
are also available:
Contribution of $19.95 (+$2 p/h).

For further information write:
FACT, Box 90140, Arlington, TX 76010, USA

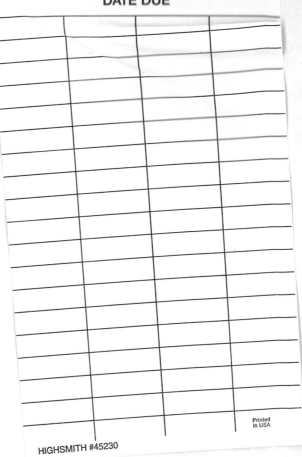

DATE DUE

Printed
in USA

HIGHSMITH #45230